THE NETTER COLLECTION

OF MEDICAL ILLUSTRATIONS

3rd Edition

Musculoskeletal System

Part I—Upper Limb

VOLUME 6

A compilation of paintings prepared by **FRANK H. NETTER, MD**

Edited by

Joseph P. Iannotti, MD, PhD
Lang Family Distinguished Chair in Orthopedics
Chief of Staff
Chief Academic and Innovations Officer
Cleveland Clinic Weston Hospital
Weston, Florida

Richard D. Parker, MD
Professor of Surgery
Cleveland Clinic Lerner College of Medicine
President, Hillcrest Hospital and East Region
Past Chairman, Department of Orthopaedic Surgery
Cleveland Clinic
Cleveland, Ohio

Additional Illustrations by

Carlos A.G. Machado, MD

CONTRIBUTING ILLUSTRATORS
John A. Craig, MD
Tiffany S. DaVanzo, MA, CMI
DragonFly Media
Paul Kim, MS
Kristen W. Marzejon, CMI
James A. Perkins, MS, MFA

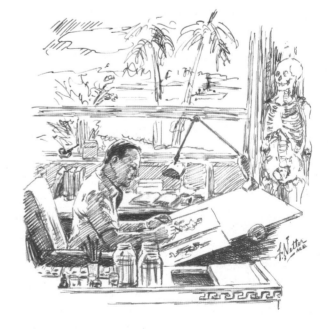

Self portrait by Dr. Netter

ELSEVIER

ELSEVIER
1600 John F. Kennedy Blvd.
Suite 1600
Philadelphia, Pennsylvania

THE NETTER COLLECTION OF MEDICAL ILLUSTRATIONS:
MUSCULOSKELETAL SYSTEM, PART I: UPPER LIMB, VOLUME 6,
THIRD EDITION

ISBN: 978-0-323-88088-6

Publisher: Elyse O'Grady
Senior Content Strategist: Marybeth Thiel
Publishing Services Manager: Catherine Jackson
Project Manager: Rosanne Toroian
Book Design: Patrick Ferguson

Printed in India

Last digit is the print number: 9 8 7 6 5 4 3 2 1

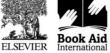

Working together
to grow libraries in
developing countries

www.elsevier.com • www.bookaid.org

"Clarification is the goal. No matter how beautifully it is painted, a medical illustration has little value if it does not make clear a medical point."

—Frank H. Netter, MD

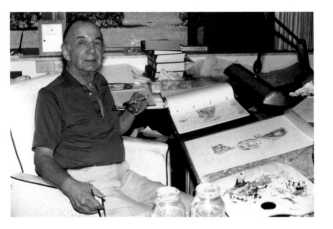

Dr. Frank Netter at work.

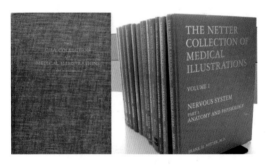

The single-volume "Blue Book" that preceded the multivolume *Netter Collection of Medical Illustrations* series, affectionately known as the "Green Books."

The Netter Collection
OF MEDICAL ILLUSTRATIONS
3rd Edition

Volume 1 **Reproductive System**
Volume 2 **Endocrine System**
Volume 3 **Respiratory System**
Volume 4 **Integumentary System**
Volume 5 **Urinary System**
Volume 6 **Musculoskeletal System**
Volume 7 **Nervous System**
Volume 8 **Cardiovascular System**
Volume 9 **Digestive System**

Dr. Frank Netter created an illustrated legacy unifying his perspectives as physician, artist, and teacher. Both his greatest challenge and greatest success was charting a middle course between artistic clarity and instructional complexity. That success is captured in *The Netter Collection,* beginning in 1948 when the first comprehensive book of Netter's work was published by CIBA Pharmaceuticals. It met with such success that over the following 40 years the collection was expanded into an 8-volume series—with each title devoted to a single body system. Between 2011 and 2016, these books were updated and rereleased. Now, after another decade of innovation in medical imaging, renewed focus on patient-centered care, conscious efforts to improve inequities in healthcare and medical education, and a growing understanding of many clinical conditions, including multisystem effects of COVID-19, we are happy to make available a third edition of Netter's timeless work enhanced and informed by modern medical knowledge and context.

Inside the classic green covers, students and practitioners will find hundreds of original works of art. This is a collection of the human body in pictures—Dr. Netter called them *pictures,* never paintings. The latest expert medical knowledge is anchored by the sublime style of Frank Netter that has guided physicians' hands and nurtured their imaginations for more than half a century.

Noted artist-physician Carlos Machado, MD, the primary successor responsible for continuing the Netter tradition, has particular appreciation for the Green Book series. *The Reproductive System* is of special significance for those who, like me, deeply admire Dr. Netter's work. In this volume, he masters the representation of textures of different surfaces, which I like to call 'the rhythm of the brush,' since it is the dimension, the direction of the strokes, and the interval separating them that create the illusion of given textures: organs have their external surfaces, the surfaces of their cavities, and texture of their parenchymas realistically represented. It set the style for the subsequent volumes of *The Netter Collection*—each an amazing combination of painting masterpieces and precise scientific information.

This third edition could not exist without the dedication of all those who edited, authored, or in other ways contributed to the second edition or the original books, nor, of course, without the excellence of Dr. Netter. For this third edition, we also owe our gratitude to the authors, editors, and artists whose relentless efforts were instrumental in adapting these classic works into reliable references for today's clinicians in training and in practice. From all of us with the Netter Publishing Team at Elsevier, thank you.

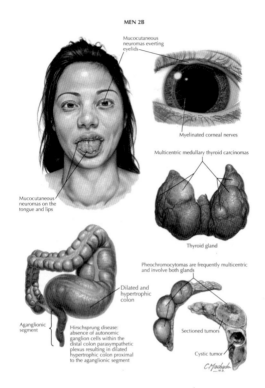

An illustrated plate painted by Carlos Machado, MD.

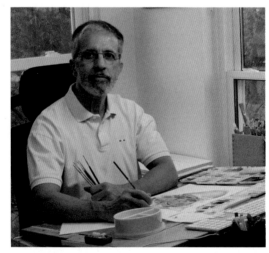

Dr. Carlos Machado at work.

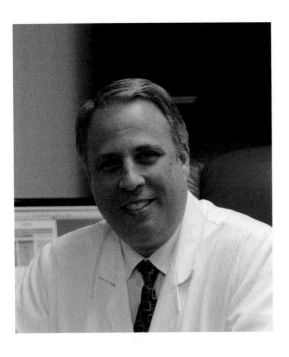

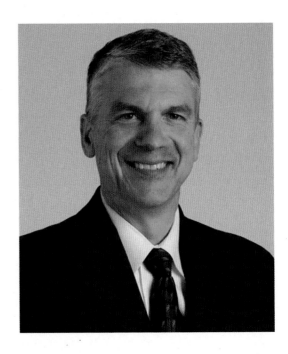

EDITORS-IN-CHIEF

Joseph P. Iannotti, MD, PhD, is Lang Family Distinguished Chair of Orthopaedics and Chief of Staff and Chief Academic and Innovation Officer for Cleveland Clinic Florida. He has a joint appointment in the Department of Bioengineering at the Lerner Research Institute.

Dr. Iannotti joined the Cleveland Clinic in 2000 as Chair of Orthopaedic Surgery (2000–2009) and Chair of the Orthopaedic and Rheumatology Institute (2008–2019). He came to the Cleveland Clinic from the University of Pennsylvania, leaving there as a tenured professor of orthopaedic surgery and Head of the Shoulder and Elbow Service. Dr. Iannotti received his medical degree from Northwestern University in 1979, completed his orthopedic residency training at the University of Pennsylvania in 1984, and earned his doctorate in cell biology from the University of Pennsylvania in 1987.

Dr. Iannotti's clinical and basic science research program focuses on innovative treatments for tendon repair and tendon tissue engineering, prosthetic design, software planning, and patient-specific instrumentation. Dr. Iannotti has had continuous extramural funding for his research since 1981. He has been the principal or co-principal investigator of dozens of research grants. He has been an invited lecturer and visiting professor at nearly 100 national and international academic institutions and societies, delivering more than 800 lectures both nationally and internationally.

Dr. Iannotti has published two textbooks on the shoulder, one in its second edition and the other in its third edition. He has authored over 350 original peer-reviewed articles, review articles, and book chapters. Dr. Iannotti has more than 100 US and international patents related to shoulder prosthetics, surgical instruments, and tissue-engineered implants. He is member of the National Academy of Innovators.

He has received awards for his academic work from the American Orthopaedic Association, including the North American and American-British-Canadian traveling fellowships and the Neer Research Award in 1996, 2001, and 2015 from the American Shoulder and Elbow Surgeons. He won the orthopedic resident teaching award in 2006 for his role in research education. He was awarded the Mason Sones Innovator of the Year award in 2012 and the Lifetime Achievement Award for Innovation in 2019 from the Cleveland Clinic.

He has served in many leadership roles at the national level, including as past Chair of the Academic Affairs Council and the Board of Directors of the American Academy of Orthopaedic Surgery. In addition, he has served and chaired several committees of the American Shoulder and Elbow Surgeons and was President of the International Society of Shoulder and Elbow Surgeons from 2005 to 2006 and Chairman of the Board of Trustees of the *Journal of Shoulder and Elbow Surgery*. He currently serves on several not-for-profit boards.

Richard D. Parker, MD, is President of Hillcrest Hospital and East Region President of Cleveland Clinic Ohio. He is Professor of Surgery at the Cleveland Clinic Lerner College of Medicine and Past Chairman of the Department of Orthopaedic Surgery at the Cleveland Clinic. Dr. Parker is an expert on the knee, ranging from nonoperative treatment to all aspects of surgical procedures, including articular cartilage, meniscus, ligament, and joint replacement. He has published more than 200 peer-reviewed manuscripts and numerous book chapters, and has presented his work throughout the world. Dr. Parker received his undergraduate degree at Walsh College in Canton, Ohio, and his medical education at The Ohio State University College of Medicine, and he completed his orthopedic residency at The Mount Sinai Medical Center in Cleveland, Ohio. He received his fellowship training with subspecialization in sports medicine through a clinical research fellowship in sports medicine, arthroscopy, knee and shoulder surgery in Salt Lake City, Utah. He obtained his Certificate of Subspecialization in orthopedic sports medicine in 2008, which was the first year it was available.

Before joining the Cleveland Clinic in 1993, Dr. Parker acted as head of the section of sports medicine at The Mount Sinai Medical Center. His current research focuses on clinical outcomes focusing on articular cartilage, meniscal transplantation, posterior cruciate ligament, and the Multicenter Orthopaedic Outcomes Network (MOON) ACL registry. In addition to his clinical and administrative duties, he also serves as the assistant team physician for the Cleveland Cavaliers and serves as a knee consultant to the Cleveland Guardians. He lives in the Chagrin Falls area with his wife, Jana, and enjoys biking, golfing, and walking in his free time.

Frank Netter produced nearly 20,000 medical illustrations spanning the entire field of medicine over a five-decade career. There is no physician who has not used his work as part of their education. Many educators use his illustrations to teach others. One of the editors of this series had the privilege and honor to be an author of portions of the original "Green Book" of musculoskeletal medical illustrations as a junior faculty member and considers it a special honor to be part of this updated series.

Many of Frank Netter's original illustrations have stood the test of time. His work depicting basic musculoskeletal anatomy and relevant surgical anatomy and exposures have remained unaltered in the current series. His illustrations demonstrated the principles of treatment or the manifestation of musculoskeletal diseases and were rendered in a manner that only a physician-artist could render.

This edition of musculoskeletal illustrations has been updated with modern text and our current understanding of the pathogenesis, diagnosis, and treatment of a wide array of diseases and conditions. We have added new illustrations and radiographic and advanced imaging to supplement the original art. We expect that this series will prove to be useful to a wide spectrum of both students and teachers at every level.

Part I covers specific disorders of the upper limb, including anatomy, trauma, and degenerative and acquired disorders. Part II covers these same areas in the lower limb and spine. Part III covers the basic science of the musculoskeletal system, metabolic bone disease, rheumatologic diseases, musculoskeletal tumors, the sequelae of trauma, and congenital deformities.

The series is jointly produced by the clinical and research staff of the Orthopaedic and Rheumatologic Institute of the Cleveland Clinic and Elsevier. The editors thank each of the many talented contributors to this three-volume series. Their expertise in each of their fields of expertise has made this publication possible. We are both very proud to work with these colleagues. We are thankful to Elsevier for the opportunity to work on this series and for their support and expertise throughout the long development and editorial process.

Joseph P. Iannotti, MD, PhD
Richard D. Parker, MD

INTRODUCTION TO PART I—ANATOMY, PHYSIOLOGY, AND METABOLIC DISORDERS

I had long looked forward to undertaking this volume on the musculoskeletal system. It deals with the most humanistic, the most soul-touching, of all the subjects I have portrayed in THE CIBA COLLECTION OF MEDICAL ILLUSTRATIONS. People break bones, develop painful or swollen joints, are handicapped by congenital, developmental, or acquired deformities, metabolic abnormalities, or paralytic disorders. Some are beset by tumors of bone or soft tissue; some undergo amputations, either surgical or traumatic; some occasionally have reimplantation; and many have joint replacement. The list goes on and on. These are people we see about us quite commonly and are often our friends, relatives, or acquaintances. Significantly, such ailments lend themselves to graphic representation and are stimulating subject matter for an artist.

When I undertook this project, however, I grossly underestimated its scope. This was true also in regard to the previous volumes of the CIBA COLLECTION, but in the case of this book, it was far more marked. When we consider that this project involves every bone, joint, and muscle of the body, as well as all the nerves and blood vessels that supply them and all the multitude of disorders that may affect each of them, the magnitude of the project becomes enormous. In my naiveté, I originally thought I could cover the subject in a single book, but it soon became apparent that this was impossible. Even two books soon proved inadequate for such an extensive undertaking and, accordingly, three books are now planned. This book, Part I, Volume 8 of the CIBA COLLECTION, covers basic gross anatomy, embryology, physiology, and histology of the musculoskeletal system, as well as its metabolic disorders. Part II, now in press, covers rheumatic and other arthritic disorders, as well as their conservative and surgical management (including joint replacement), congenital and developmental disorders, and both benign and malignant neoplasms of bones and soft tissues. Part III, on which I am still at work, will include fractures and dislocations and their emergency and definitive care, amputations (both surgical and traumatic) and prostheses, sports injuries, infections, peripheral nerve and plexus injuries, burns, compartment syndromes, skin grafting, arthroscopy, and care and rehabilitation of handicapped patients.

But classification and organization of this voluminous material turned out to be no simple matter, since many disorders fit equally well into several of the above groups. For example, osteogenesis imperfecta might have been classified as metabolic, congenital, or developmental. Baker's cyst, ganglion, bursitis, and villonodular synovitis might have been considered with rheumatic, developmental, or in some instances even with traumatic disorders. Pathologic fractures might be covered with fractures in general or with the specific underlying disease that caused them. In a number of instances, therefore, empiric decisions had to be made in this connection, and some subjects were covered under several headings. I hope that the reader will be considerate of these problems. In addition, there is much overlap between the fields of orthopedics, neurology, and neurosurgery, so that the reader may find it advantageous to refer at times to my atlases on the nervous system.

I must express herewith my thanks and appreciation for the tremendous help which my very knowledgeable collaborators gave to me so graciously. In this Part I, there was first of all Dr. Russell Woodburne, a truly great anatomist and professor emeritus at the University of Michigan. It is interesting that during our long collaboration I never actually met with Dr. Woodburne, and all our communications were by mail or phone. This, in itself, tells of what a fine understanding and meeting of the minds there was between us. I hope and expect that in the near future I will have the pleasure of meeting him in person.

Dr. Edmund S. Crelin, professor at Yale University, is a long-standing friend (note that I do not say "old" friend because he is so young in spirit) with whom I have collaborated a number of times on other phases of embryology. He is a profound student and original investigator of the subject, with the gift of imparting his knowledge simply and clearly, and is in fact a talented artist himself.

Dr. Frederick Kaplan (now Freddie to me), assistant professor of orthopaedics at the University of Pennsylvania, was invaluable in guiding me through the difficult subjects of musculoskeletal physiology and metabolic bone disease. I enjoyed our companionship and friendship as much as I appreciated his knowledge and insight into the subject.

I was delighted to have the cooperation of Dr. Henry Mankin, the distinguished chief of orthopaedics at Massachusetts General Hospital and professor at Harvard University, for the complex subject of rickets in its varied forms—nutritional, renal, and metabolic. He is a great but charming and unassuming man.

There were many others, too numerous to mention here individually, who gave to me of their knowledge and time. They are all credited elsewhere in this book but I thank them all very much herewith. I will write about the great people who helped me with other parts of Volume 8 when those parts are published.

Finally, I give great credit and thanks to the personnel of the CIBA-GEIGY Company and to the company itself for having done so much to ease my burden in producing this book. Specifically, I would like to mention Mr. Philip Flagler, Dr. Milton Donin, Dr. Roy Ellis, and especially Mrs. Regina Dingle, all of whom did so much more in that connection than I can tell about here.

Frank H. Netter, 1987

INTRODUCTION TO PART II—DEVELOPMENTAL DISORDERS, TUMORS, RHEUMATIC DISEASES, AND JOINT REPLACEMENT

In my introduction to Part I of this atlas, I wrote of how awesome albeit fascinating I had found the task of pictorializing the fundamentals of the musculoskeletal system, both its normal structure as well as its multitudinous disorders and diseases. As compactly, simply, and succinctly as I tried to present the subject matter, it still required three full books (Parts I, II, and III of Volume 8 of The Ciba Collection of Medical Illustrations). Part I of this trilogy covered the normal anatomy, embryology, and physiology of the musculoskeletal system as well as its diverse metabolic diseases, including the various types of rickets. This book, Part II, portrays its congenital and developmental disorders, neoplasms—both benign and malignant—of bone and soft tissue, and rheumatic and other arthritic diseases, as well as joint replacement. Part III, on which I am still at work, will cover trauma, including fractures and dislocations of all the bones and joints, soft-tissue injuries, sports injuries, burns, infections including osteomyelitis and hand infections, compartment syndromes, amputations, both traumatic and surgical, replantation of limbs and digits, prostheses, and rehabilitation, as well as a number of related subjects.

As I stated in my above-mentioned previous introduction, some disorders, however, do not fit exactly into a precise classification and are therefore covered piece-meal herein under several headings. Furthermore, a considerable number of orthopedic ailments involve also the fields of neurology and neurosurgery, so readers may find it helpful to refer in those instances to my atlases on the anatomy and pathology of the nervous system (Volume 1, Parts I and II of The Ciba Collection of Medical Illustrations).

Most meaningfully, however, I herewith express my sincere appreciation of the many great physicians, surgeons, orthopedists, and scientists who so graciously shared with me their knowledge and supplied me with so much material on which to base my illustrations. Without their help I could not have created this atlas. Most of these wonderful people are credited elsewhere in this book under the heading of "Acknowledgments" but I must nevertheless specifically mention a few who were not only collaborators and consultants in this undertaking but who have become my dear and esteemed friends. These are Dr. Bob Hensinger, my consulting editor, who guided me through many puzzling aspects of the organization and subject matter of this atlas; Drs. Alfred and Genevieve Swanson, pioneers in the correction of rheumatically deformed hands with Silastic implants, as well as in the classification and study of congenital limb deficits; Dr. William Enneking, who has made such great advances in the diagnosis and management of bone tumors; Dr. Ernest ("Chappy") Conrad III; the late Dr. Charley Frantz, who first set me on course for this project, and Dr. Richard Freyberg, who became the consultant on the rheumatic diseases plates; Dr. George Hammond; Dr. Hugo Keim; Dr. Mack Clayton; Dr. Philip Wilson; Dr. Stuart Kozinn; and Dr. Russell Windsor.

Finally, I also sincerely thank Mr. Philip Flagler, Ms. Regina Dingle, and others of the CIBA-GEIGY organization who helped in more ways than I can describe in producing this atlas.

Frank H. Netter, MD, 1990

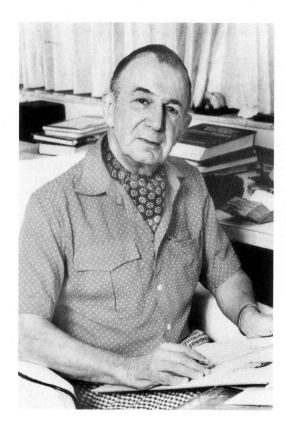

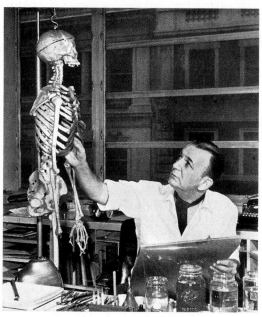

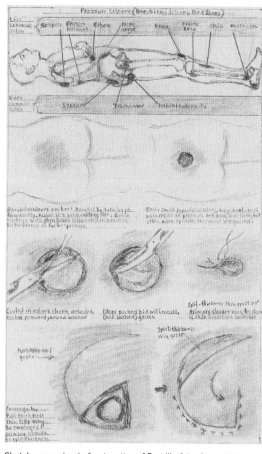

Sketch appearing in front matter of Part III of the first edition.

EDITORS-IN-CHIEF

Joseph P. Iannotti, MD, PhD
Lang Family Distinguished Chair in Orthopedics
Chief of Staff
Chief Academic and Innovations Officer
Cleveland Clinic Weston Hospital
Weston, Florida

Richard D. Parker, MD
Professor of Surgery
Cleveland Clinic Lerner College of Medicine
President, Hillcrest Hospital and East Region
Past Chairman, Department of Orthopaedic Surgery
Cleveland Clinic
Cleveland, Ohio
Associate Editors

Abby G. Abelson, MD, FACR
Clinical Assistant Professor of Medicine
Chair, Department of Rheumatic and Immunologic
    Diseases
Cleveland Clinic Lerner College of Medicine at Case
    Western Reserve University
Cleveland, Ohio
EDITOR: PART III: SECTIONS 3, 5
AUTHOR: PART III: PLATES 3.26–3.29, 3.34–3.37,
    3.45–3.47, 5.45, 5.52–5.54

Thomas E. Mroz, MD
Chair, Enterprise Orthopaedic Surgery and
    Rehabilitation
Cervical Spine Surgery
Director, Spine Research
Cleveland Clinic
Cleveland, Ohio
PART II: SECTION 1

Brendan M. Patterson, MD, MBA
Chair, Department of Orthopaedic Surgery
Cleveland Clinic Health Care System
Professor, Orthopaedic Surgery
Case Western Reserve University School of Medicine
Cleveland, Ohio
EDITOR: PART II: SECTIONS 2, 3, 4, 5;
    PART III: SECTIONS 1, 2, 4, 6, 7, 8, 9
AUTHOR: PART II: PLATES 2.63–2.77, 3.1–3.26,
    3.42–3.43, 4.1–4.13; PART III: PLATES 1.1–1.21,
    2.1–2.15, 2.27–2.41, 7.1–7.11, 9.2, 9.3, 9.9, 9.10

CONTRIBUTORS

Vahid Entezari, MD, MMSc
Assistant Professor, Orthopaedic Surgery
Cleveland Clinic
Cleveland, Ohio
PLATES 1.27–1.57, 1.60–1.65

Peter J. Evans, MD, PhD
Institute Chair, Orthopaedics and Rheumatology
Cleveland Clinic Florida
Weston, Florida
PLATES 4.1–4.66

Jason Ho, MD
Department of Orthopaedic Surgery
Cleveland Clinic
Cleveland, Ohio
PLATES 1.21–1.26, 1.58–1.59

Steven D. Maschke, MD
Director, Hand and Upper Limb Center
Cleveland Clinic
Cleveland, Ohio
PLATES 3.1–3.38

Eric T. Ricchetti, MD
Maynard Madden Arthritis Endowed Professorship
Director, Shoulder Center and Shoulder and Elbow
    Surgery Fellowship
Department of Orthopaedic Surgery
Cleveland Clinic
Cleveland, Ohio
PLATES 1.1–1.20, 1.27–1.57, 1.60–1.65

Joseph Styron, MD, PhD
Staff Surgeon
Department of Orthopaedic Surgery
Cleveland Clinic
Cleveland, Ohio
PLATES 2.1–2.47

CONTENTS OF COMPLETE VOLUME 6— MUSCULOSKELETAL SYSTEM: THREE-PART SET

PART I   **Upper Limb**

SECTION   1   Shoulder

SECTION   2   Upper Arm and Elbow

SECTION   3   Forearm and Wrist

SECTION   4   Hand and Finger

ISBN: 978-0-3238-8088-6

PART II   **Spine and Lower Limb**

SECTION   1   Spine

SECTION   2   Pelvis, Hip, and Thigh

SECTION   3   Knee

SECTION   4   Lower Leg

SECTION   5   Ankle and Foot

ISBN: 978-0-3238-8128-9

PART III   **Biology and Systemic Diseases**

SECTION   1   Embryology

SECTION   2   Physiology

SECTION   3   Metabolic Disorders

SECTION   4   Congenital and Development Disorders

SECTION   5   Rheumatic Diseases

SECTION   6   Tumors of Musculoskeletal System

SECTION   7   Injury to Musculoskeletal System

SECTION   8   Soft Tissue Infections

SECTION   9   Fracture Complications

ISBN: 978-0-3238-8087-9

CONTENTS

SECTION 1 SHOULDER

Anatomy

1.1 Scapula and Humerus: Posterior View, 2
1.2 Scapula and Humerus: Anterior View, 3
1.3 Clavicle, 4
1.4 Ligaments, 5
1.5 Glenohumeral Arthroscopic Anatomy, 6
1.6 Glenohumeral Arthroscopic Anatomy (Continued), 7
1.7 Anterior Muscles, 8
1.8 Anterior Muscles: Cross Section, 9
1.9 Posterior Muscles, 10
1.10 Posterior Muscles: Cross Section, 11
1.11 Muscles of Rotator Cuff, 12
1.12 Muscles of Rotator Cuff: Cross Sections, 13
1.13 Axilla Dissection: Anterior View, 14
1.14 Axilla: Posterior Wall and Cord, 15
1.15 Deep Neurovascular Structures and Intervals, 16
1.16 Axillary and Brachial Arteries, 17
1.17 Axillary Artery and Anastomoses Around Scapula, 18
1.18 Brachial Plexus, 19
1.19 Peripheral Nerves: Dermatomes, 20
1.20 Peripheral Nerves: Sensory Distribution and Neuropathy in Shoulder, 21

Clinical Problems and Correlations
Fractures and Dislocation

1.21 Proximal Humeral Fractures: Neer Classification, 22
1.22 Proximal Humeral Fractures: Two-Part Tuberosity Fracture, 23
1.23 Proximal Humeral Fractures: Two Part Surgical Neck Fracture and Humeral Head Dislocation, 24
1.24 Proximal Humeral Fractures: Valgus-Impacted Four-Part Fracture, 25
1.25 Proximal Humeral Fractures: Displaced Four-Part Fractures with Articular Head Fracture, 26
1.26 Proximal Humeral Fractures: Reverse Total Shoulder Replacement, 27
1.27 Anterior Dislocation of Glenohumeral Joint: Anterior Dislocation Types and Stimson Maneuver, 28
1.28 Anterior Dislocation of Glenohumeral Joint: Pathologic Lesions, 29
1.29 Anterior Dislocation of Glenohumeral Joint: Imaging, 30
1.30 Posterior Dislocation of Glenohumeral Joint, 31
1.31 Posterior Dislocation of Glenohumeral Joint (Continued), 32
1.32 Acromioclavicular and Sternoclavicular Dislocation, 33
1.33 Fractures of the Clavicle, 34
1.34 Fractures of the Clavicle and Scapula, 35

Common Soft Tissue Disorders

1.35 Calcific Tendonitis, 36
1.36 Frozen Shoulder: Clinical Presentation, 37
1.37 Frozen Shoulder: Risk Factors and Diagnostic Tests, 38
1.38 Biceps, Tendon Tears, and SLAP Lesions: Presentation and Physical Examination, 39
1.39 Biceps, Tendon Tears, and SLAP Lesions: Types of Tears, 40
1.40 Acromioclavicular Joint Arthritis, 41
1.41 Impingement Syndrome and the Rotator Cuff: Presentation and Diagnosis, 42
1.42 Impingement Syndrome and the Rotator Cuff: Radiologic and Arthroscopic Imaging, 43
1.43 Rotator Cuff Tears: Physical Examination, 44
1.44 Supraspinatus and Infraspinatus Rotator Cuff Tears: Imaging, 45
1.45 Supraspinatus and Infraspinatus Rotator Cuff Tears: Surgical Management, 46
1.46 Supraspinatus and Infraspinatus Cuff Tear: Surgical Management Superior Capsular Reconstruction and Balloon Arthroplasty, 47
1.47 Supraspinatus and Infraspinatus Cuff Tear: Surgical Management Latissimus and Trapezius Transfers, 48
1.48 Management of Subscapularis Rotator Cuff Tears, 49
1.49 Management of Irreparable Subscapularis Tears: Pectoralis and Latissimus Transfers, 50
1.50 Osteoarthritis of the Glenohumeral Joint, 51
1.51 Osteoarthritis of the Glenohumeral Joint: Surgical Imaging, 52
1.52 Avascular Necrosis of the Humeral Head, 53
1.53 Rheumatoid Arthritis of the Glenohumeral Joint: Radiographic Presentations and Treatment Options, 54
1.54 Rheumatoid Arthritis of the Glenohumeral Joint: Conservative Humeral Head Surface Replacement, 55
1.55 Rotator Cuff–Deficient Arthritis (Rotator Cuff Tear Arthropathy): Physical Findings and Appearance, 56
1.56 Rotator Cuff–Deficient Arthritis (Rotator Cuff Tear Arthropathy): Radiographic Findings, 57
1.57 Rotator Cuff–Deficient Arthritis (Rotator Cuff Tear Arthropathy): Radiographic Findings (Continued), 58
1.58 Neurologic Conditions of the Shoulder: Suprascapular Nerve, 59
1.59 Neurologic Conditions of the Shoulder: Long Thoracic and Spinal Accessory Nerves, 60

Amputation

1.60 Amputation of Upper Arm and Shoulder, 61

Injections, Basic Rehabilitation, and Surgical Approaches

1.61 Shoulder Injections, 62
1.62 Basic, Passive, and Active-Assisted Range of Motion Exercises, 63
1.63 Basic Shoulder-Strengthening Exercises, 64
1.64 Basic Shoulder Strengthening Exercises (Continued), 65
1.65 Common Surgical Approaches to the Shoulder, 66

SECTION 2 UPPER ARM AND ELBOW

Anatomy

2.1 Topographic Anatomy, 68
2.2 Anterior and Posterior Views of Humerus, 69
2.3 Elbow Joint: Bones, 70
2.4 Elbow Joint: Radiographs, 71
2.5 Elbow Ligaments: Anterior Views, 72
2.6 Elbow Ligaments: Lateral and Medial Views, 73
2.7 Muscles Origins and Insertions, 74
2.8 Muscles: Anterior Views, 75
2.9 Muscles: Posterior Views, 76
2.10 Cross Sectional Anatomy of Upper Arm, 77
2.11 Cross Sectional Anatomy of Elbow, 78
2.12 Cutaneous Nerves and Superficial Veins, 79
2.13 Cutaneous Innervation, 80
2.14 Musculocutaneous Nerve of Upper Arm and Elbow, 81
2.15 Radial Nerve, 82
2.16 Brachial Artery In Situ, 83
2.17 Brachial Artery and Anastomoses around Elbow, 84

Clinical Problems and Correlations

2.18 Physical Examination and Range of Motion, 85

Fractures and Dislocation

2.19 Humeral Shaft Fractures, 86
2.20 Injury to the Elbow, 87
2.21 Fracture of Distal Humerus, 88
2.22 Fracture of Distal Humerus: Total Elbow Arthroplasty, 89
2.23 Fracture of Distal Humerus: Capitellum, 90
2.24 Fracture of Head and Neck of Radius, 91
2.25 Fracture of Head and Neck of Radius: Imaging, 92
2.26 Fracture of Olecranon, 93
2.27 Dislocation of Elbow Joint, 94
2.28 Dislocation of Elbow Joint (Continued), 95
2.29 Injuries in Children: Supracondylar Humerus Fractures, 96
2.30 Injuries in Children: Elbow, 97
2.31 Injuries in Children: Subluxation of Radial Head, 98
2.32 Complications of Fracture, 99

Common Soft Tissue Disorders

2.33 Arthritis: Open and Arthroscopic Elbow Debridement, 100
2.34 Arthritis: Elbow Arthroplasty Options, 101
2.35 Arthritis: Imaging of Total Elbow Arthroplasty Designs, 102
2.36 Cubital Tunnel Syndrome: Sites of Compression, 103
2.37 Cubital Tunnel Syndrome: Clinical Signs and Treatment, 104
2.38 Epicondylitis and Olecranon Bursitis, 105
2.39 Rupture of Biceps and Triceps Tendon, 106
2.40 Medial Elbow and Posterolateral Rotatory Instability Tests, 107
2.41 Osteochondritis Dissecans of the Elbow, 108
2.42 Osteochondrosis of the Elbow (Panner Disease), 109
2.43 Congenital Dislocation of Radial Head, 110
2.44 Congenital Radioulnar Synostosis, 111

Injections, Basic Rehabilitation, and Surgical Approaches

2.45 Common Elbow Injections and Basic Rehabilitation, 112
2.46 Surgical Approaches to the Upper Arm and Elbow, 113
2.47 Surgical Approaches to the Upper Arm and Elbow (Continued), 114 ·

SECTION 3 FOREARM AND WRIST

Anatomy

3.1 Topographic Anatomy, 116
3.2 Bones of Forearm, 117
3.3 Bones of Wrist, 118
3.4 Radiologic Findings of Wrist, 119
3.5 Ligaments of Wrist, 120
3.6 Arthroscopy of Wrist, 121
3.7 Muscles of Forearm (Superficial Layer): Anterior View, 122
3.8 Muscles of Forearm (Intermediate and Deep Layers): Anterior View, 123
3.9 Muscles of Forearm (Superficial and Deep Layers): Posterior View, 124
3.10 Cross-Sectional Anatomy of Right Forearm, 125
3.11 Cross-Sectional Anatomy of Wrist, 126
3.12 Muscles of Forearm: Origins and Insertions, 127
3.13 Blood Supply of Forearm, 128
3.14 Median Nerve of Forearm, 129
3.15 Ulnar Nerve of Forearm, 130
3.16 Cutaneous Nerves of Forearm, 131

Clinical Problems and Correlations

3.17 Carpal Tunnel Syndrome, 132
3.18 Cubital Tunnel Syndrome, 133
3.19 Fracture of Distal Radius: Colles Fracture, 134
3.20 Fracture of Distal Radius: Radiology, 135
3.21 Fracture of Distal Radius: Closed Reduction and Plaster Cast Immobilization of Colles Fracture, 136
3.22 Fracture of Distal Radius: Radiology of Open Reduction and Internal Fixation, 137
3.23 Fracture of Scaphoid: Presentation and Classification, 138
3.24 Fracture of Scaphoid: Blood Supply and Treatment, 139
3.25 Fracture of Scaphoid: Radiology, 140
3.26 Fracture of Hamulus of Hamate, 141
3.27 Dislocation of Carpus: Presentation and Treatment, 142

3.28 Dislocation of Carpus: Radiology, 143
3.29 Fracture of Both Forearm Bones, 144
3.30 Fracture of Shaft of Ulna, 145
3.31 Fracture of Shaft of Radius, 146
3.32 Ganglion of Wrist, 147
3.33 De Quervain Disease, 148
3.34 Rheumatoid Arthritis of Wrist, 149
3.35 Arthritis of Wrist, 150
3.36 Kienböck Disease, 151
3.37 Radial Longitudinal Deficiency: Forearm Manifestations, 152
3.38 Radial Longitudinal Deficiency: Type II Hypoplastic Thumb, 153

SECTION 4 HAND AND FINGER

Anatomy

4.1 Topographic Anatomy: Anterior View, 156
4.2 Topographic Anatomy: Posterior View, 157
4.3 Metacarpophalangeal and Interphalangeal Ligaments, 158
4.4 Definitions of Hand Motion, 159
4.5 Flexor and Extensor Tendons in Fingers, 160
4.6 Flexor and Extensor Zones and Lumbrical Muscles, 161
4.7 Wrist and Hand: Deep Dorsal Dissection, 162
4.8 Wrist and Hand: Intrinsic Muscles, 163
4.9 Spaces, Bursae, and Tendon and Lumbrical Sheaths of Hand, 164
4.10 Wrist and Hand: Palmar Dissections, 165
4.11 Vascular Supply of the Hand and Finger, 166
4.12 Ulnar Nerve of Hand, 167
4.13 Median Nerve of Hand, 168
4.14 Radial Nerve of Hand, 169
4.15 Skin and Subcutaneous Fascia: Anterior View, 170
4.16 Skin and Subcutaneous Fascia: Posterior View, 171
4.17 Lymphatic Drainage, 172
4.18 Digits: Sectional Anatomy, 173
4.19 Thumb: Sectional Anatomy, 174

Degenerative and Systemic Disorders

4.20 Hand Involvement in Osteoarthritis, 175
4.21 Hand Involvement in Rheumatoid Arthritis and Psoriatic Arthritis, 176
4.22 Hand Involvement in Gouty Arthritis and Reiter Syndrome, 177
4.23 Deformities of Thumb Joints: Metacarpophalangeal Deformities, 178
4.24 Deformities of Thumb Joints: Carpometacarpal Osteoarthritis, 179
4.25 Deformities of Thumb Joints: Ligament Replacement and Tendon Interposition Arthroplasty, 180
4.26 Deformities of the Metacarpophalangeal Joints: Implant Resection Arthroplasty, 181
4.27 Deformities of the Metacarpophalangeal Joints: Implant Resection Arthroplasty (Continued), 182
4.28 Deformities of the Metacarpophalangeal Joints: Implant Resection Arthroplasty (Continued), 183
4.29 Deformities of the Metacarpophalangeal Joints: Modular versus Implant Resection Arthroplasty, 184
4.30 Deformities of Interphalangeal Joint: Radiographic Findings, 185
4.31 Deformities of Interphalangeal Joint: Swan Neck and Boutonniere, 186
4.32 Deformities of Interphalangeal Joint: Implant Resection Arthroplasty, 187
4.33 Deformities of Interphalangeal Joint: Modular Versus Implant Resection Arthroplasty, 188
4.34 Dupuytren Contracture: Presentation and Treatment, 189
4.35 Dupuytren Contracture: Surgical Approach to Finger, 190

Infections and Tendon Disorders

4.36 Cellulitis and Abscess, 191
4.37 Tenosynovitis and Infection of Fascial Space, 192
4.38 Tenosynovitis and Infection of Fascial Space (Continued), 193
4.39 Infected Wounds, 194
4.40 Infection of Deep Compartments of Hand, 195
4.41 Lymphangitis, 196
4.42 Bier Block Anesthesia, 197
4.43 Thumb Carpometacarpal Injection, Digital Block, and Flexor Sheath Injection, 198
4.44 Tendon Disorders: Trigger Finger and Jersey Finger, 199
4.45 Tendon Disorders: Repair of Tendon, 200

Fractures and Dislocations

4.46 Fracture of Metacarpal Neck and Shaft, 201
4.47 Fracture of Thumb Metacarpal Base, 202
4.48 Fracture of Proximal and Middle Phalanges, 203
4.49 Management of Fracture of Proximal and Middle Phalanges, 204
4.50 Special Problems in Fracture of Middle and Proximal Phalanges, 205
4.51 Thumb Ligament Injury and Dislocation, 206
4.52 Carpometacarpal and Metacarpophalangeal Joint Injury, 207
4.53 Dorsal and Palmar Interphalangeal Joint Dislocations, 208
4.54 Treatment of Dorsal Interphalangeal Joint Dislocation, 209
4.55 Injuries to the Fingertip, 210
4.56 Rehabilitation after Injury to Hand and Fingers, 211

Amputation and Replantation

4.57 Amputation of Phalanx, 212
4.58 Amputation of Thumb and Deepening of Thenar Web Cleft, 213
4.59 Thumb Lengthening Post Amputation, 214
4.60 Microsurgical Instrumentation for Replantation, 215
4.61 Debridement, Incisions, and Repair of Bone in Replantation of Digit, 216
4.62 Repair of Blood Vessels and Nerves, 217
4.63 Postoperative Dressing and Monitoring of Blood Flow, 218
4.64 Replantation of Avulsed Thumb and Midpalm, 219
4.65 Lateral Arm Flap for Defect of Thumb Web, 220
4.66 Transfer of Great Toe to Thumb Site, 221

Selected References, 223
Index, 225

SHOULDER

Plate 1.1

Upper Limb: PART I

SCAPULA AND HUMERUS: POSTERIOR VIEW

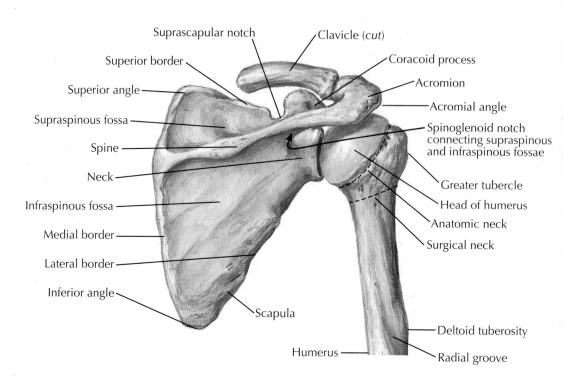

Suprascapular notch
Superior border
Superior angle
Supraspinous fossa
Spine
Neck
Infraspinous fossa
Medial border
Lateral border
Inferior angle
Scapula
Humerus
Clavicle (cut)
Coracoid process
Acromion
Acromial angle
Spinoglenoid notch connecting supraspinous and infraspinous fossae
Greater tubercle
Head of humerus
Anatomic neck
Surgical neck
Deltoid tuberosity
Radial groove

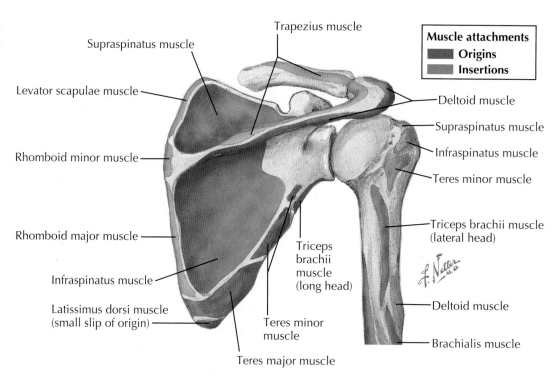

Trapezius muscle
Supraspinatus muscle
Levator scapulae muscle
Rhomboid minor muscle
Rhomboid major muscle
Infraspinatus muscle
Latissimus dorsi muscle (small slip of origin)
Teres major muscle
Triceps brachii muscle (long head)
Teres minor muscle

Muscle attachments	
■	Origins
■	Insertions

Deltoid muscle
Supraspinatus muscle
Infraspinatus muscle
Teres minor muscle
Triceps brachii muscle (lateral head)
Deltoid muscle
Brachialis muscle

SCAPULA AND HUMERUS

The function of the upper extremity is highly dependent on correlated motion in the four articulations of the shoulder. These include the glenohumeral (GH) joint, the acromioclavicular (AC) joint, the sternoclavicular joint, and the scapulothoracic articulation. The GH joint has minimal bony constraints, thus allowing for an impressive degree of motion.

SCAPULA

Ossification centers of the scapula begin to form during the eighth week of intrauterine life, but complete fusion does not occur until the end of the second decade. The acromial apophysis develops from four separate centers of ossification: the basi-acromion, meta-acromion, meso-acromion, and pre-acromion. Failure of complete fusion in a skeletally mature individual, referred to as an *os acromiale,* is estimated to occur in 8% of the population, with one-third of cases being bilateral. The proximal humeral epiphysis is composed of three primary ossification centers (the humeral head, the greater tuberosity, and the lesser tuberosity) that coalesce at approximately age 6 years. Eighty percent of longitudinal growth of the humerus is achieved through the proximal physis. Physeal closure occurs at the end of the second decade.

The top of the humerus has a large, nearly spherical articular surface surrounded at its articular margin (anatomic neck of the humerus) by two tuberosities. The humeral head articulates with the glenoid surface, which is only a little more than one-third of its size. The great freedom of movement of the GH joint is inevitably accompanied by a considerable loss of stability.

The insertion of the supraspinatus portion of the rotator cuff is superiorly on the greater tuberosity, and the infraspinatus and teres minor insert on the posteriormost part of the greater tuberosity. All four rotator cuff muscles take origin from the body of the scapula. The scapula is a thin sheet of bone that provides the site of attachment for several important muscles of the shoulder girdle. The lateral end of the clavicle articulates with the medial aspect of the acromion to form the AC joint.

The large deltoid muscle has its broad origin from the spine of the scapula posteriorly around the lateral acromion and then from the lateral third of the clavicle. Likewise, the trapezius muscle takes its insertion over a very similar area superior and medial to the deltoid origin. The trapezius has its primary function in scapula retraction and elevation of the scapula. The deltoid origin on the humerus at the deltoid tuberosity is approximately one-third the distance from the shoulder to the elbow. The levator scapulae and rhomboid major

and minor insert on the medial border of the scapula and function to retract the scapula toward the spine.

Between the anterior portion of the scapula and the chest wall (not shown) is the scapulothoracic articulation. This articulation is another important component of proper shoulder function. In addition to its contribution to overall shoulder motion, rotation of the scapula brings the glenoid underneath the humeral head so it can bear a portion of the weight of the upper extremity, thus decreasing the necessary force generated by the

Plate 1.2

Shoulder

SCAPULA AND HUMERUS: ANTERIOR VIEW

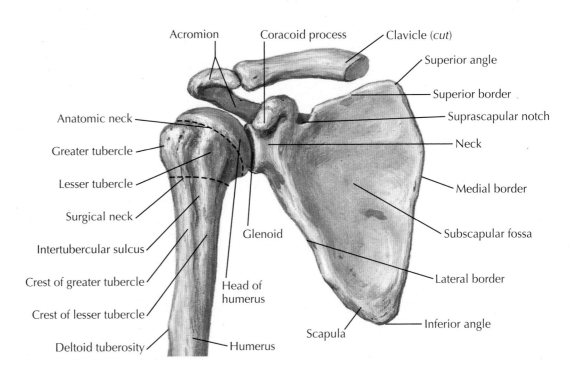

Acromion — Coracoid process — Clavicle (*cut*)

Superior angle

Superior border

Anatomic neck — Suprascapular notch

Greater tubercle — Neck

Lesser tubercle — Medial border

Surgical neck — Glenoid

Subscapular fossa

Intertubercular sulcus — Lateral border

Crest of greater tubercle — Head of humerus

Crest of lesser tubercle — Inferior angle

Scapula

Deltoid tuberosity — Humerus

SCAPULA AND HUMERUS
(Continued)

muscles of the shoulder girdle. Bony and soft tissue pathologic processes can result in bursitis and possibly crepitus at this articulation, leading to a "snapping scapula."

The body of the scapula has a large concavity on its costal surface, the subscapular fossa, for the subscapularis muscle. The dorsum is convex and is separated by the prominent spinous process into a supraspinous fossa above, for the supraspinatus muscle, and an infraspinous fossa below, for the infraspinatus muscle. The suprascapular notch is immediately medial to the coracoid process at the superior aspect of the scapular body. The spinous process is a large triangular projection of the dorsum of the bone, extending from the medial border to just short of the glenoid process. It increases its elevation and weight as it progresses laterally and ends in a concave border, the origin of which is the neck of the scapula. The spinous process continues freely to arch above the head of the humerus as the acromion, which overhangs the shoulder joint. Its lateral surface provides the origin for the posterior and middle thirds of the deltoid muscle.

The coracoid process projects anteriorly and laterally from the neck of the scapula. It gives attachment to the pectoralis minor, the short head of the biceps brachii, the coracobrachialis, the coracoacromial (CA) ligament, and the coracoclavicular ligaments. The lateral angle of the scapula broadens to form the glenoid, which has minimal bony concavity. It is pear shaped, with a wider inferior aspect. The fibrocartilaginous glenoid labrum attaches circumferentially to the margin of the glenoid, and the long head of the biceps brachii attaches directly to the supraglenoid tubercle.

HUMERUS

The humerus is a long bone composed of a shaft and two articular extremities. Proximally, the head is roughly one-third of a sphere, although the anteroposterior (AP) dimension is slightly less than the superoinferior distance. The anatomic neck is the slight indentation at the margin of the articular surface where the capsule

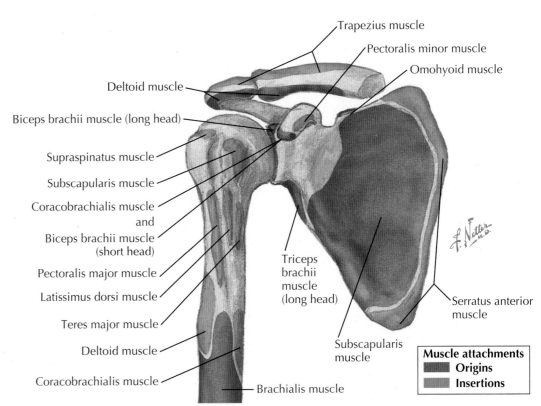

Trapezius muscle

Pectoralis minor muscle

Omohyoid muscle

Deltoid muscle

Biceps brachii muscle (long head)

Supraspinatus muscle

Subscapularis muscle

Coracobrachialis muscle and
Biceps brachii muscle (short head)

Pectoralis major muscle

Latissimus dorsi muscle

Teres major muscle

Deltoid muscle

Coracobrachialis muscle

Triceps brachii muscle (long head)

Serratus anterior muscle

Subscapularis muscle

Brachialis muscle

Muscle attachments
■ Origins
■ Insertions

attaches. The surgical neck is the narrowed area just distal to the tubercles, where fractures frequently occur. The greater tubercle serves as the attachments for the supraspinatus, infraspinatus, and teres minor tendons. The lesser tubercle is the insertion of the subscapularis tendon. Each of the tubercles is prolonged downward by bony crests, with the crest of the greater tubercle receiving the tendon of the pectoralis major (PM) muscle and the crest of the lesser tubercle receiving the tendon of

the teres major muscle. The intertubercular groove, lodging the long tendon of the biceps brachii muscle, also receives the tendon of the latissimus dorsi (LD) muscle into its floor. The shaft of the humerus is somewhat rounded above and prismatic in its lower portion. The deltoid tuberosity is prominent laterally over the midportion of the shaft, with a groove for the radial nerve that indents the bone posteriorly, spiraling lateralward as it descends.

Plate 1.3

Upper Limb: PART I

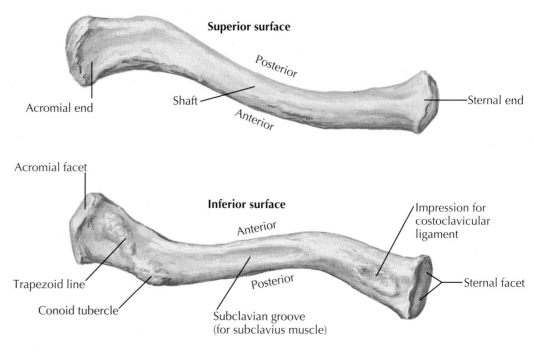

Right clavicle

Superior surface

Posterior

Acromial end · Shaft · Sternal end

Anterior

Acromial facet

Inferior surface

Anterior

Impression for costoclavicular ligament

Trapezoid line · Conoid tubercle

Posterior

Subclavian groove (for subclavius muscle)

Sternal facet

Trapezius muscle

Superior surface

Muscle origins
Muscle insertions
Ligament attachments

Posterior

Sterno-cleidomastoid muscle

Anterior

Deltoid muscle

Pectoralis major muscle

Inferior surface

Anterior

Costoclavicular ligament

Coraco-clavicular ligament { Trapezoid ligament / Conoid ligament }

Posterior

Subclavius muscle

Sternohyoid muscle

CLAVICLE

The clavicle is the first bone to ossify in the developing embryo; however, complete ossification does not occur until the third decade of life. When viewed from above, the clavicle has a gentle S shape with a larger medial curve that is convex anteriorly and a smaller lateral curve that is convex posteriorly. The medial two-thirds of the bone is roughly triangular in section, whereas the lateral third is flattened. Several bony prominences are present on the inferior surface of the clavicle. The undersurface of the lateral third of the bone demonstrates the conoid tubercle and trapezoid line, which correspond to the attachment of the two parts of the coraco-clavicular ligament. Centrally, the subclavius groove receives the subclavius muscle. Medially, there is an impression where the costoclavicular ligament attaches. The sternal extremity of the bone is triangular and exhibits a saddle-shaped articular surface, which is received into the clavicular fossa of the manubrium of

the sternum. The acromial extremity has an oval articular facet, directed lateralward and slightly downward, for the acromion.

In addition to functioning as a strut that keeps the shoulder in a more lateral position, it also serves as a point of attachment for several muscles. Medially, the clavicular head of the PM originates anteriorly, whereas the sternohyoid muscle originates posteriorly. The subclavius muscle originates from the inferior surface of the middle third of the clavicle. Laterally, the anterior third of the deltoid originates anteriorly, a portion of

the sternocleidomastoid originates superiorly, and a portion of the trapezius inserts posteriorly. Resection of portions of the clavicle is typically well tolerated as long as the integrity of the muscular attachments is not compromised. The sternoclavicular joint represents the only true articulation between the trunk and the upper limb. Rotation of the clavicle at this joint allows the arm to be placed in an over-the-head position. An articular disc is interposed between the joint surfaces, which greatly increases the capacity for movement. Joint stability is conveyed through static stabilizers.

Plate 1.4

Shoulder

LIGAMENTS

Glenohumeral joint and ligaments

Anterior view

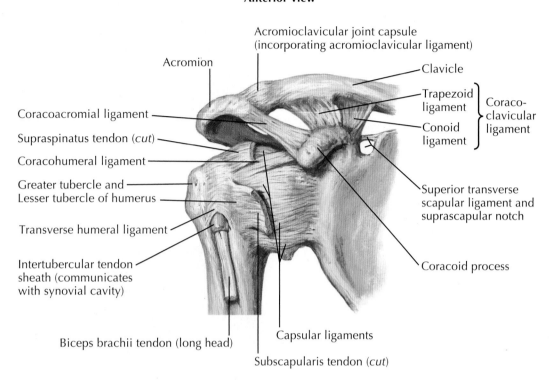

Acromioclavicular joint capsule
(incorporating acromioclavicular ligament)

Acromion

Clavicle

Coracoacromial ligament

Trapezoid
ligament

Coraco-
clavicular
ligament

Supraspinatus tendon (*cut*)

Conoid
ligament

Coracohumeral ligament

Greater tubercle and
Lesser tubercle of humerus

Superior transverse
scapular ligament and
suprascapular notch

Transverse humeral ligament

Intertubercular tendon
sheath (communicates
with synovial cavity)

Coracoid process

Biceps brachii tendon (long head)

Capsular ligaments

Subscapularis tendon (*cut*)

LIGAMENTS

Stability of the shoulder is highly dependent on numerous static stabilizers. The superior, middle, and inferior GH ligaments are thickenings in the anterior wall of the articular capsule. Visible only on the inner aspect of the capsule, they radiate from the anterior glenoid margin adjacent to and extending downward from the supraglenoid tubercle of the scapula. These ligaments are best seen on arthroscopic photographs.

SUPERIOR GLENOHUMERAL LIGAMENT

The superior glenohumeral ligament (SGL) is slender, arises immediately anterior to the attachment of the tendon of the long head of the biceps brachii muscle, and parallels that tendon to end near the upper end of the lesser tubercle of the humerus. The anterior biceps sling is formed by the confluence of the SGL and the coracohumeral ligament, which stabilizes the long head of the biceps brachii tendon as it enters the bicipital groove.

MIDDLE GLENOHUMERAL LIGAMENT

The middle glenohumeral ligament (MGL) arises next to the SGL and reaches the humerus at the front of the lesser tubercle and just inferior to the insertion of the subscapularis muscle. It has an oblique course immediately inferior to the opening of the subscapular bursa. When present, the middle glenoid humeral ligament inserts on the glenoid rim posterior to the labrum. The MGL may be cord-like, thin, or even absent. A thin MGL is seen in the arthroscopic pictures of the shoulder, allowing intraarticular visualization of most of the articular side of the subscapularis tendon.

Sternoclavicular joint and ligaments

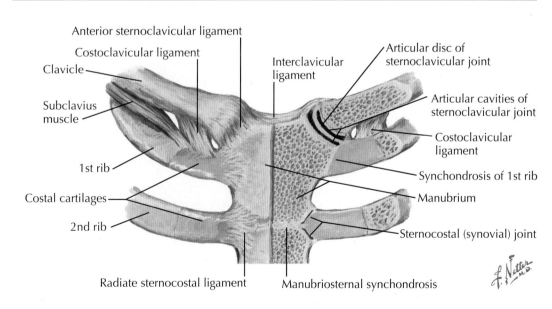

Anterior sternoclavicular ligament

Costoclavicular ligament

Clavicle

Subclavius
muscle

Interclavicular
ligament

Articular disc of
sternoclavicular joint

Articular cavities of
sternoclavicular joint

Costoclavicular
ligament

1st rib

Synchondrosis of 1st rib

Costal cartilages

Manubrium

2nd rib

Sternocostal (synovial) joint

Radiate sternocostal ligament

Manubriosternal synchondrosis

INFERIOR GLENOHUMERAL LIGAMENT

The inferior GH ligament arises from the scapula directly below the notch (comma of the glenoid) in the anterior border of the glenoidal process of the scapula and descends to the underside of the neck of the humerus at the inferior fold of the inferior capsular pouch. The latter two ligaments may be poorly separated. The inferior GH ligament inserts into the anteroinferior and posteroinferior labrum.

CORACOHUMERAL LIGAMENT

The coracohumeral ligament, partly continuous with the articular capsule, is a broad band arising from the lateral border of the coracoid process. Flattening, it blends with the upper and posterior part of the capsule and ends in the anatomic neck of the humerus adjacent to the greater tubercle.

There are two openings in the capsule. The opening at the upper end of the intertubercular groove allows

Plate 1.5

Upper Limb: PART I

GLENOHUMERAL ARTHROSCOPIC ANATOMY

Long head of the biceps tendon

Anterior edge of the supraspinatus tendon forming the lateral pulley for the medial wall of the biceps groove

Confluence of the superior glenohumeral ligaments, coraco-humeral ligament to form the medial pulley for the medial wall of the biceps groove

Rotator interval containing the coracohumeral and superior glenohumeral ligaments

Upper half of the articular surface of the glenoid fossa

Upper border of the subscapularis tendon

Articular surface of the humeral head

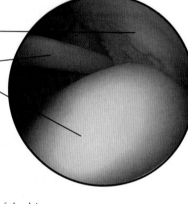

Crescent of the supraspinatus surrounded by the cable of the supraspinatus tendon

Long head of the biceps tendon

Articular surface of the humeral head

Insertion of the long head of the bicep into the superior labrum at the superior glenoid tubercle

Anterior to posterior limits of the superior labrum. Pathology of this portion of the labrum between these two points is defined as a SLAP lesion.

This region of anatomy constitutes the superior labrum biceps tendon complex and is a common site of shoulder pathology as it relates to degenerative and traumatic injuries to these tissues.

LIGAMENTS (Continued)

for the passage of the tendon of the long head of the biceps brachii muscle. The other opening is an anterior communication of the joint cavity with the subcoracoid bursa. The synovial membrane extends from the margin of the glenoid cavity and lines the capsule to the limits of the articular cartilage of the humerus. It also forms the intertubercular synovial sheath on the tendon of the biceps brachii muscle.

CORACOCLAVICULAR LIGAMENTS

The coracoclavicular ligaments arise from the superior aspect of the base of the coracoid. The conoid portion is more posterior and medial, whereas the trapezoid portion is more anterior and lateral. In conjunction with the AC joint capsule, they prevent superior displacement of the clavicle.

CORACOACROMIAL LIGAMENT

The CA ligament arises from the tip of the coracoid process and attaches to the most anterior aspect of the acromion. Traction spurs may develop at the acromial attachment, giving the acromion a more hooked shape. This ligament plays an important role in the rotator cuff–deficient shoulder, where it becomes the only remaining restraint to superior migration of the humeral head.

STERNOCLAVICULAR JOINT

The sternoclavicular joint represents the only true articulation between the trunk and the upper limb. Rotation of the clavicle at this joint allows the arm to be

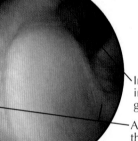

Upper border of the subscapularis tendon. There is wide variation in the presence and insertion of the middle glenohumeral ligaments in the normal population. The thin tissue over the tendon is the middle glenohumeral ligament, which is thin and almost translucent in this example. This tissue can be, in other patients, a very thick and robust ligament.

Anterior superior band of the inferior glenohumeral ligament inserting onto the anterior inferior glenoid labrum

Articular surface of the midportion of the humeral head

Inferior glenoid labrum

Midpoint of the anterior glenoid articular surface of the fossa in which there is a change. The medial lateral dimension of the fossa results in a curvature called the comma of the glenoid, also seen as a C shape along the articular surface of the glenoid.

placed in an over-the-head position. An articular disc is interposed between the joint surfaces, which greatly increases the capacity for movement. Joint stability is conveyed through static stabilizers. The articular capsule is relatively weak but is reinforced by the capsular ligaments. The anterior sternoclavicular ligament is a broad anterior band of fibers attached to the upper and anterior borders of the sternal end of the clavicle; below, it is attached to the upper anterior surface of the

manubrium of the sternum. This strong band is reinforced by the tendinous origin of the sternocleidomastoid muscle. The posterior sternoclavicular ligament has a similar orientation on the back of the capsule and has similar bony attachments. The costoclavicular ligament is a short, flat band of fibers running between the cartilage of the first rib and the costal tuberosity on the undersurface of the clavicle. The interclavicular ligament strengthens the capsule above. It passes between

Plate 1.6   Shoulder

GLENOHUMERAL ARTHROSCOPIC ANATOMY (CONTINUED)

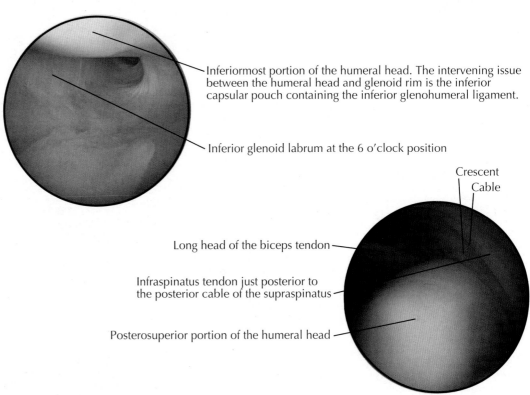

Inferiormost portion of the humeral head. The intervening issue between the humeral head and glenoid rim is the inferior capsular pouch containing the inferior glenohumeral ligament.

Inferior glenoid labrum at the 6 o'clock position

Crescent
Cable

Long head of the biceps tendon

Infraspinatus tendon just posterior to the posterior cable of the supraspinatus

Posterosuperior portion of the humeral head

The change in coloration of the posterior portion of the humeral head near the posteriormost insertion of the rotator cuff is the upper portion of the bare area of the humeral head, which is normally devoid of articular cartilage.

LIGAMENTS (Continued)

the right and left clavicles with additional attachment to the upper border of the sternum. The anterior supraclavicular nerve gives the sternoclavicular joint its nerve supply. Blood supply is derived from branches of the internal thoracic artery, the superior thoracic artery, and the clavicular branch of the thoracoacromial artery.

GLENOHUMERAL JOINT

Given the lack of bony constraint, the GH joint is circumferentially surrounded by static and dynamic stabilizers. Arthroscopic examination of these structures is essential to accurately identify a pathologic process in a symptomatic shoulder. The anatomic structures and their relationship can be visualized by arthroscopy of the joint (Plates 1.5 and 1.6). The long head of the biceps must be visualized along its entire intraarticular course. The integrity of the biceps anchor should be examined, as should the stability of the biceps sling at the superior aspect of the bicipital groove. The attachment of the glenoid labrum should be inspected circumferentially, although a sublabral foramen in the anterosuperior quadrant can be a normal variant. An attached labrum is seen in the arthroscopic views. The condition of the articular cartilage on the glenoid and humeral head can be characterized according to its appearance on arthroscopic examination. Grade 1 changes are seen as softening of the cartilage without loss of the smooth cartilage surface. Grade 2 changes show loss of the smooth cartilage surface and luster with a cobblestone appearance yet no loss of cartilage thickness. Grade 3 indicates loss of cartilage thickness and fissuring of the cartilage, giving it a velvet

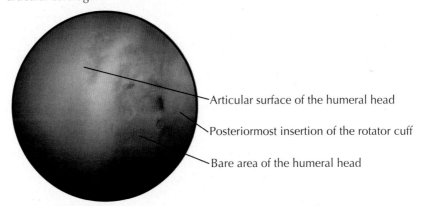

Articular surface of the humeral head

Posteriormost insertion of the rotator cuff

Bare area of the humeral head

Posteriormost portion of the glenohumeral joint showing the posteriormost aspect of the articular surface of the humeral head and the posteriormost insertion of the rotator cuff, between which is the bare area of the humeral head in which articular cartilage is not covering the humeral head. All pits in the bare area represent the remnants of the vascular channels of the epiphysis vessels that were present during development prior to closure of the growth plate. The blood supply to the epiphysis of the humeral head came from these vessels. After growth plate closures, these vessels involute, leaving behind the empty vascular channels. After growth plate closure, the epiphysis receives its blood supply from the metaphyseal vessels that cross over the area of the closed growth plate. The humeral head also receives blood supply from the terminal vessel of Liang, from the ascending branch of the anterior humeral circumflex artery, and from the posterior humeral circumflex artery (see Plate 1.16).

appearance when mild and the end of a mop appearance when severe. Grade 4 is characterized by complete loss of cartilage down to the subchondral bone. The axillary pouch must be visualized because this is a common location of loose bodies within the joint.

The insertion sites of the four rotator cuff tendons should be noted. Superiorly the footprint is adjacent to the articular margin, but posteriorly there is a bare area of bone between the articular cartilage and

infraspinatus/teres minor insertion. The subscapularis tendon is located anteriorly, and complete visualization of its insertion can be challenging when there is a well-defined MGL. Medial subluxation of the long head of the biceps brachii tendon from being centered in the bicipital groove is a sign that the insertion of the subscapularis is compromised or there is damage to the medial pulley and soft tissue wall of the biceps groove.

Plate 1.7

Upper Limb: PART I

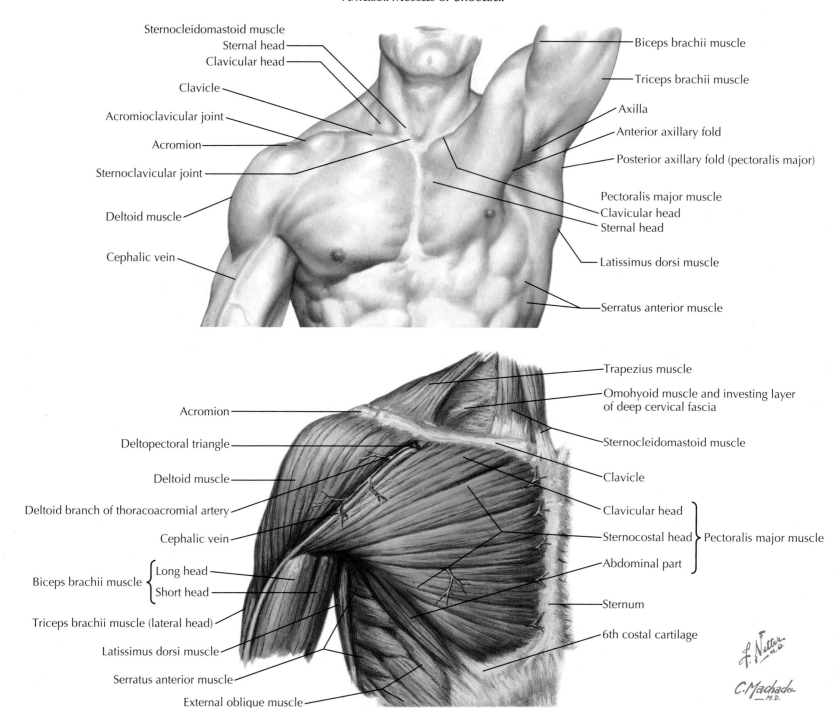

ANTERIOR MUSCLES OF SHOULDER

Sternocleidomastoid muscle
Sternal head
Clavicular head
Clavicle
Acromioclavicular joint
Acromion
Sternoclavicular joint
Deltoid muscle
Cephalic vein

Biceps brachii muscle
Triceps brachii muscle
Axilla
Anterior axillary fold
Posterior axillary fold (pectoralis major)
Pectoralis major muscle
Clavicular head
Sternal head
Latissimus dorsi muscle
Serratus anterior muscle

Acromion
Deltopectoral triangle
Deltoid muscle
Deltoid branch of thoracoacromial artery
Cephalic vein
Biceps brachii muscle { Long head / Short head
Triceps brachii muscle (lateral head)
Latissimus dorsi muscle
Serratus anterior muscle
External oblique muscle

Trapezius muscle
Omohyoid muscle and investing layer of deep cervical fascia
Sternocleidomastoid muscle
Clavicle
Clavicular head
Sternocostal head } Pectoralis major muscle
Abdominal part
Sternum
6th costal cartilage

MUSCLES OF SHOULDER

DELTOID MUSCLE

The deltoid muscle is triangular with a semicircular origin along the lateral third of the clavicle, the lateral border of the acromion, and the lower lip of the crest of the spine of the scapula. All fasciculi converge to be inserted on the deltoid tuberosity of the humerus. The deltoid muscle is a principal abductor of the humerus, an action produced primarily by its powerful central portion. Because of their position and greater fiber length, the clavicular and scapular portions of the deltoid muscle have different actions from those of the central portion of the muscle. The clavicular portion assists in flexion and internal rotation of the arm,

whereas the scapular portion assists in extension and external rotation.

The axillary nerve (C5, C6) from the posterior cord of the brachial plexus supplies the deltoid muscle. An upper branch curves around the posterior surface of the humerus and courses from behind forward on the deep surface of the muscle, sending offshoots into the muscle. A lower branch supplies the teres minor muscle by ascending onto its lateral and superficial surface. It then becomes the superior lateral brachial cutaneous nerve. The posterior circumflex humeral artery serves this muscle.

PECTORALIS MUSCLE

The PM muscle originates from the medial half of the clavicle on its anterior surface and the anterior surface

of the manubrium and body of the sternum. Additional fascicles arise from the cartilages of the second to sixth ribs as well as from the anterior layer of the sheath of the rectus abdominis muscle. The muscular fibers converge to insert on the crest immediately distal to the greater tubercle, lateral to the bicipital groove. The tendon folds on itself to form a bilaminar, U-shaped tendon with the fold of the tendon below. Thus the fibers of the clavicular part insert as the upper part of the anterior lamina; the lower sternal and abdominal fibers reach up into the superior part of the posterior limb; and the sternal fibers distribute into the anterior lamina, the fold, and the lower part of the posterior lamina.

The PM muscle flexes and adducts the humerus; it is also capable of medial rotation of the arm but usually becomes active only when this action is resisted. The

Plate 1.8   Shoulder

ANTERIOR MUSCLES OF SHOULDER: CROSS SECTIONS

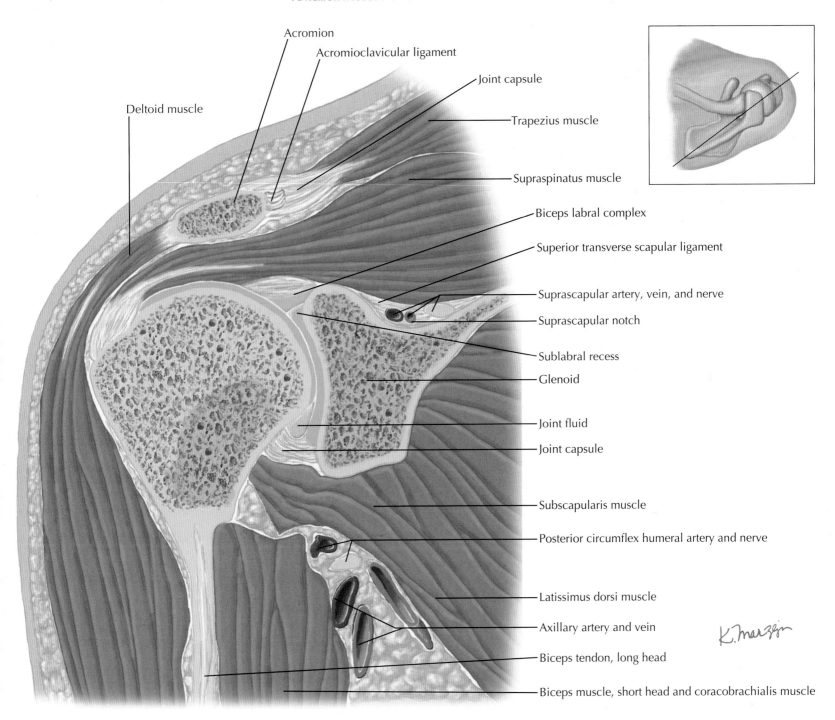

Acromion

Acromioclavicular ligament

Joint capsule

Deltoid muscle

Trapezius muscle

Supraspinatus muscle

Biceps labral complex

Superior transverse scapular ligament

Suprascapular artery, vein, and nerve

Suprascapular notch

Sublabral recess

Glenoid

Joint fluid

Joint capsule

Subscapularis muscle

Posterior circumflex humeral artery and nerve

Latissimus dorsi muscle

Axillary artery and vein

Biceps tendon, long head

Biceps muscle, short head and coracobrachialis muscle

K. Marzejon

MUSCLES OF SHOULDER (Continued)

clavicular portion of the PM muscle elevates the shoulder and flexes the arm, whereas the sternocostal portion draws the shoulder downward. The muscle is innervated by the lateral and medial pectoral nerves from both the lateral and medial cords of the brachial plexus, involving all the roots (C5 to T1). The pectoral branches of the thoracoacromial artery accompany the nerves to the muscle.

The deltopectoral triangle is a separation just below the clavicle of the upper and adjacent fibers of the deltoid and PM muscles. Distally, the separation

of these adjacent fibers is made by the cephalic vein and the deltoid branch of the thoracoacromial artery.

The pectoralis minor muscle arises from the outer surfaces of the third, fourth, and fifth ribs near their costal cartilages, with a slip from the second rib a frequent addition. The muscle fibers converge to an insertion on the medial border and upper surface of the coracoid process. The pectoralis minor muscle draws the scapula forward, medially, and strongly downward. With the scapula fixed, the muscle assists in forced inspiration. The muscle is innervated by the medial pectoral nerve (C8, T1), which completely penetrates the muscle to pass across the interpectoral space into the PM muscle. Pectoral branches of the thoracoacromial artery are distributed with the nerve.

Deep to the tendon of the pectoralis minor muscle pass the axillary artery and the cords of the brachial plexus.

SERRATUS MUSCLE

The serratus anterior muscle originates laterally from the first eight ribs. The muscle fibers converge to insert on the deep surface of the lateral border of the scapular body. Contraction of the muscle protracts the scapula and participates in upward rotation of the scapula. Weakness results in scapula winging (see Plates 1.20 and 1.59). Innervation is supplied by the long thoracic nerve (C5 to C8), which can easily be injured during axillary lymph node dissection. The blood supply is primarily through the lateral thoracic artery.

Plate 1.9

Upper Limb: PART I

POSTERIOR MUSCLES OF SHOULDER

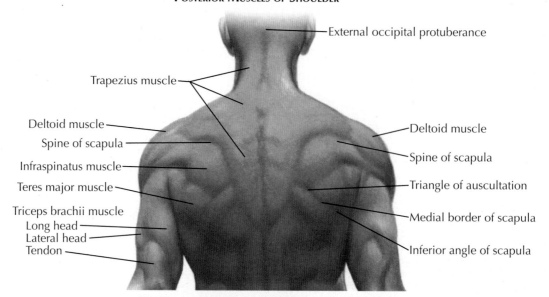

External occipital protuberance

Trapezius muscle

Deltoid muscle

Spine of scapula

Infraspinatus muscle

Teres major muscle

Triceps brachii muscle
Long head
Lateral head
Tendon

Deltoid muscle

Spine of scapula

Triangle of auscultation

Medial border of scapula

Inferior angle of scapula

Posterior view: superficial layer

Posterior view: deeper layer

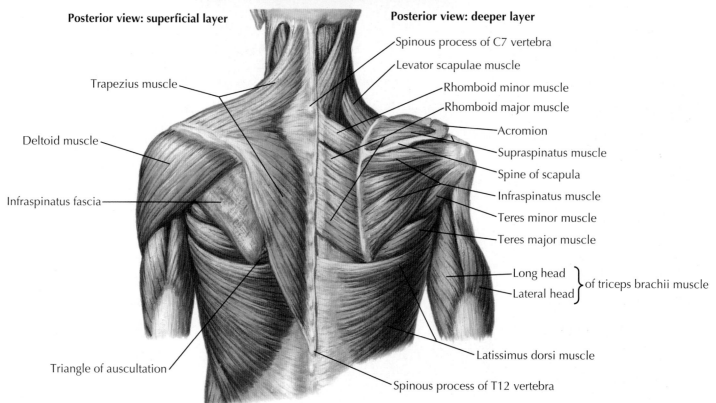

Trapezius muscle

Deltoid muscle

Infraspinatus fascia

Triangle of auscultation

Spinous process of C7 vertebra

Levator scapulae muscle

Rhomboid minor muscle

Rhomboid major muscle

Acromion

Supraspinatus muscle

Spine of scapula

Infraspinatus muscle

Teres minor muscle

Teres major muscle

Long head
Lateral head } of triceps brachii muscle

Latissimus dorsi muscle

Spinous process of T12 vertebra

MUSCLES OF SHOULDER (Continued)

SUBCLAVIUS MUSCLE

The subclavius muscle is a small, pencil-like muscle that arises from the junction of the first rib and its cartilage. It lies parallel to the underside of the clavicle and inserts in a groove on the underside of the clavicle, between the attachments of the conoid ligament laterally and the costoclavicular ligament medially. The muscle assists by its traction on the clavicle in drawing the shoulder forward and downward. The nerve to the subclavius muscle is a branch of the superior trunk of the

brachial plexus, with fibers from the fifth cervical nerve, which reaches the upper posterior border of the muscle. There is a small, special clavicular branch of the thoracoacromial artery to the muscle.

TRAPEZIUS MUSCLE

The trapezius muscle is divided into upper, middle, and lower divisions with a broad origin from the occipital protuberance superiorly to the spinous process of the T12 vertebrae inferiorly. It inserts onto the posterior border of the lateral third of the clavicle, the medial border of the acromion, and the upper border of the crest of the spine of the scapula. The directionality of the upper and lower divisions allows it to rotate the scapula so the glenoid faces superiorly, which allows

full elevation of the upper extremity. The middle division serves to retract the scapula. When the function of the trapezius is absent, the scapula wings laterally owing to unopposed contraction of the serratus anterior (see Plate 1.59). The nerves reaching the trapezius muscle are the spinal accessory (cranial nerve XI) and direct branches of ventral rami of the second, third, and fourth cervical nerves. The accessory nerve perforates and supplies the sternocleidomastoid muscle and then crosses the posterior triangle of the neck directly under its fascial covering, coursing diagonally downward to reach the underside of the trapezius muscle. The transverse cervical artery of the subclavian system supplies the trapezius muscle; it is supplemented in the lower third of the muscle by a muscular perforating branch of the dorsal scapular artery.

Plate 1.10

Shoulder

POSTERIOR MUSCLES OF SHOULDER: CROSS SECTIONS

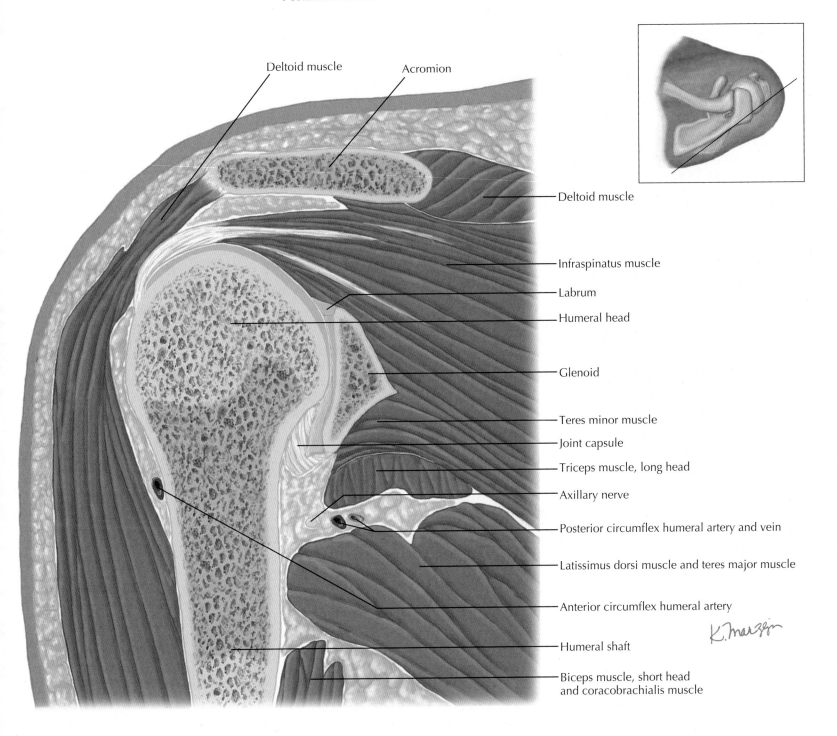

Deltoid muscle

Acromion

Deltoid muscle

Infraspinatus muscle

Labrum

Humeral head

Glenoid

Teres minor muscle

Joint capsule

Triceps muscle, long head

Axillary nerve

Posterior circumflex humeral artery and vein

Latissimus dorsi muscle and teres major muscle

Anterior circumflex humeral artery

Humeral shaft

Biceps muscle, short head and coracobrachialis muscle

K. marzejn

MUSCLES OF SHOULDER (Continued)

LEVATOR SCAPULAE MUSCLE

The levator scapulae originates from the transverse processes of the first three or four cervical vertebrae. It inserts into the medial border of the scapula from the superior angle to the spine. It is overlapped and partially obscured by the sternocleidomastoid and trapezius muscles. It functions to elevate and adduct the scapula. Innervation is provided by the dorsal scapular nerve (C3 to C5), and blood supply is from the dorsal scapular artery.

RHOMBOIDEUS MUSCLE

The rhomboideus minor muscle originates from the lower part of the ligamentum nuchae and the spinous processes of C7 to T1. It lies parallel to the rhomboideus major muscle, directed downward and lateralward, and it is inserted on the medial border of the scapula at the root of the scapular spine. The rhomboideus major muscle arises from the spinous processes of T2 to T5 and inserts on the medial border of the scapula below its spine. Both rhomboideus muscles draw the scapula upward and medially and assist the serratus anterior muscle in holding it firmly to the chest wall. Their oblique traction aids in depressing the point of the shoulder. The innervation and blood supply are the same as for the levator scapulae.

LATISSIMUS DORSI MUSCLE

The LD muscle originates from the inferior thoracic vertebrae, the thoracolumbar fascia, the iliac crest, and the lower third to fourth ribs. It inserts onto the floor of the intertubercular groove of the humerus. Contraction of this muscle extends the humerus, drawing the arm downward and backward and rotating it internally. The muscle is innervated by the thoracodorsal nerve from the posterior cord of the brachial plexus, with fibers from the seventh and eighth cervical nerves. The thoracodorsal artery, a branch of the subscapular artery, and a vein of the same name accompany the nerve.

Plate 1.11

Upper Limb: PART I

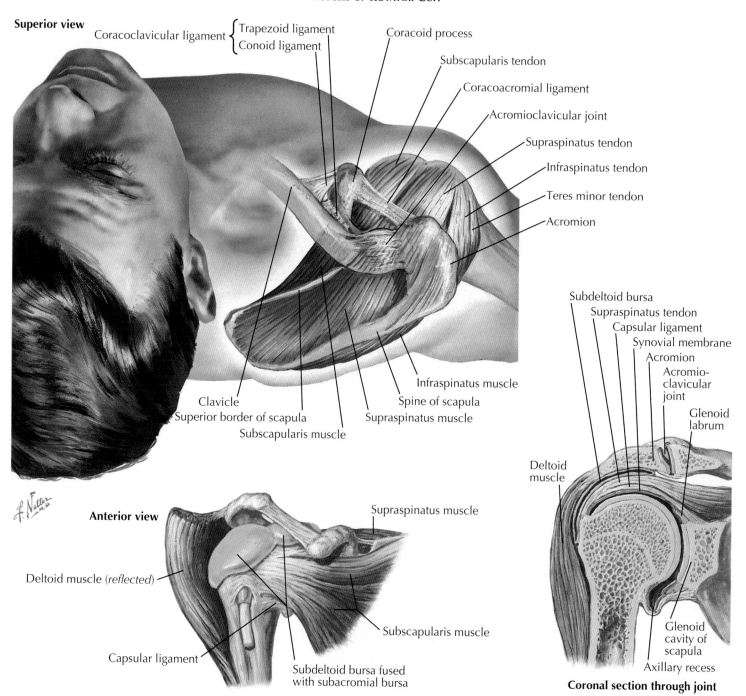

MUSCLES OF ROTATOR CUFF

Superior view

Coracoclavicular ligament { Trapezoid ligament / Conoid ligament

Coracoid process

Subscapularis tendon

Coracoacromial ligament

Acromioclavicular joint

Supraspinatus tendon

Infraspinatus tendon

Teres minor tendon

Acromion

Infraspinatus muscle

Spine of scapula

Supraspinatus muscle

Clavicle

Superior border of scapula

Subscapularis muscle

Subdeltoid bursa

Supraspinatus tendon

Capsular ligament

Synovial membrane

Acromion

Acromio-clavicular joint

Glenoid labrum

Deltoid muscle

Glenoid cavity of scapula

Axillary recess

Coronal section through joint

Anterior view

Supraspinatus muscle

Deltoid muscle (*reflected*)

Subscapularis muscle

Capsular ligament

Subdeltoid bursa fused with subacromial bursa

MUSCLES OF SHOULDER AND UPPER ARM

ROTATOR CUFF

The main function of the four musculotendinous units that contribute to the rotator cuff is to compress the humeral head into the glenoid to provide a fulcrum for rotation. Whereas each muscle aids in specific motions, it is this concavity compression that is essential for the proper function of the other muscles that affect the GH joint.

Supraspinatus Muscle

The supraspinatus muscle occupies the supraspinous fossa of the scapula. It takes its origin from the medial two-thirds of the bony walls of this fossa. The tendon blends deeply with the capsule of the shoulder joint and inserts on the highest of the three facets of the greater tubercle of the humerus. The supraspinatus muscle aids the deltoid in the first 90 degrees of forward flexion and abduction. Partial- or full-thickness tears of this tendon are not uncommon and may be well tolerated if the remaining intact cuff can compensate. This is particularly true if the tear involves the crescent portion of the supraspinatus tendon rather than the cable portion of the tendon. Tears involving the anteriormost portion of the supraspinatus and, in particular, the anterior cable result in a larger amount of muscle weakness, tendon retraction, and muscle atrophy than tears isolated to the central crescent portion of the tendon. Large two-tendon tears involving more than the supraspinatus can lead to superior migration of the humeral head, owing

to the unopposed contraction of the deltoid. The supraspinatus muscle is innervated by the suprascapular nerve (SSN) (C5, C6) from the superior trunk of the brachial plexus. The nerve may become entrapped as it enters the supraspinous fossa through the scapular notch, where it passes under the superior transverse scapular ligament. The suprascapular artery accompanies the nerve, but it passes over the transverse scapular ligament.

Infraspinatus Muscle

The infraspinatus muscle arises from the infraspinous fossa of the scapula and inserts on the middle facet of the greater tubercle of the humerus. Deeply, its fibers blend with those of the capsule of the shoulder joint. This muscle acts to externally rotate the arm. Pronounced weakness is demonstrated by the external

Plate 1.12   Shoulder

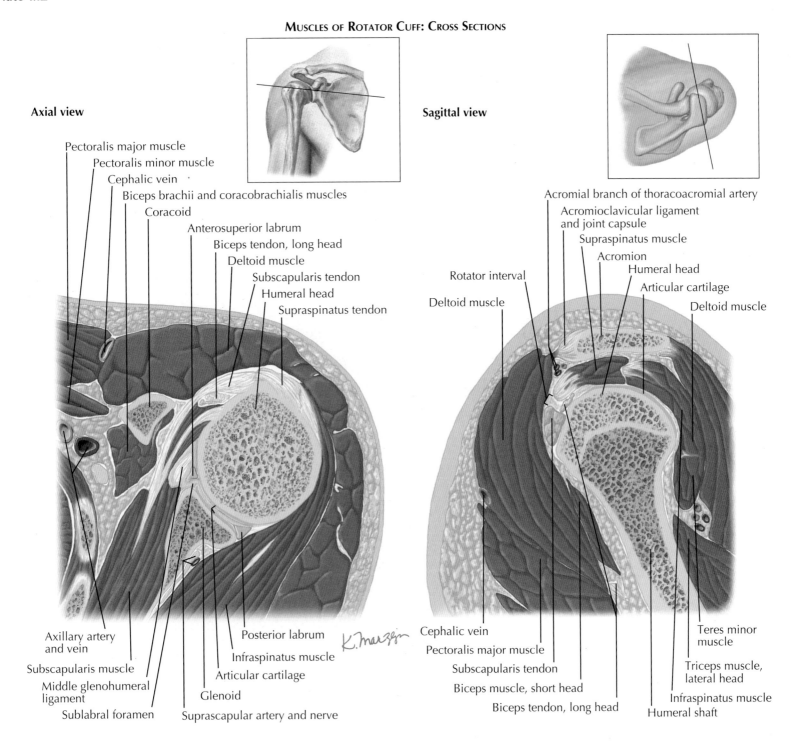

MUSCLES OF ROTATOR CUFF: CROSS SECTIONS

Axial view

- Pectoralis major muscle
- Pectoralis minor muscle
- Cephalic vein
- Biceps brachii and coracobrachialis muscles
- Coracoid
- Anterosuperior labrum
- Biceps tendon, long head
- Deltoid muscle
- Subscapularis tendon
- Humeral head
- Supraspinatus tendon

- Axillary artery and vein
- Subscapularis muscle
- Middle glenohumeral ligament
- Sublabral foramen
- Posterior labrum
- Infraspinatus muscle
- Articular cartilage
- Glenoid
- Suprascapular artery and nerve

Sagittal view

- Acromial branch of thoracoacromial artery
- Acromioclavicular ligament and joint capsule
- Supraspinatus muscle
- Acromion
- Humeral head
- Articular cartilage
- Deltoid muscle

- Rotator interval
- Deltoid muscle

- Cephalic vein
- Pectoralis major muscle
- Subscapularis tendon
- Biceps muscle, short head
- Biceps tendon, long head
- Teres minor muscle
- Triceps muscle, lateral head
- Infraspinatus muscle
- Humeral shaft

K. Marzen

MUSCLES OF SHOULDER AND UPPER ARM (Continued)

rotation lag sign, in which the patient cannot maintain passive external rotation at the side (see Plate 1.43). The SSN and artery continue through the spinoglenoid notch after giving off branches to the supraspinatus. Ganglion cysts can be seen in this area in conjunction with GH labral tears and may compress the nerve (see Plate 1.58).

Teres Minor Muscle

The teres minor muscle arises from the upper two-thirds of the lateral border of the scapula. Its tendon passes upward and lateralward to insert in the lower facet of the greater tubercle and surgical neck of the humerus. It also blends deeply with the capsule of the shoulder joint. The muscle is invested by the infraspinatus fascia and is sometimes inseparable from the infraspinatus muscle. The teres minor muscle contracts with the infraspinatus to aid in external rotation of the humerus. A branch of the axillary nerve ascends onto its lateral margin at about its midlength. The teres minor muscle is separated from the teres major by the long head of the triceps brachii and by the axillary nerve and posterior circumflex humeral vessels. It is pierced by branches of the circumflex scapular vessels along the lateral border of the scapula.

Subscapularis Muscle

The subscapularis muscle originates from the medial two-thirds of the subscapularis fossa on the anterior surface of the scapular body. The tendon passes across the anterior surface of the capsule of the shoulder joint to end in the lesser tubercle of the humerus. The tendon is separated from the neck of the scapula by the large subscapular bursa. The subscapularis muscle is the principal internal rotator of the arm but also acts in adduction. The upper half of the subscapularis has been shown to carry over 70% of the muscle fibers, tension, and strength of the entire muscle. As a result of this, distribution tears of the upper portion of the subscapularis are associated with more disability than tears involving the inferior half of the muscle. Dysfunction of the subscapularis muscle results in weakness best defined with the abdominal compression test and the internal rotation lift-off test (see Plate 1.48). The muscle is innervated on its costal surface by the upper and lower subscapular nerves.

Plate 1.13

Upper Limb: PART I

AXILLA DISSECTION: ANTERIOR VIEW

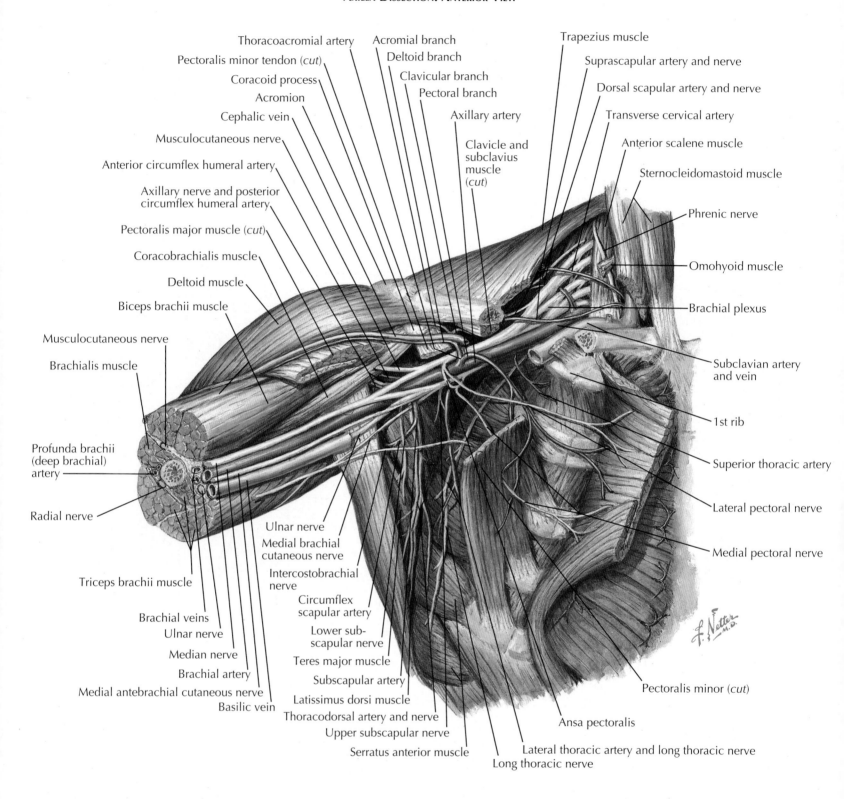

Thoracoacromial artery
Pectoralis minor tendon (cut)
Coracoid process
Acromion
Cephalic vein
Musculocutaneous nerve
Anterior circumflex humeral artery
Axillary nerve and posterior circumflex humeral artery
Pectoralis major muscle (cut)
Coracobrachialis muscle
Deltoid muscle
Biceps brachii muscle
Musculocutaneous nerve
Brachialis muscle
Profunda brachii (deep brachial) artery
Radial nerve
Triceps brachii muscle
Brachial veins
Ulnar nerve
Median nerve
Brachial artery
Medial antebrachial cutaneous nerve
Basilic vein
Ulnar nerve
Medial brachial cutaneous nerve
Intercostobrachial nerve
Circumflex scapular artery
Lower subscapular nerve
Teres major muscle
Subscapular artery
Latissimus dorsi muscle
Thoracodorsal artery and nerve
Upper subscapular nerve
Serratus anterior muscle
Long thoracic nerve

Acromial branch
Deltoid branch
Clavicular branch
Pectoral branch
Axillary artery
Clavicle and subclavius muscle (cut)

Trapezius muscle
Suprascapular artery and nerve
Dorsal scapular artery and nerve
Transverse cervical artery
Anterior scalene muscle
Sternocleidomastoid muscle
Phrenic nerve
Omohyoid muscle
Brachial plexus
Subclavian artery and vein
1st rib
Superior thoracic artery
Lateral pectoral nerve
Medial pectoral nerve
Pectoralis minor (cut)
Ansa pectoralis
Lateral thoracic artery and long thoracic nerve

NEUROVASCULAR RELATIONSHIPS

Brachial plexus anatomy and its relationship to the surrounding bone and muscle structure can vary. The most common anatomic relationships of the brachial plexus are shown in Plate 1.13. The brachial plexus is formed through the coalescence of the anterior rami of the C5, C6, C7, C8, and T1 spinal nerves, although variable contributions from C4 and T2 can occur. The roots combine to form trunks that, along with the subclavian

artery, exit the cervical spine between the anterior scalene (scalenus anticus) and middle scalene (scalenus medius) muscles. The plexus is posterior and superior to the artery at this level owing to the inferior tilt of the first rib. The peripheral nerves of the plexus supply motor and sensory nerve function to all the scapula musculature (except the trapezius muscle, which is innervated by the spinal accessory nerve) and the rest of the upper extremity.

Interscalene injection of a local anesthetic is commonly performed for all surgery on the upper

extremity. Dispersal of medication is minimized outside the area surrounding the nerves because the nerves become enclosed in prevertebral fascia as they pass between the scalene muscles. The brachial plexus passes through the scalene muscles over the first rib and under the clavicle and pectoralis minor before entering the axilla. In any of these locations there can be compression of the neurovascular structures from congenital or acquired conditions, resulting in vascular or neurovascular symptoms, particularly when using the arm above shoulder level or with repetitive tasks in any arm

Plate 1.14

Shoulder

AXILLA: POSTERIOR WALL AND CORD

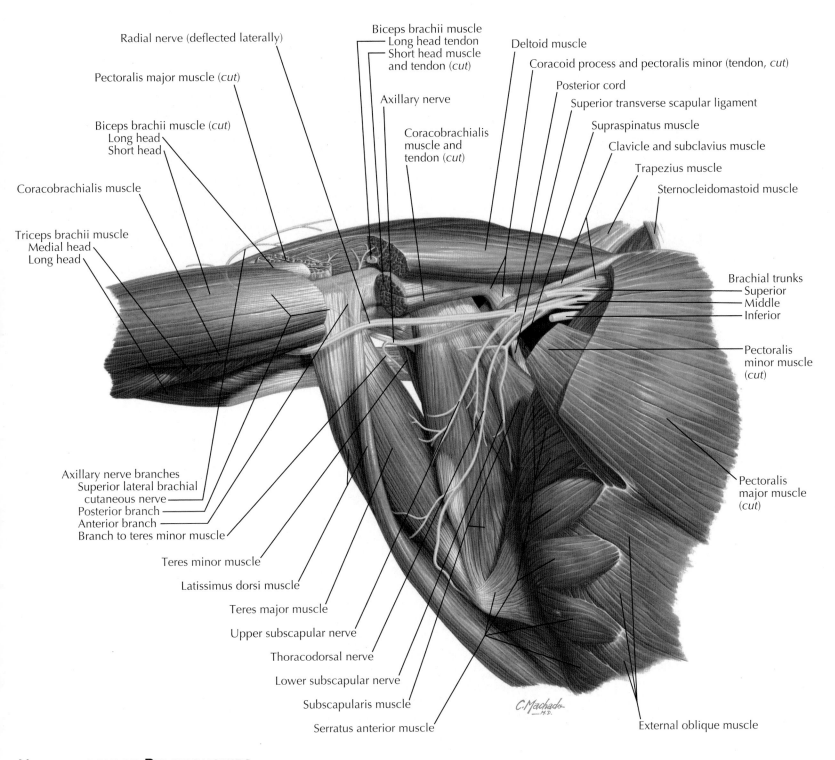

Radial nerve (deflected laterally)

Pectoralis major muscle (*cut*)

Biceps brachii muscle (*cut*)
Long head
Short head

Coracobrachialis muscle

Triceps brachii muscle
Medial head
Long head

Axillary nerve branches
Superior lateral brachial
cutaneous nerve
Posterior branch
Anterior branch
Branch to teres minor muscle

Teres minor muscle

Latissimus dorsi muscle

Teres major muscle

Upper subscapular nerve

Thoracodorsal nerve

Lower subscapular nerve

Subscapularis muscle

Serratus anterior muscle

Biceps brachii muscle
Long head tendon
Short head muscle
and tendon (*cut*)

Axillary nerve

Coracobrachialis
muscle and
tendon (*cut*)

Deltoid muscle

Coracoid process and pectoralis minor (tendon, *cut*)

Posterior cord

Superior transverse scapular ligament

Supraspinatus muscle

Clavicle and subclavius muscle

Trapezius muscle

Sternocleidomastoid muscle

Brachial trunks
Superior
Middle
Inferior

Pectoralis
minor muscle
(*cut*)

Pectoralis
major muscle
(*cut*)

C. Machado
_M.D.

External oblique muscle

NEUROVASCULAR RELATIONSHIPS (Continued)

position. These symptoms are noted in thoracic outlet syndrome.

The plexus splits into cords at or before it passes below the clavicle. The cords are named according to their position relative to the axillary artery: lateral, posterior, and medial. Upon formation of the terminal branches, the median, ulnar, and radial nerves continue with the artery into the arm. Injury or entrapment of these peripheral nerves can result in symptoms of sensory or motor deficits based on the innervation of the involved nerve.

Knowledge of the transition of the posterior neurovascular structures from their anterior origin is essential. The divergence of the teres minor and teres major muscles produces a long horizontal triangular opening laterally (see Plate 1.15). The triangle is bisected vertically by the long head of the triceps brachii muscle and is closed laterally by the shaft of the humerus. This forms a small triangular space medial to the long head of the triceps brachii, in which the circumflex scapular vessels curve onto the dorsum of the scapula, and a quadrangular space lateral to the triceps brachii muscle (see Plate 1.17). The latter space is bounded by the teres muscles above and below, by the triceps brachii medially, and by the humerus laterally. In the quadrangular space, the axillary nerve and posterior circumflex humeral vessels pass around the shaft of the humerus. Distally, the triangular interval (sometimes referred to as the lateral or lower triangular space), which transmits the radial nerve, is bounded by the teres major proximally, the long head of the triceps brachii medially, and the shaft of the humerus laterally.

Plate 1.15

Upper Limb: PART I

DEEP NEUROVASCULAR STRUCTURES AND INTERVALS

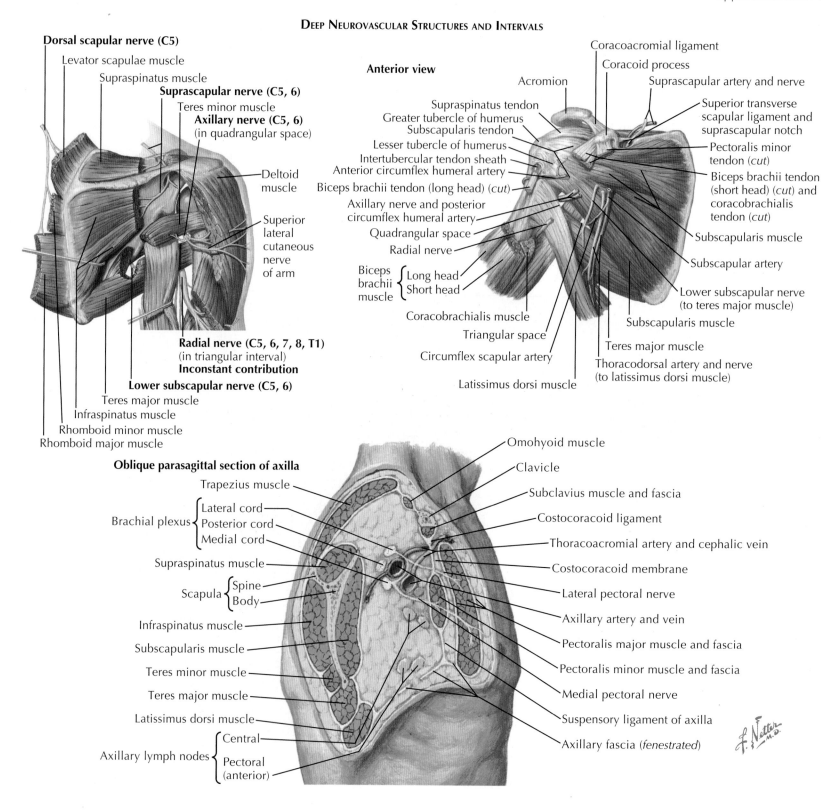

Dorsal scapular nerve (C5)
Levator scapulae muscle
Supraspinatus muscle
Suprascapular nerve (C5, 6)
Teres minor muscle
Axillary nerve (C5, 6)
(in quadrangular space)
Deltoid muscle
Superior lateral cutaneous nerve of arm

Radial nerve (C5, 6, 7, 8, T1)
(in triangular interval)
Inconstant contribution
Lower subscapular nerve (C5, 6)
Teres major muscle
Infraspinatus muscle
Rhomboid minor muscle
Rhomboid major muscle

Anterior view

Coracoacromial ligament
Coracoid process
Acromion
Suprascapular artery and nerve
Superior transverse scapular ligament and suprascapular notch
Supraspinatus tendon
Greater tubercle of humerus
Subscapularis tendon
Lesser tubercle of humerus
Intertubercular tendon sheath
Anterior circumflex humeral artery
Biceps brachii tendon (long head) (cut)
Axillary nerve and posterior circumflex humeral artery
Quadrangular space
Radial nerve
Biceps brachii muscle { Long head / Short head }
Coracobrachialis muscle
Triangular space
Circumflex scapular artery
Latissimus dorsi muscle
Pectoralis minor tendon (cut)
Biceps brachii tendon (short head) (cut) and coracobrachialis tendon (cut)
Subscapularis muscle
Subscapular artery
Lower subscapular nerve (to teres major muscle)
Subscapularis muscle
Teres major muscle
Thoracodorsal artery and nerve (to latissimus dorsi muscle)

Oblique parasagittal section of axilla
Trapezius muscle
Brachial plexus { Lateral cord / Posterior cord / Medial cord }
Supraspinatus muscle
Scapula { Spine / Body }
Infraspinatus muscle
Subscapularis muscle
Teres minor muscle
Teres major muscle
Latissimus dorsi muscle
Axillary lymph nodes { Central / Pectoral (anterior) }

Omohyoid muscle
Clavicle
Subclavius muscle and fascia
Costocoracoid ligament
Thoracoacromial artery and cephalic vein
Costocoracoid membrane
Lateral pectoral nerve
Axillary artery and vein
Pectoralis major muscle and fascia
Pectoralis minor muscle and fascia
Medial pectoral nerve
Suspensory ligament of axilla
Axillary fascia (fenestrated)

NEUROVASCULAR RELATIONSHIPS (Continued)

AXILLA

The axilla is a space at the junction of the upper limb, chest, and neck. It is shaped like a truncated pyramid and serves as the passageway for nerves, blood vessels, and lymphatics into or from the limb. Its walls are musculofascial. The base is the concave armpit, the actual floor being the axillary fascia. The anterior wall is composed of the two planes of pectoral muscles and the associated pectoral and clavipectoral fasciae. The lateral border of the PM muscle forms the anterior axillary fold. The posterior wall of the axilla is made up of the scapula, the scapular musculature, and the associated fasciae. The lower members of this group, together with the tendon of the LD muscle, form the posterior axillary fold. The chest wall, covered by the serratus anterior muscle and its fascia, forms the medial wall. The lateral wall is formed by the convergence of the tendons of the anterior and posterior axillary fold muscles onto the greater tubercular crest, the intertubercular groove, and the lesser tubercular crest of the humerus. The apex of the axilla is formed by the convergence of the bony members of the three major walls—the clavicle, the scapula, and the first rib.

Plate 1.16   Shoulder

AXILLARY AND BRACHIAL ARTERIES

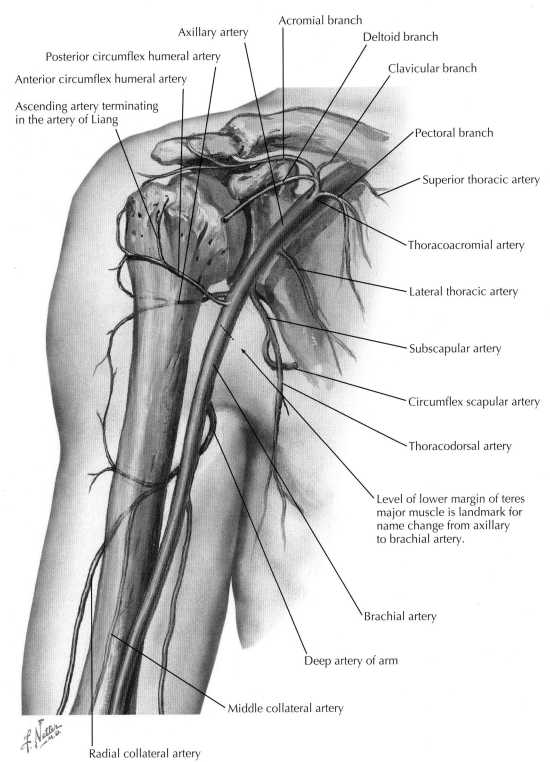

Axillary artery

Posterior circumflex humeral artery

Anterior circumflex humeral artery

Ascending artery terminating in the artery of Liang

Acromial branch

Deltoid branch

Clavicular branch

Pectoral branch

Superior thoracic artery

Thoracoacromial artery

Lateral thoracic artery

Subscapular artery

Circumflex scapular artery

Thoracodorsal artery

Level of lower margin of teres major muscle is landmark for name change from axillary to brachial artery.

Brachial artery

Deep artery of arm

Middle collateral artery

Radial collateral artery

VASCULAR ANATOMY OF SHOULDER

The blood supply to the upper extremity is derived from the subclavian artery, which travels with the brachial plexus between the anterior and middle scalene muscles. The first important branch relevant to shoulder anatomy is the thyrocervical trunk, which gives rise to the transverse cervical and suprascapular arteries. The next branch encountered is the dorsal scapular artery, which occasionally comes off the transverse cervical artery, as opposed to the subclavian artery.

The axillary artery is the continuation of the subclavian artery beyond the lateral border of the first rib. The artery is divided into three sections based on the position of the pectoralis minor tendon. The first division is proximal to the tendon and has only one branch, the superior thoracic. It descends behind the axillary vein to the intercostal muscles of the first and second intercostal spaces and to the upper portion of the serratus anterior muscle. The second division is deep to the tendon and has two branches, the thoracoacromial artery and the lateral thoracic artery. The thoracoacromial branch gives off four branches: acromial, deltoid, pectoral, and clavicular. The acromial branch passes lateralward across the coracoid process to the acromion. It gives branches to the deltoid muscle and participates with branches of the anterior and

posterior circumflex humeral and suprascapular vessels in the formation of the acromial network of small vessels on the surface of the acromion. The deltoid branch (often arising not separately but as a branch of the acromial artery) occupies the interval between the deltoid and PM muscles in company with the cephalic vein. It sends branches into these muscles. The pectoral

branch is large and descends between the PM and minor muscles. It gives branches to these muscles, anastomoses with intercostal and lateral thoracic arteries, and, in the female, supplies the mammary gland in its deep aspect. The clavicular branch is a slender vessel ascending medialward to supply the subclavius muscle and the sternoclavicular joint. The lateral thoracic

Plate 1.17

Upper Limb: PART I

AXILLARY ARTERY AND ANASTOMOSES AROUND SCAPULA

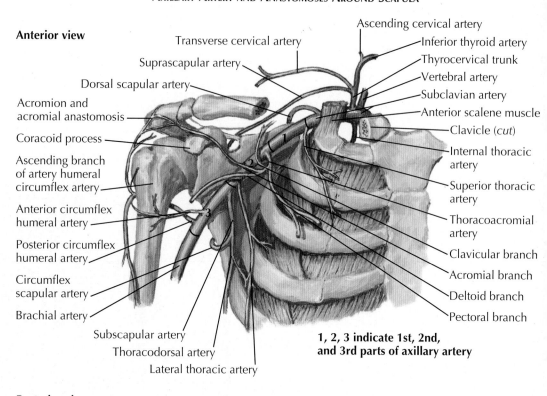

Anterior view

Transverse cervical artery

Suprascapular artery

Dorsal scapular artery

Acromion and acromial anastomosis

Coracoid process

Ascending branch of artery humeral circumflex artery

Anterior circumflex humeral artery

Posterior circumflex humeral artery

Circumflex scapular artery

Brachial artery

Subscapular artery

Thoracodorsal artery

Lateral thoracic artery

Ascending cervical artery

Inferior thyroid artery

Thyrocervical trunk

Vertebral artery

Subclavian artery

Anterior scalene muscle

Clavicle (cut)

Internal thoracic artery

Superior thoracic artery

Thoracoacromial artery

Clavicular branch

Acromial branch

Deltoid branch

Pectoral branch

1, 2, 3 indicate 1st, 2nd, and 3rd parts of axillary artery

Posterior view

Levator scapulae muscle

Dorsal scapular artery

Supraspinatus muscle (cut)

Transverse scapular ligament and supra- scapular foramen

Spine of scapula

Infraspinatus muscle (cut)

Teres minor muscle (cut)

Teres major muscle

Omohyoid muscle (inferior belly)

Suprascapular artery

Acromial branch of thoracoacromial artery

Acromion and acromial plexus

Infraspinous branch of suprascapular artery

Posterior circum- flex humeral artery (in quadrangular space) and ascending and descending branches

Lateral head ⎫ of triceps
Long head ⎭ brachii muscle

Circumflex scapular artery

VASCULAR ANATOMY OF SHOULDER (Continued)

artery is variable. It may arise directly from the axillary artery, from the thoracoacromial artery, or from the subscapular artery; it is frequently represented by several vessels. Typically (in 65% of cases), it arises from the axillary artery, descends along the lateral border of the pectoralis minor muscle, and sends branches to the serratus anterior and pectoral muscles and axillary lymph nodes.

The third division of the axillary artery is distal to the pectoralis minor tendon and gives off three branches: the subscapular, anterior humeral circumflex, and posterior humeral circumflex arteries. The subscapular artery is the largest branch of the axillary artery. It divides into the circumflex scapular and thoracodorsal branches. The circumflex scapular artery, the larger branch, passes posteriorly through the triangular space, turns onto the dorsum of the scapula, and ramifies in the infraspinous fossa. Here, it supplies the muscles of the dorsum of the scapula and anastomoses with the dorsal scapular artery and the terminals of the suprascapular artery. By branches given off in the triangular space, it supplies the subscapularis and the two teres muscles. The thoracodorsal artery is the principal supply of the LD muscle, entering it on its deep surface in company with the

thoracodorsal nerve. It frequently has a thoracic branch that substitutes for the inferior portion of the distribution of the lateral thoracic artery.

The two circumflex humeral arteries branch next. The anterior vessel gives off an ascending branch that continues to become the arcuate artery. This vessel provides most of the blood supply to the humeral head. The posterior circumflex artery passes posteriorly with the axillary nerve through the quadrangular space. It encircles the surgical neck of the humerus

and anastomoses with the anterior circumflex humeral artery.

The axillary artery becomes the brachial artery as it crosses the inferior limit of the axilla at the lower border of the teres major. It enters the arm accompanied by two brachial veins and the median, ulnar, and radial nerves. The axillary vein is anterior and inferior to the artery in normal posture but rises and is more completely anterior to the artery when the arm is abducted.

Plate 1.18

Shoulder

Note: Usual composition shown. Prefixed plexus has large C4 contribution but lacks T1. Postfixed plexus lacks C5 but has T2 contribution.

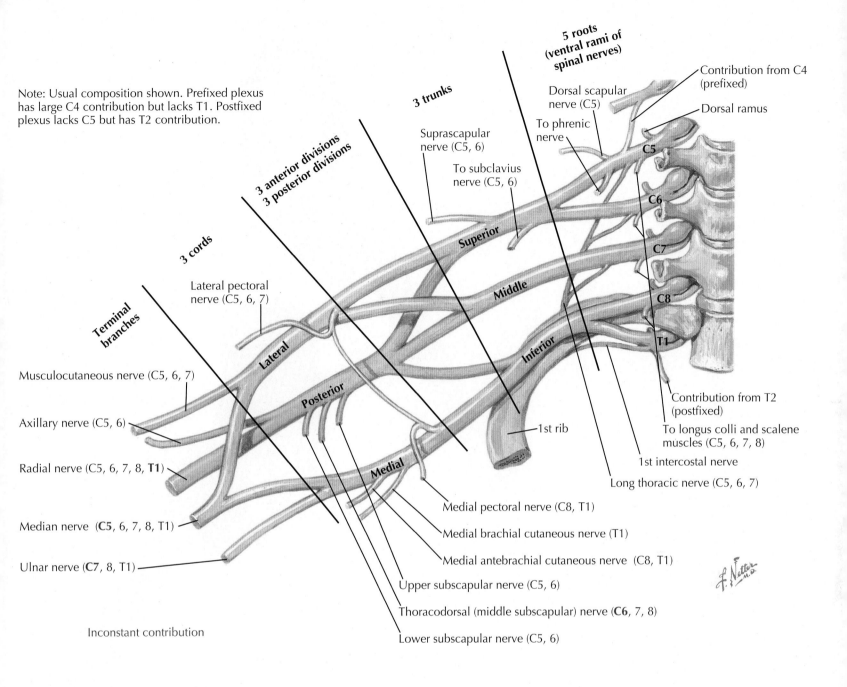

5 roots (ventral rami of spinal nerves)

Contribution from C4 (prefixed)

Dorsal scapular nerve (C5)

Dorsal ramus

3 trunks

Suprascapular nerve (C5, 6)

To phrenic nerve

C5

To subclavius nerve (C5, 6)

3 anterior divisions
3 posterior divisions

C6

Superior

C7

Middle

3 cords

Lateral pectoral nerve (C5, 6, 7)

C8

Inferior

Lateral

Terminal branches

Musculocutaneous nerve (C5, 6, 7)

Posterior

T1

Axillary nerve (C5, 6)

1st rib

Contribution from T2 (postfixed)

To longus colli and scalene muscles (C5, 6, 7, 8)

Radial nerve (C5, 6, 7, 8, **T1**)

1st intercostal nerve

Medial

Long thoracic nerve (C5, 6, 7)

Median nerve (**C5**, 6, 7, 8, T1)

Medial pectoral nerve (C8, T1)

Medial brachial cutaneous nerve (T1)

Ulnar nerve (**C7**, 8, T1)

Medial antebrachial cutaneous nerve (C8, T1)

Upper subscapular nerve (C5, 6)

Thoracodorsal (middle subscapular) nerve (**C6**, 7, 8)

Inconstant contribution

Lower subscapular nerve (C5, 6)

F. Netter

Brachial Plexus

The innervation of the upper extremity is provided by the branches of the brachial plexus. This large nerve complex does not originate in the axilla, although the greater part of its branching and the formation of the definitive nerves of the limb do take place in this region. Although anatomic variants are not uncommon, a thorough understanding of the classic description of this network is essential.

The brachial plexus is formed by the ventral rami (roots) of the fifth to the eighth cervical nerves (C5 to C8) and the greater part of the first thoracic nerve (T1). Small contributions may come from the fourth cervical nerve (C4) and the second thoracic nerve (T2). The sympathetic fibers conducted by each root are added as

they pass between the scalene muscles. Each of the ventral rami of C5 and C6 receives a gray ramus communicans from the middle cervical ganglion. The cervicothoracic ganglion (inferior cervical plus first thoracic ganglia) contributes gray rami to the C7, C8, and T1 roots of the plexus.

The ventral rami of C5 and C6 unite to form the superior trunk, the ramus of C7 continues alone as the middle trunk, and the rami of C8 and T1 form the inferior trunk. Each trunk separates into an anterior and a posterior division. The anterior division supplies the originally ventral parts of the limb, and the posterior division supplies the dorsal parts. All the posterior divisions unite to form the posterior cord of the plexus, the anterior divisions of the superior and middle trunks form the lateral cord, and the medial cord is the continuation of the anterior division of the inferior trunk. Thus the posterior cord contains nerve bundles from

C5 to T1 destined for the back of the limb, the lateral cord is formed of nerve bundles from C5 to C7 for the anterior portion of the limb, and the medial cord carries anterior nerve components from C8 and T1. The cords are named to show their relationships to the axillary artery.

The terminal branches regroup further and form the terminal nerves of the plexus. Large portions of the lateral and medial cords form the median nerve. The remainder of the lateral cord constitutes the musculocutaneous nerve; the rest of the medial cord is the ulnar nerve. The posterior cord gives off the axillary nerve at the lower border of the subscapularis muscle, and the remainder continues distally as the radial nerve.

In addition to these terminal branches, several nerves arise from the roots and cords of the plexus (T10). These are grouped according to the portion of plexus that gives them origin.

Plate 1.19

Upper Limb: PART I

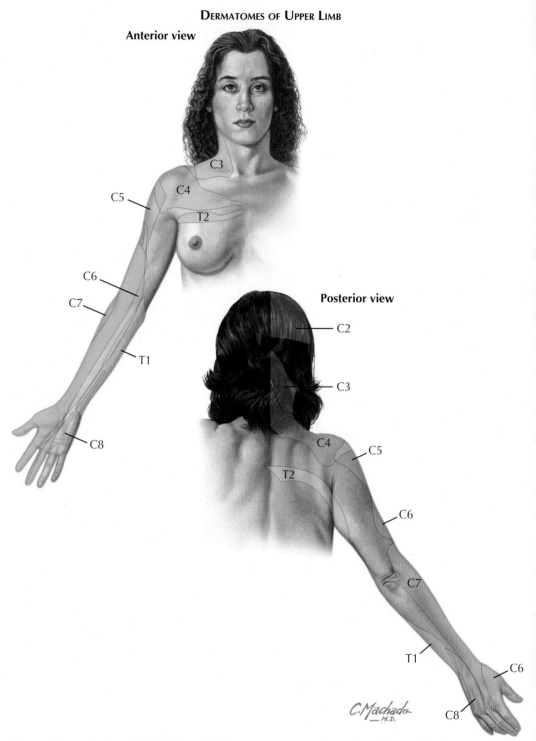

DERMATOMES OF UPPER LIMB

Anterior view

Posterior view

Schematic based on Lee MW, McPhee RW, Stringer MD. An evidence-based approach to human dermatomes. Clin Anat. 2008;21(5):363–373. doi: 10.1002/ca.20636. PMID: 18470936. Note that these areas are not absolute and vary from person to person. S3, S4, S5, and Co supply the perineum but are not shown for reasons of clarity. Of note, the dermatomes are larger than illustrated, as the figure is based on best evidence; gaps represent areas in which the data are inconclusive.

PERIPHERAL NERVES

The cutaneous nerves of the upper limb are for the most part derived from the brachial plexus, although the uppermost nerves to the shoulder are derived from the cervical plexus. The supraclavicular nerves (C3, C4) become superficial at the posterior border of the sternocleidomastoid muscle within the posterior triangle of the neck. They pierce the superficial layer of the cervical fascia and the platysma muscle, radiating in three lines: (1) the medial supraclavicular nerves over the clavicle; (2) the intermediate supraclavicular nerves toward the acromion; and (3) the lateral, or posterior, supraclavicular nerves over the scapula.

The superior lateral cutaneous nerve of the arm (C5, C6) is the termination of the lower branch of the axillary nerve of the brachial plexus. Leaving the axillary nerve, it turns superficially around the posterior border of the lower third of the deltoid muscle to pierce the

brachial fascia. Its cutaneous distribution is the lower half of the deltoid muscle and the long head of the triceps brachii.

The inferior lateral cutaneous nerve of the arm (C5, C6) is derived from the posterior antebrachial cutaneous nerve shortly after this nerve branches from the radial nerve. The inferior lateral brachial cutaneous

nerve becomes superficial in line with the lateral intermuscular septum a little below the insertion of the deltoid muscle. It accompanies the lower part of the cephalic vein and distributes in the lower lateral and the anterior surface of the arm.

The posterior cutaneous nerve of the arm (C5–C8) arises within the axilla as a branch of the radial nerve.

Plate 1.20   Shoulder

SENSORY DISTRIBUTION AND NEUROPATHY IN SHOULDER

Sensory distribution

Anterior (palmar) view

Posterior (dorsal) view

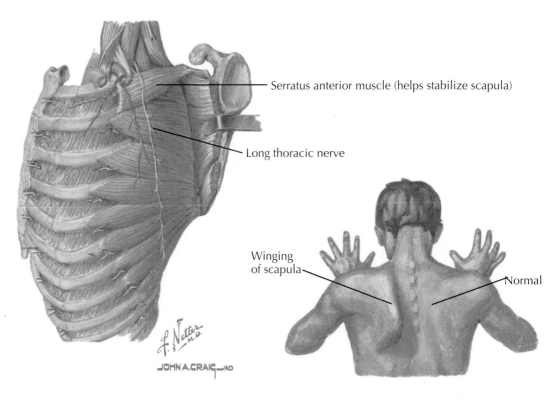

Supraclavicular nerves (from cervical plexus—C3, 4)

Axillary nerve
Superior lateral cutaneous nerve of arm (C5, 6)

Radial nerve
Inferior lateral cutaneous nerve of arm (C5, 6)

Intercostobrachial nerve (T2) and medial cutaneous nerve of arm (C8, T1, 2)

Supraclavicular nerves (from cervical plexus—C3, 4)

Axillary nerve
Superior lateral cutaneous nerve of arm (C5, 6)

Radial nerve
Posterior cutaneous nerve of arm (C5, 6, 7, 8)
Inferior lateral cutaneous nerve of arm
Posterior cutaneous nerve of forearm (C[5], 6, 7, 8)

Intercostobrachial nerve (T2) and medial cutaneous nerve of arm (C8, T1, 2)

Neuropathy about shoulder: long thoracic nerve

Serratus anterior muscle (helps stabilize scapula)

Long thoracic nerve

Winging of scapula

Normal

JOHN A. CRAIG—AD

PERIPHERAL NERVES (Continued)

Traversing the medial side of the long head of the triceps brachii muscle, the nerve penetrates the brachial fascia to distribute in the middle third of the back of the arm above and behind the distribution of the medial brachial cutaneous nerve and the intercostobrachial nerve.

The medial cutaneous nerve of the arm (C8, T1) arises from the medial cord of the brachial plexus in the lower axilla. It descends along the medial side of the brachial artery to the middle of the arm, where it pierces the brachial fascia and supplies the skin of the posterior surface of the lower third of the arm as far as the olecranon.

The intercostobrachial nerve (T2) is the larger part of the lateral cutaneous branch of the second thoracic nerve. In the second intercostal space at the axillary line, it pierces the serratus anterior muscle to enter the axilla. Here it usually anastomoses with the medial brachial cutaneous nerve and then pierces the brachial fascia just beyond the posterior axillary fold. Its cutaneous distribution is along the medial and posterior surfaces of the arm from the axilla to the elbow.

A complete neurologic examination of the shoulder tests the just-mentioned dermatomes as well as the coordinated contraction of the shoulder girdle musculature (T11). One commonly encountered neuropathy is long thoracic nerve dysfunction, which can result from axillary lymph node dissection. Physical examination reveals medial winging of the scapula when the arm is placed anterior to the plane of the body, which is exaggerated by pushing against a wall.

Plate 1.21

Upper Limb: PART I

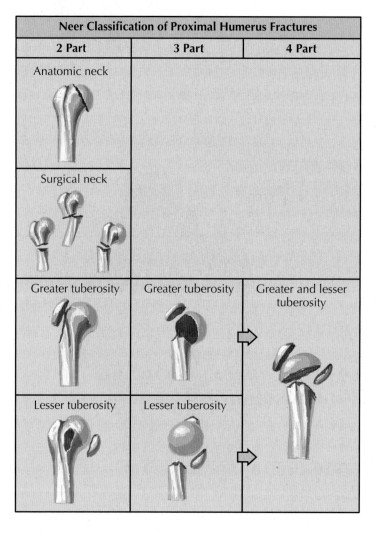

Supraspinatus and external rotator muscles
Rotator interval
Anatomic neck
Greater tuberosity
Surgical neck
Long tendon of biceps brachii muscle
Lesser tuberosity
Subscapularis muscle

Neer four-part classification of fractures of proximal humerus:
1. Articular fragment (humeral head)
2. Lesser tuberosity
3. Greater tuberosity
4. Shaft. If none of the fragments is displaced, the fracture is considered stable (most common) and treated with minimal external immobilization and early range-of-motion exercise. Displacement of 1 cm or angulation of 45 degrees of one or more fragments is usually an indication for surgical reduction and internal fixation or prosthetic replacement.

PROXIMAL HUMERAL FRACTURES: NEER CLASSIFICATION

Fractures of the proximal humerus are common, occurring most frequently in older patients from a fall on the outstretched hand.

The fragment is considered significantly displaced as it may relate to surgical indications if the displacement is greater than 1 cm or the angulation is greater than 45 degrees. The four-part classification proposed by Neer requires identification of the following four major fracture fragments and their relationships to one another on initial radiographs: (1) articular fragment, (2) greater tuberosity with the attached supraspinatus muscle, (3) lesser tuberosity with the attached subscapularis muscle, and (4) humeral shaft. The fractures can be associated with dislocation of the humeral head segment, in which case they are classified as a fracture and dislocation. For example, the fracture may involve the greater tuberosity and the humeral head may be dislocated anteriorly. This is called a two-part fracture-dislocation. These injuries have clinical importance regarding the nature of the tissue damage treatment and prognosis. For example, a common fracture-dislocation involves the greater tuberosity and anterior dislocation of the humeral head. In these cases, closed reduction of the humeral head may result in persistence of significant displacement of the greater tuberosity, requiring surgery for reduction of the fractures. In contrast, if the closed reduction of the humeral head results in a close approximation of the greater tuberosity, then surgery is not needed but, more importantly, recurrent dislocations of the humeral head after the fracture is healed are rare because tearing of the GH ligaments does not occur because the fracture of the greater tuberosity and the soft tissue damage to the rotator cuff allow for dislocation to occur with treatment of the GH ligaments.

Likewise, variations of proximal humeral fractures include damage to the articular head segment (see Plate 1.25). When damage occurs to the humeral head segment, then this is a variant of the classic four-part classification. In most cases, replacement of the humeral head is required to manage both the long-term sequelae of avascular necrosis (AVN) (loss of blood supply) to the humeral head and the posttraumatic arthritis resulting from trauma to the articular cartilage.

The Neer classification of proximal humeral fractures includes two-part, three-part, and four-part fractures. Two-part fractures may involve the anatomic neck or the surgical neck or the greater tuberosity or lesser tuberosity. Three-part fractures include the humeral head segment and either the greater or lesser tuberosity. Four-part fractures include both tuberosities, the humeral head segment, and the humeral shaft. In four-part fractures with wide displacement, the humeral head is isolated from its blood supply and there is a higher incidence of AVN.

Diagnosis, and resulting classification, of proximal humeral fractures is confirmed from radiographs taken in at least two orthogonal planes (90 degrees from one another) and should include an AP view and a transscapular Y-view of the shoulder. When possible, a modified axillary view should be obtained. In many cases with acute fracture an axillary view is difficult to obtain because of pain associated with fracture and the arm position needed to obtain this view. Computed tomography (CT) with multiplanar reconstruction or three-dimensional reconstruction allows for better determination of the number of parts and their displacement. In some fractures, each of the major segments of the proximal humerus may have more than one fracture line (i.e., comminution). In these cases, the fractures are classified using the four-part classification with the added modification of the term *comminution* to the segment involved. In other words, these are not called five- or six-part fractures. In the cases in which one or more segments of the proximal humerus are fractured but there is minimal displacement of any of the segments, then these fractures are considered one-part fractures to indicate that none of the fragments is displaced or requires surgical reduction. For example, an isolated fracture of the greater tuberosity without significant displacement would be called a one-part fracture involving the greater tuberosity or a minimally displaced fracture of the greater tuberosity.

Neer Classification of Proximal Humerus Fractures		
2 Part	**3 Part**	**4 Part**
Anatomic neck		
Surgical neck		
Greater tuberosity	Greater tuberosity	Greater and lesser tuberosity
Lesser tuberosity	Lesser tuberosity	

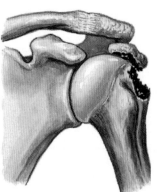

Displaced fracture of greater tuberosity is surgically repaired using wires through small drill holes and suturing of the rotator cuff tears. Very small fragments may be excised and the supraspinatus tendon reattached.

Plate 1.22

Shoulder

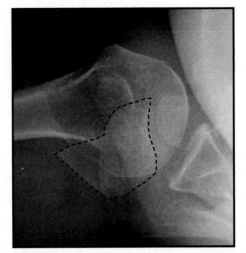
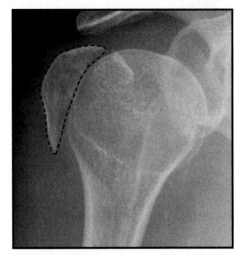

Axillary radiograph (*left*) and AP radiograph (*right*) of a two-part greater tuberosity fracture fragment (*dotted line*), which is displaced posteriorly and laterally

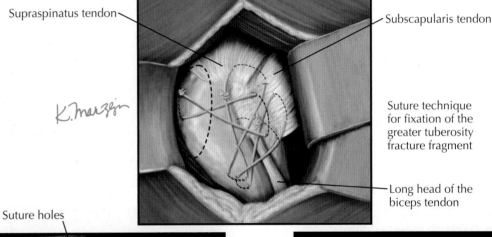

Supraspinatus tendon

Subscapularis tendon

Suture technique for fixation of the greater tuberosity fracture fragment

Long head of the biceps tendon

Suture holes

PROXIMAL HUMERAL FRACTURES: TWO-PART GREATER TUBEROSITY FRACTURE

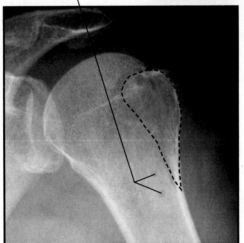
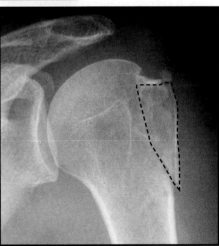

Reduction and internal fixation using suture technique for the greater tuberosity fracture or fragment (*dotted line*) demonstrating AP (*left*) and internal rotation AP radiographic (*right*) views

A displaced fracture of the greater tuberosity as described previously requires isolated involvement of the greater tuberosity with displacement of more than 1 cm. In the example shown, the displacement is posterior as seen on the axillary view and superior as seen on the AP view. This finding represents disruption of the surrounding soft tissue and tearing of the rotator cuff tissue to allow this fragment to displace. The supraspinatus, infraspinatus, and teres minor are attached to the greater tuberosity. These rotator cuff muscles function to elevate and externally rotate the arm. A fracture of the greater tuberosity of this large-sized fragment will result in the ability of these rotator cuff muscles to pull the fragment superiorly and posteriorly. Surgery is required for placing the fragment in its proper location to restore proper rotator cuff strength and to avoid loss of motion due to malunion of the fragment. Malunion will cause impingement of the malunited fragment on the posterior aspect of the glenoid when attempting external rotation of the arm or impingement on the undersurface of the acromion when attempting elevation of the shoulder. Posterior displacement will also result in shortening of the posterior capsule, resulting in loss of internal rotation and external rotation weakness. Treatment of the late sequelae of a malunion is

very difficult and often results in a less than ideal functional outcome. Early recognition of these displaced fractures is important for early surgical intervention. If an anatomic reduction is achieved with stable fixation, then healing and rehabilitation can result in normal shoulder function and no pain. Several types of surgery can be performed to achieve this goal. In the case shown, the fracture was treated with open reduction and internal fixation with heavy suture material. This technique is best used in the older patient with osteoporosis when fixation using screws may fail owing to

poor fixation of the screw due to osteoporosis between the bone fragments. Suture fixation between the tendon insertions of the rotator cuff is much stronger than fixation isolated to the bone fragments. Suture fixation is also better when there are multiple small fragments of the greater tuberosity (see Plate 1.22).

With isolated fracture of the greater tuberosity in patients with good-quality bone, minimally invasive reduction under fluoroscopy and screw fixation can be done as an effective, less invasive alternative to open reduction and suture fixation (see Plate 1.23).

Plate 1.23

Upper Limb: PART I

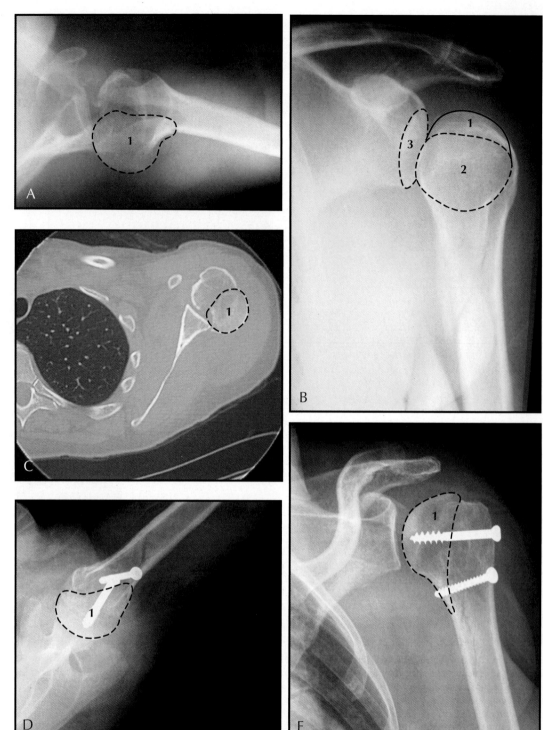

PROXIMAL HUMERAL FRACTURES: TWO-PART SURGICAL NECK FRACTURE AND DISLOCATION OF THE HUMERAL HEAD

A fracture along with dislocation of the humeral head segment is a common variation of the four-part classification of proximal humeral fractures. The clinical significance is related to the additional damage caused to the articular cartilage of the humeral head, the additional trauma to the blood supply to the humeral head, and the additional trauma to the glenoid and GH ligaments. Each of these can result in additional long-term adverse clinical sequelae, specifically posttraumatic arthritis, AVN of the humeral head, glenoid arthritic changes, or instability of the joint. Each of these additional problems makes surgery necessary to manage this problem and increases the urgency for early surgical invention. It should be noted that the difficulty in diagnosis of the dislocated part of the fracture pattern on the AP radiograph reinforces the need for the axillary radiographic view and an axial CT image. It is also difficult to see the fracture of the humeral head segment on the AP radiograph. These types of fractures are often missed in the office or emergency department setting if imaging is inadequate. When this occurs, early surgical invention is not performed, and in some cases the patient is treated without surgery, resulting in a very poor outcome. Late reconstructive surgery for management of the late sequelae of malunion of this fracture often results in improvement but a less than favorable outcome compared with early fracture management.

Axillary radiograph (**A**) of a two-part fracture-dislocation. The fracture extends through the anatomic neck into the humeral shaft. The humeral head is dislocated posteriorly. The same fracture is shown in an AP radiograph, also showing an "empty" glenoid fossa (**B**) and in an axial CT scan (**C**). Open reduction and internal fixation with two interfragmentary cancellous and corticoid screws (**D** and **E**). Anatomic reduction achieved with minimal internal fixation. **1,** Humeral head articular surface; **2,** greater tuberosity humerus in extreme internal rotation; **3,** empty glenoid.

In this case of a young middle-aged and active person who fell from a horse, open surgery for an anatomic reduction of the fracture and reduction of the dislocation resulted in the ability to use minimal fixation devices because of the high-quality bone tissue and an anatomic reduction allowing for interfragment compression fixation using the lag screw concept. The distal screw was a cortical screw for the cortical bone using overdrilling of the lateral fragment, resulting in compression at the fracture site. The screw orientation was perpendicular to the fracture line, thus resulting in compression of the fracture. The superior screw is a partially threaded cancellous screw placed into cancellous bone of the humeral head. The larger threads of the cancellous screw achieve better fixation in cancellous bone. The smooth part of the cancellous screw allows for the lag screw again effecting compression across the fracture site. Again the screw is placed perpendicular to the fracture line, maximizing the compression effect and fracture fragment stability with the use of a minimal implant and avoiding a large plate.

Plate 1.24

Shoulder

PROXIMAL HUMERAL FRACTURES: VALGUS-IMPACTED FOUR-PART FRACTURE

Valgus-impacted open reduction and internal fixation

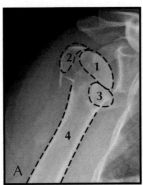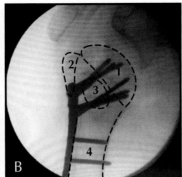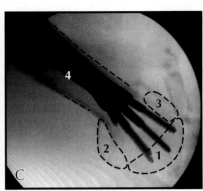

AP radiograph (**A**) showing a valgus-impacted four-part fracture. Fracture was treated by open reduction and internal fixation using a locking plate. Postoperative radiograph (**B**) and postoperative axillary radiograph (**C**).

A valgus-impacted four-part fracture is a variation of a classic four-part fracture-dislocation. In a classic four-part fracture-dislocation the humeral head segment is completely separated from the other three segments of the proximal humerus (greater and lesser tuberosity and the humeral shaft). In many of these classic four-part fractures, the humeral head segment is also dislocated from the joint and is not articulating with the glenoid. When the articular segment is separated from its blood supply (see Plate 1.16), there is a high incidence of AVN. In most cases these fractures occur in the elderly, and humeral head replacement using a stemmed prosthesis as shown in Plate 1.25 is the preferred treatment for reduction and fixation of the tuberosities and replacement of the avascular articular segment. In some cases, use of a reverse total shoulder arthroplasty is preferred because healing of the tuberosities with anatomic arthroplasty is highly variable, and loss of fixation with an anatomic arthroplasty will generally lead to a poor outcome (see Plate 1.26). The adverse outcome is less common with reverse total shoulder arthroplasty when failure to heal the tuberosity occurs.

The valgus-impacted four-part fracture results in rotation of the humeral head articular segment into a horizontal position with impaction of this segment between the fractures of the greater and lesser tuberosities that become split and widened to accommodate the impacted humeral head. With this fracture, the humeral head segment is oriented with the articular surface facing superiorly toward the undersurface of the acromion. The humeral head is not in contact with the glenoid and is shrouded by the displaced tuberosities. In many of these fractures the periosteum on the medial side of the humeral shaft and humeral head segment remains intact and forms a soft tissue bridge between the two, adding to the stability of the head segment and to its blood supply. This results in a much lower incidence of AVN than that seen with classic four-part fracture-dislocations. Both the greater and lesser tuberosity fracture fragments are displaced laterally but keep an intact soft tissue attachment to the humeral shaft. As a result of these soft tissue attachments, this fracture configuration allows for keeping the humeral head and fracture in reduction and fixation rather than displacement. It is important to recognize this specific fracture pattern both for the ability to keep the humeral head segment and more importantly to not confuse this with a minimally displaced fracture that would otherwise be treated nonoperatively. If the medial soft tissue hinge is present and providing some stability of the head segment, then a more minimally invasive method of fracture reduction and internal fixation can be accomplished as shown at the bottom of Plate 1.24. When there is more instability of the fragment, comminution of the segments, or poor bone quality secondary to osteoporosis, then a more formal operation with open incision and plate fixation as shown at the top of Plate 1.24 is preferred.

Percutaneous method of reduction of the humeral head fracture fragment

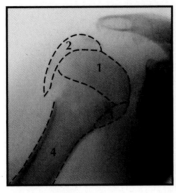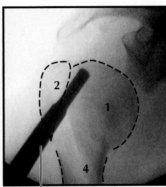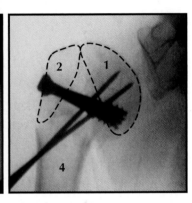

Bone tamp

An instrument is placed through a small incision laterally, and under fluoroscopic guidance the humeral head segment is reduced into a more normal neck shaft angle of approximately 135 degrees. With traction on the arm, both the greater and lesser tuberosities are reduced by tensioning the intact soft tissues. Percutaneous placement of two cannulated cancellous screws through the greater tuberosity fracture fragment thereby completes the internal fixation using minimally invasive techniques. Articular segment is in slight 10–15 degrees of valgus malposition compared with an anatomic neck shaft angle, which is clinically acceptable.

1, Humeral head articular surface; **2,** greater tuberosity; **3,** lesser tuberosity; and **4,** humeral shaft.

Open reduction and internal fixation provide more rigid internal fixation but require a larger open procedure. When a minimally invasive reduction and fixation procedure is performed, a small incision (1–2 cm) is placed distal to the fracture site, and, under fluoroscopic control, the humeral head segment is elevated into an anatomic position using a blunt instrument placed under the humeral head segment at its superior part, thereby rotating it out of its valgus position. As a result of the soft tissue attachments to each of the fragments, elevation of the head fragment with traction on the arm easily realigns the tuberosities under the humeral head segment. Percutaneous pinning and screw fixation provide sufficient fixation of the segments to maintain the reduction. This is not ridged fixation, and removal of the pins at 6 weeks after surgery allows for sufficient healing to begin rehabilitation. Because of the minimally invasive approach, delay in rehabilitation does not result in significant stiffness of the shoulder; most patients achieve good range of motion, assuming the fracture fragments heal in a good position.

Patients treated in plate fixation generally have better fixation and should start rehabilitation range-of-motion exercises soon after surgery.

Plate 1.25

Upper Limb: PART I

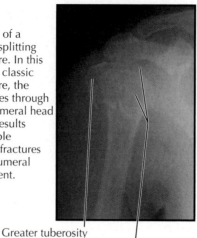

AP radiographs of a complex head-splitting four-part fracture. In this variation of the classic four-part fracture, the fracture line goes through the articular humeral head segment. This results in a very unstable fracture. These fractures often require humeral head replacement.

Greater tuberosity

Humeral head split

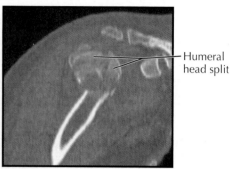

Humeral head split

CT reconstruction in the antero-posterior view showing the articular head segment fracture

PROXIMAL HUMERAL FRACTURES: HUMERAL HEAD SPLIT WITH A CLASSIC FOUR-PART FRACTURE-DISLOCATION

The classic four-part fracture-dislocation can be associated with a fracture through the articular surface of the humeral head. These fractures generally occur in higher-velocity and higher-energy trauma. The fracture through the humeral head segment results in a much more difficult fracture to manage and generally requires humeral head replacement. In addition, the likelihood for posttraumatic arthritis and AVN in this fracture configuration is certain, again making humeral head replacement the treatment of choice. With humeral head replacement, the stem of the prosthetic is securely placed into the shaft of the humerus, in most cases using bone cement. One of the most difficult parts of the surgery is to place the stem in the correct height and rotation to reproduce the normal prefracture anatomy. When done correctly, there will be the same amount of space between the metallic humeral head and the shaft as there was before the fracture to place all the fracture fragments of the greater and lesser tuberosities within this interval so that the fragments are below the metallic humeral head and above the humeral shaft. Fixation of these fragments is aided by use of the metallic stem as an internal fixation device, around which the fragments are reduced with the humeral head in place. Very heavy and strong nonresorbable sutures are placed through the humeral shaft bone and prosthetic, as well as through the rotator cuff tendons that are attached to the tuberosity fragments. Despite the multiple fractures and fragments of bone, when an anatomic reduction is achieved with good fixation, long-term outcome is excellent.

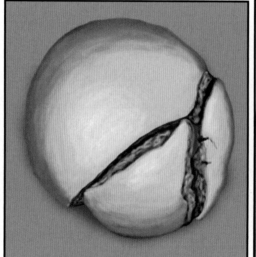

Complex humeral head fracture in the articular head

Greater tuberosity

Humeral shaft
Long head of biceps tendon
Lesser tuberosity
Humeral head

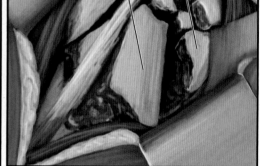

Multiple fracture fragments are present in this fracture, which occurred by high-energy, high-velocity trauma in a skiing accident.

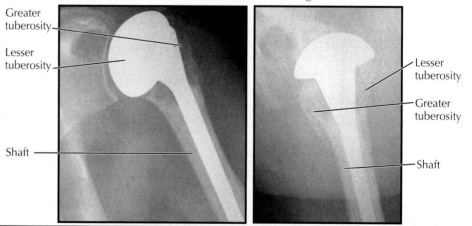

Greater tuberosity
Lesser tuberosity
Shaft

Lesser tuberosity
Greater tuberosity
Shaft

Humeral head replacement in which the humeral head is replaced with a stemmed humeral prosthetic while performing a hemiarthroplasty. The humeral stem acts as an intramedullary strut for fixation of an anatomically sized humeral head. It also acts as a means for fixation of both the greater and lesser tuberosities around the proximal portion of the stem as shown. Sutures are used to fix the tuberosities to the stem. In this case, both tuberosities are anatomically reduced under the humeral head and healed in an anatomic position. When these results are achieved, the clinical results are often excellent in terms of function and pain relief.

Plate 1.26

Shoulder

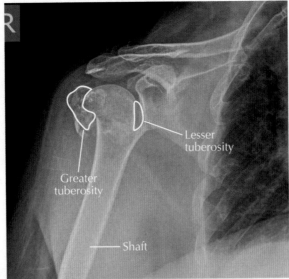

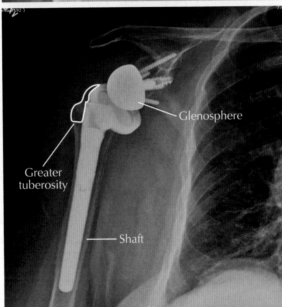

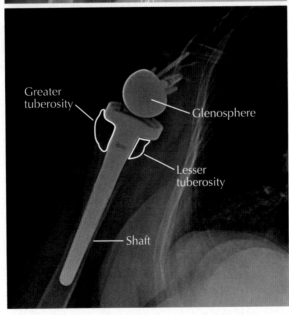

PROXIMAL HUMERAL FRACTURES: REVERSE TOTAL SHOULDER REPLACEMENT

Reverse total shoulder replacement has been gaining widespread use in patients who were previously treated with anatomic humeral head replacement. This implant allows for more reliable outcomes as perfect tuberosity healing is not necessary for a good functional outcome. Fixation of the stem and tuberosities to the stem is similar to that of humeral head replacement, and the addition of glenoid preparation for a baseplate and glenosphere placement is also required.

Reverse total shoulder replacement has become the predominant arthroplasty treatment of choice for many complex proximal humerus fractures. The ball (glenosphere) is placed on the glenoid and the stem in the humerus. The tuberosity fragments are repaired around the humeral stem similar to humeral head hemiarthroplasty with heavy suture. This case shows the tuberosities repaired in a good position.

Plate 1.27

Upper Limb: PART I

ANTERIOR DISLOCATION TYPES AND STIMSON MANEUVER

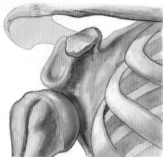

Subcoracoid dislocation (most common)

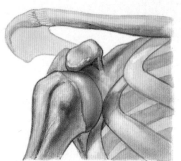

Subglenoid dislocation

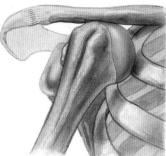

Subclavicular dislocation (uncommon). Very rarely, humeral head penetrates between ribs, producing intrathoracic dislocation.

ANTERIOR DISLOCATION OF GLENOHUMERAL JOINT

About 95% of shoulder dislocations are anterior and are chiefly due to an indirect mechanism. The most common anterior dislocation type is a subcoracoid dislocation; the most uncommon is a subclavicular dislocation. Anterior dislocations are seen in all age groups and are most commonly seen in adolescents and young adults. They are often due to athletic injuries in which there is trauma to the shoulder, generally from a fall or contact to the more distal aspect of the arm, where the arm is placed into abduction and external rotation (i.e., a cocked arm position for overhead throwing). It is also in this position that patients are most likely to have a recurrent dislocation of the shoulder or have a sense of instability of the shoulder. The clinical appearance of anterior dislocation demonstrates a prominent acromion and a flattened area of the lateral deltoid region with a prominence of the humeral head anteriorly. The arm is often in an abducted and internally rotated position with loss of passive external rotation. The axillary nerve is located anteriorly immediately outside the anterior inferior axillary portion of the capsular ligaments. With a traumatic anterior dislocation of the shoulder there is often a traction-type injury to the axillary nerve. In many cases the nerve injury is transient and resolves with relocation of the shoulder. This nerve injury can result in an area of decreased sensation in the lateral aspect of the arm as well as a weakness of deltoid function. In addition, the musculocutaneous nerve is located 5 to 7 cm distal to the tip of the coracoid process and can be injured by compression or traction in the anterior shoulder dislocation. This will often result in decreased sensation in the preaxial border of

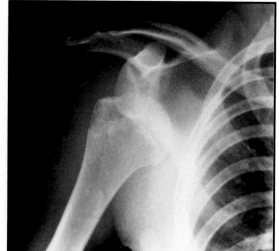

Anteroposterior radiograph. Subcoracoid dislocation.

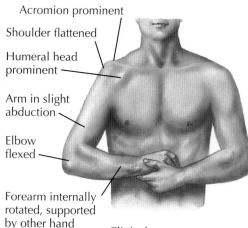

Acromion prominent

Shoulder flattened

Humeral head prominent

Arm in slight abduction

Elbow flexed

Forearm internally rotated, supported by other hand

Clinical appearance

Testing sensation in areas of (1) axillary and (2) musculocutaneous nerves

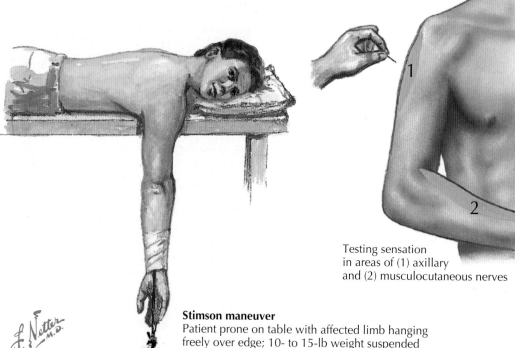

Stimson maneuver
Patient prone on table with affected limb hanging freely over edge; 10- to 15-lb weight suspended from wrist. Gradual traction overcomes muscle spasm and in most cases achieves reduction in 20–25 minutes.

Plate 1.28

Shoulder

HILL-SACHS, BANKART, AND CAPSULAR LESIONS

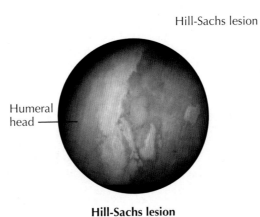

Bankart lesion

Anterior inferior capsule
Humeral head
Glenoid

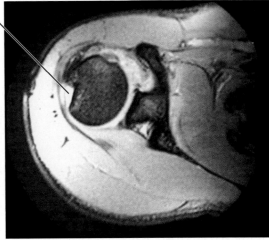

Capsular lesion

Humeral head
Anterior inferior capsule reattached to the glenoid rim—Bankart repair
Glenoid

Hill-Sachs lesion

Humeral head

Hill-Sachs lesion

Axial CT showing a Hill-Sachs lesions in the upper aspect of the humeral head

ANTERIOR DISLOCATION OF GLENOHUMERAL JOINT (Continued)

the forearm and will result in weakness of elbow flexion.

Closed reduction of the shoulder is most commonly performed at the location of the dislocation if a trained person is available or in an emergency department setting. First-time dislocations are often the most difficult to reduce. The sooner a dislocation can be safely reduced, the least likely further damage could occur to the cartilage of the joint, to the posterior aspect of the humeral head (Hill-Sachs lesion), or to axillary and/or musculocutaneous nerves. In all methods of closed reduction, relaxation of the patient and the muscles around the shoulder and axial traction are components of the successful reduction. The less rotational manipulation, the less likely it is to create further trauma as a result of the reduction. A commonly used method of reduction is the Stimson maneuver. The patient is placed prone and given conscious sedation or pain medication. The arm is gently placed over the edge of the bed and traction applied either manually or by a static weight, as shown in Plate 1.27. In most cases, when the patient becomes relaxed the humeral head becomes disengaged from the anterior glenoid and the shoulder reduces into the glenoid fossa.

PATHOLOGIC LESIONS

Commonly seen in traumatic anterior dislocation of the shoulder is a Bankart lesion, which is an avulsion of the anterior inferior GH ligaments along with the anterior inferior labrum. In most cases of recurrent anterior instability associated with an avulsion of the anterior inferior labrum and GH ligaments, when surgery is

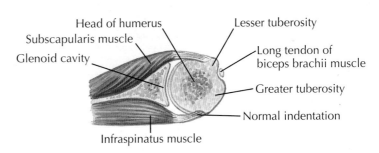

Head of humerus
Subscapularis muscle
Glenoid cavity
Lesser tuberosity
Long tendon of biceps brachii muscle
Greater tuberosity
Normal indentation
Infraspinatus muscle

Section through normal glenohumeral joint

— **Stages in formation of Hill-Sachs lesion** —

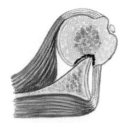

Anterior dislocation. Anterior rim of glenoid indents posterolateral part of humeral head.

Anterior dislocation continues; indentation in humeral head enlarges.

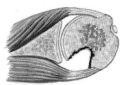

After reduction. Defect persists, causing instability and predisposing to recurrent dislocation.

Plate 1.29

Upper Limb: PART I

IMAGING OF GLENOHUMERAL JOINT ANTERIOR DISLOCATION

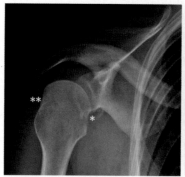
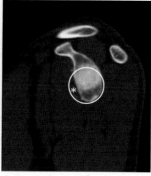
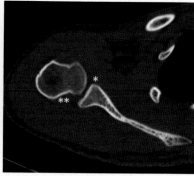

Radiographs and CT scan demonstrating a patient with anterior dislocation of the humeral head with concomitant bony injuries to the glenoid (*asterisk*) and humeral head (Hill-Sachs lesion; *double asterisks*). The glenoid bone loss is better appreciated on CT scan in the sagittal plane demonstrating bone loss when drawing a best-fit circle on the face of the glenoid and in the axial cuts showing anterior glenoid bone loss. The Hill-Sachs lesion is also clearly visible on the axial CT cuts (*double asterisks*). With injuries of both humeral head and glenoid, soft tissue–only repairs may be inadequate to prevent recurrent instability, and bony reconstructions such as the Latarjet coracoid transfer procedure may be necessary.

ANTERIOR DISLOCATION OF GLENOHUMERAL JOINT (Continued)

indicated, a Bankart-type procedure is performed in which these tissues are sewn back to the original attachment site along the anterior and inferior rim of the glenoid. If there is an acute fracture of the glenoid rim associated with a first-time or recurrent dislocation, then reduction and internal fixation of the fragment can restore both the glenoid fossa surface area and the attached ligaments. If there is bone deficiency that is not associated with a bone fragment that can be reduced and fixed to achieve these surgical goals, then a bone graft procedure is preferred. Several types of bone substitution procedures are available for these types of surgery. The most popular of these bone transfer procedures uses the coracoid process and the associated tendons (short head of the biceps and the coracobrachialis) placed along the anterior inferior glenoid defect and held in place with screw fixation. This procedure (Bristow or Latarjet) provides both restoration of the bone loss of the glenoid and a dynamic stabilization by the sling effect of the transferred tendon and muscle tissue. All these types of shoulder stabilization procedures can be done by either open or arthroscopic methods. In addition, there is, in many cases, a variably sized impaction-type fracture in the posterosuperior aspect of the humeral head that is termed a *Hill-Sachs lesion.* This lesion occurs in anterior dislocation when the softer bone of the humeral head is impacted against the harder bone of the anterior glenoid rim. These lesions may be large and are occasionally treated with placement of a humeral head allograft or small partial head prosthetic replacement into this defect. Hill-Sachs lesions can also be treated by suturing the posterior rotator cuff and capsule tissue into the defect.

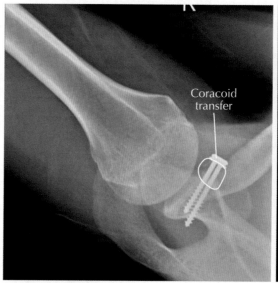
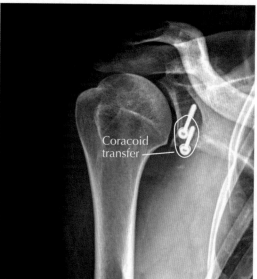

Postoperative radiographs of a patient who underwent a Latarjet coracoid transfer with screw fixation. Note the transferred coracoid fragment filling in the anterior glenoid defect.

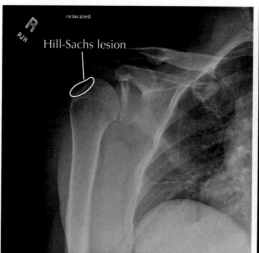
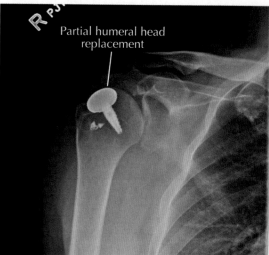

Preoperative (*left*) and postoperative (*right*) radiographs showing a large Hill-Sachs lesion from recurrent dislocations and the use of a partial humeral head resurfacing implant to fill in the Hill-Sachs lesion.

Plate 1.30

Shoulder

Posterior (subacromial) dislocation

Antero-posterior view

Lateral view

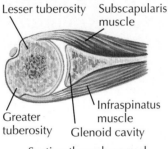

Anteroposterior radiograph. Difficult to determine if humeral head is within, anterior, or posterior to glenoid cavity.

Lateral radiograph (parallel to plane of body of scapula). Humeral head clearly seen to be posterior to glenoid cavity.

Glenoid "Reverse" Hill-Sachs lesion Humeral head

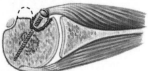

True axillary view. Also shows humeral head posterior to glenoid cavity.

Lesser tuberosity Subscapularis muscle

Greater tuberosity Glenoid cavity Infraspinatus muscle

Section through normal glenohumeral joint

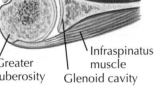

Posterior dislocation. Posterior rim of glenoid cavity causes depression of anteromedial part of humeral head (reverse Hill-Sachs lesion).

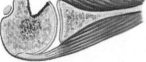

Closed reduction. Persistent defect, instability, and tendency to redislocate.

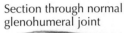

Open reduction. Subscapularis tendon or lesser tuberosity with tendon transplanted into defect.

Closed reduction. Downward traction applied to humerus plus downward and forward pressure to humeral head to reduce it into glenoid cavity. Forced external rotation must be avoided as fracture of head or shaft may result.

POSTERIOR DISLOCATION OF GLENOHUMERAL JOINT

Posterior dislocations account for approximately 5% of shoulder dislocations. In most cases, posterior instability is traumatic. Like anterior dislocation, posterior dislocation can also be atraumatic. Atraumatic or minimally traumatic causes are more common in posterior instability. This type of instability is often recurrent subluxation or partial dislocation and can be associated with generalized ligamentous laxity, developmental glenoid hypoplasia resulting in posterior inferior glenoid bone deficiency as shown in Plate 1.30, or muscle imbalance often seen with scapula winging or abnormal scapula motion. Atraumatic posterior instability is not usually associated with a defect or injury to the posterior capsule or labrum. Complete traumatic dislocation of the shoulder, with the humeral head posterior to the glenoid rim, is most commonly associated with posterior ligament and posterior labrum tears as one would see with anterior instability (e.g., a Bankart lesion). Traumatic posterior dislocation can require physician-assisted reduction. In these cases, a reverse Hill-Sachs lesion on the anterior aspect of the humeral head can been seen and occurs by the same mechanism as the more common posterior Hill-Sachs lesions. Unlike anterior dislocation, posterior dislocation is more often missed on routine shoulder AP radiographs, as seen in Plate 1.30. The posterior displacement of the humeral head is much more easily seen on the transscapular lateral or axillary view. For this reason, when evaluating a patient who has sustained a traumatic injury, it is essential that at least two if not all three of these radiographic views be included.

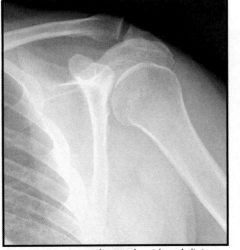

Anteroposterior radiograph with a deficient posteroinferior glenoid due to a developmental defect in the glenoid growth plate. This is called a hypoplastic glenoid and can be associated with posterior instability.

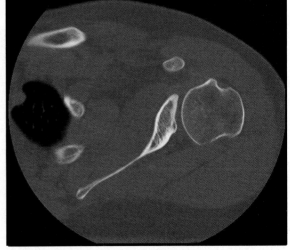

Axial CT scan showing glenoid retroversion of approximately 50 degrees in a patient with a hypoplastic glenoid.

Plate 1.31

Upper Limb: PART I

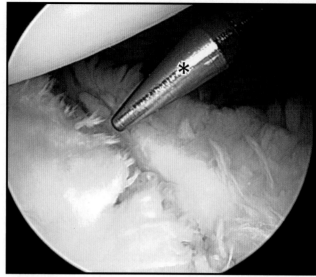

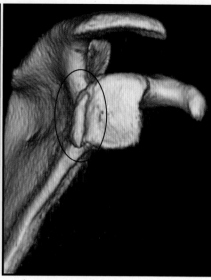

A. Arthroscopic image of a posterior labral tear with associated fracture along the posterior glenoid rim (posterior bony Bankart lesion). The metallic probe (*asterisk*) points to the site of the posterior labral tear and glenoid rim fracture.

B. The posterior glenoid rim fracture can also be seen circled on the three-dimensional CT image.

Posterior Dislocation of Glenohumeral Joint (Continued)

Traumatic posterior dislocation is more common in patients with major motor seizure disorders. Under-development of the glenoid (hypoplasia) occurs in patients with growth plate abnormalities of the glenoid; the posterior and inferior portions of the glenoid are underdeveloped, resulting in a hypoplastic glenoid.

Closed reduction of posterior dislocation follows the same principles of closed reduction of anterior disloca-tion. Axial longitudinal traction of the arm and muscle relaxation are important for a gentle nontraumatic re-duction. Direct pressure over the posterior aspect of the humeral head can also help reduce the dislocation.

Similar to recurrent anterior instability, recurrent posterior instability associated with avulsion of the posterior capsule and labrum can be treated with an arthroscopic posterior capsulolabral repair in which these tissues are sewn back to the original attachment site along the posterior rim of the glenoid (Plate 1.31, A–C). If there is a fracture of the glenoid rim associated with the recurrent instability, then the fracture frag-ment can be incorporated into the arthroscopic repair. If there is bone deficiency that is not associated with a bone fragment, then a bone graft procedure is consid-ered (Plate 1.31, D and E). In addition to management of the posterior glenoid pathology, a reverse Hill-Sachs lesion may be treated with transfer of the subscapularis tendon and/or lesser tuberosity into the defect, whereas larger reverse Hill-Sachs defects can be treated with placement of a humeral head allograft or small partial head prosthetic replacement.

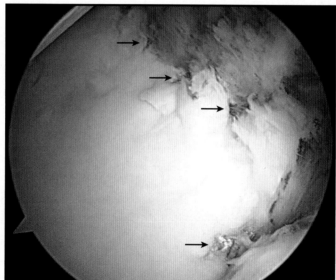

C. The posterior labral tear can be repaired arthroscopically, incorporating the bone fragment into the repair. The locations of the suture anchors repairing the labrum back to the glenoid rim are identified with *arrows*.

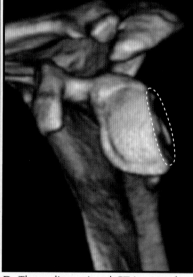

D. Three-dimensional CT image of posterior glenoid bone loss from recurrent posterior instability. The outline of the normal glenoid shape is identified by the *dotted line* to demonstrate the area of posterior glenoid bone loss.

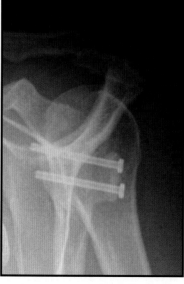

E. A postoperative lateral scapular Y radiograph shows the bone graft held in place with two screws.

(*D* and *E* from Wellmann M, Pastor MF, Ettinger M, et al. Arthroscopic posterior bone block stabilization-early results of an effective procedure for the recurrent posterior instability. Knee Surg Sports Traumatol Arthrosc. 2018;26(1):292–298. doi: 10.1007/s00167-017-4753-x. PMID: 29085981.)

Plate 1.32

Shoulder

ACROMIOCLAVICULAR AND STERNOCLAVICULAR DISLOCATION

AC dislocations, otherwise commonly called *AC separations*, are common injuries after trauma associated with landing on the superior aspect of the shoulder. These are commonly seen in football injuries and injuries sustained in bicycling or other riding accidents when someone falls from the bike or a horse and lands on the superior aspect of the shoulder. AC separation is classified into six different types depending on the amount of damage to the soft tissues and the orientation of the distal end of the clavicle:

- Grade I: Sprain of the AC capsular ligaments.
- Grade II: Complete disruption of the AC capsule ligaments and the strain of the coracoclavicular ligaments.
- Grade III: Complete disruption of the AC ligaments and coracoclavicular ligaments, resulting in an unstable clavicle segment. The distal clavicle appears to be superiorly displaced, but on more careful review of the radiographs or on physical examination, the clavicles are at the same height and the scapula and humeral are displaced distally by gravity and the weight of the arm.
- Grade IV: Grade III ligament injuries but with disruption of the trapezius fascia, thus resulting in a posterior dislocation of the distal end of the clavicle through the trapezius muscle. This type of injury is best seen on the axillary radiographic view and on physical examination.
- Grade V: Lesions with more extensive soft tissue damage. In addition to injury to the AC and coracoclavicular ligaments, there is complete disruption of the deltotrapezial fascia and very significant displacement between the clavicle and scapular bone, usually affecting two to three widths of the distal clavicle, more easily seen on stress radiographs.
- Grade VI: Rare injuries that result from complete ligamental disruption and displacement of the distal end of the clavicle under the coracoid.

Most grade I, II, and III injuries are treated by nonoperative measures. Grade IV, V, and VI injuries are generally treated by surgical reconstruction of the ligaments and reduction of the clavicle to the acromion. In some patients with grade III lesions who either have persistent symptoms of pain or fatigue or have a high physical demand, reconstruction of the AC joint and ligament attachments is performed.

Anterior sternoclavicular dislocation is often a result of high-velocity traumatic lesions resulting from a direct blow to the anterior aspect of the shoulder. Disruption of the sternoclavicular and costoclavicular ligaments results in a complete anterior dislocation of the sternoclavicular joint. In many cases, this will result in severe deformity and significant swelling. In many of these cases, closed reduction cannot be achieved with maintenance of joint reduction. These

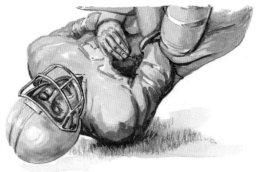

Injury to acromioclavicular joint. This is usually caused by fall on tip of shoulder, depressing acromion (shoulder separation).

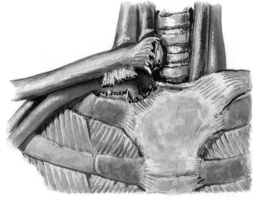

Posterior dislocation of sternoclavicular joint. This can be a serious injury because of possible injury to trachea or vessels. Both posterior and anterior dislocations can usually be reduced manually or with aid of towel clip and anesthesia.

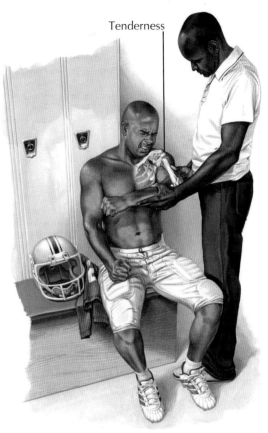

Tenderness

Patient will have tenderness over AC joint.

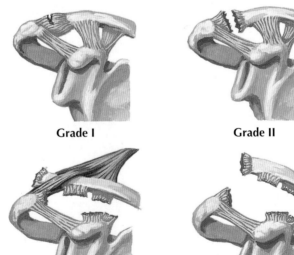

Grade I   **Grade II**   **Grade III**

Grade IV   **Grade V**   **Grade VI**

injuries are often treated nonoperatively because many of these patients, particularly those with lower functional bands, will have minimal symptoms. If there is significant residual pain or limitations of function, then later reduction and ligament reconstruction can be performed in those selected patients. Posterior dislocation of the sternoclavicular joint is a more serious traumatic lesion because there can be injury or compression of the underlying neurovascular structures. In these cases, closed reduction under

general anesthesia is performed. On occasion, an open reduction and ligament reconstruction may be required. The growth plate at the medial end of the clavicle does not close in most individuals until the early 20s. Trauma and deformity in these younger patients often result in fracture through the growth plate. These growth plate injuries heal as a fracture, the ligaments are not torn, and the clavicle after healing is not unstable. Although there may be a deformity, most of these patients are asymptomatic.

Plate 1.33

Upper Limb: PART I

FRACTURES OF CLAVICLE

Fractures of lateral third of clavicle

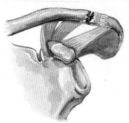

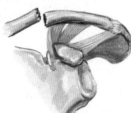

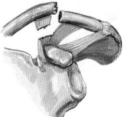

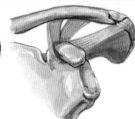

Type I. Fracture with no disruption of ligaments and therefore no displacement. Treated with simple sling for few weeks.

Type IIA. Fracture is medial to ligaments. Both ligaments are intact.

Type IIB. Fracture is between ligaments; coracoid is disrupted, trapezoid is intact. Medial fragment may elevate.

Type III. Fracture through acromioclavicular joint; no displacement. This is often missed and may later cause painful osteoarthritis requiring resection arthroplasty.

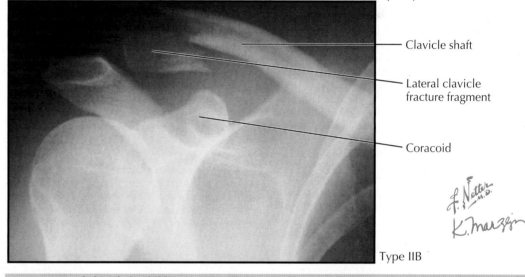

Clavicle shaft

Lateral clavicle fracture fragment

Coracoid

Type IIB

FRACTURES OF THE CLAVICLE AND SCAPULA

FRACTURES OF THE CLAVICLE

Fractures of the distal third of the clavicle are classified as those involving the lateralmost portion of the clavicle. A type I fracture involves the clavicle distal to the corticoclavicular ligaments and is without significant displacement. Type II fractures involve the distal third of the clavicle in the region of the corticoclavicular ligaments. These fractures are often displaced based on the location of the fracture relevant to the corticoclavicular ligaments. Those fractures that are medial to the corticoclavicular ligaments have a stable lateral fracture fragment, whereas those that have involvement of the fracture lateral to the ligaments with disruption of the corticoclavicular ligaments result in a displaced clavicle segment. Type III fractures involve a contusion or compression fracture of the distal third of the fracture at its articular surface. Type I fractures are often treated by nonoperative measures. Type II fractures with minimal displacement can likewise be treated with nonoperative treatment, whereas those with significant displacement will often require fixation of the fracture and reconstruction of the coracoclavicular ligaments by either direct suture or ligament substitution. Type III fractures are often treated nonoperatively, but in many cases posttraumatic arthritis will result.

Midclavicular fractures involve the middle third segment. These are very common fractures in all age groups and one of the most common fractures throughout the body. In many cases, these fractures can be treated nonoperatively. Only when there is significant comminution and displacement of the middle third fractures is early

Fracture of clavicle in children

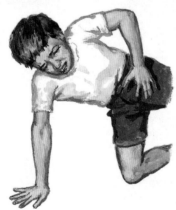

Commonly caused by fall on outstretched hand with force transmitted via shoulder to clavicle

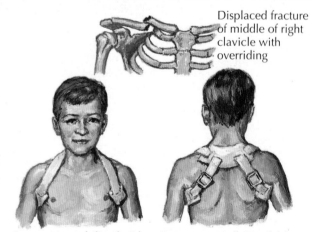

Displaced fracture of middle of right clavicle with overriding

Fracture immobilized with snug, commercially available shoulder harness or figure-of-8 bandage for 3-4 weeks

surgical treatment indicated. In severely displaced fractures, significant malunion, nonunion, or compromise of the neurovascular structures can result (see Plate 1.34). In cases in which nonoperative treatment is appropriate, use of a figure-of-eight harness or sling is an effective means to decrease the use of the shoulder and to place the shoulder in a more favorable position. A figure-of-eight harness places the shoulder in a position of scapula retraction and helps to support the fracture and lengthen the clavicle to aid in reduction of the

fracture fragments. Fracture healing without internal fixation will result in callus formation with a residual deformity in the area of the clavicle. Minor deformities often remodel over time, resulting in an acceptable appearance to the contour of the shoulder.

FRACTURES OF THE CLAVICLE IN CHILDREN

Fractures of the clavicle are among the most common fractures in children and can be caused by both direct

Plate 1.34

Shoulder

FRACTURES OF CLAVICLE AND SCAPULA

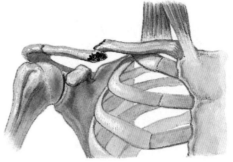

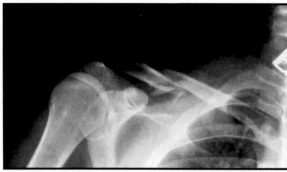

Fracture of middle third of clavicle (most common). Medial fragment displaced upward by pull of sternocleidomastoid muscle; lateral fragment displaced downward by weight of shoulder. These fractures occur most often in children.

Anteroposterior radiograph. Fracture of middle third of clavicle.

FRACTURES OF THE CLAVICLE AND SCAPULA (Continued)

trauma to the clavicle or indirect trauma from a fall onto an outstretched arm. The clavicle in children has great healing potential, and even with comminution or deformity these fractures heal and remodel better than the same fracture type in adults. Most children with a closed clavicular fracture without neurovascular injury will be successfully treated with closed nonoperative management. Use of a figure-of-eight brace maintains a comfortable position of the fracture and allows for healing. True fracture immobilization is not achieved with this type of fracture, and pain management is largely a matter of decreased activity level and analgesic medication. In the child, early fracture healing and decreased mobility of the fracture fragments occur within 4 to 6 weeks after fracture. Solid fracture healing takes considerably longer, and these patients should avoid participation in any sports for 3 months and in any contact-type sport for 4 to 6 months.

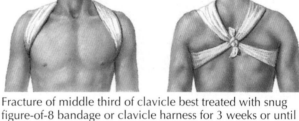

Fracture of middle third of clavicle best treated with snug figure-of-8 bandage or clavicle harness for 3 weeks or until pain subsides. Bandage or harness must be tightened occasionally because it loosens with wear.

Healed fracture of clavicle. Even with proper treatment, small lump may remain.

FRACTURES OF THE SCAPULA

Scapular fractures often result from high-velocity trauma to the chest wall. These fractures can often be associated with other visceral or thoracic trauma, including rib fractures. Glenoid rim fractures can occur as a result of traumatic dislocations of the shoulder. The anterior glenoid rim fractures often result from anterior dislocation, and posterior rim fractures occur from posterior dislocation of the shoulder. Early surgery should be performed for reduction of the fragment and internal fixation when larger in size and displaced. When these are isolated fragments, this can be done by arthroscopic surgery.

Acromial fractures often result from trauma to the superior aspect of the shoulder by direct trauma. Non-fused growth centers of the acromion can occur and appear to be fractures but are not related to trauma. This entity is more commonly associated with chronic rotator cuff problems and is called an os acromiale. These growth abnormalities are shown in Plate 1.42.

Fracture fragments can include multiple portions of the scapula body. Scapular body fractures or scapular neck fractures that are not displaced or only moderately displaced are most often treated by nonoperative measures. Those fracture fragments that involve the articular surface of the glenoid with displacement are often treated by surgical means, particularly those that are associated with anterior or posterior dislocation of the shoulder. These fracture fragments often will result in persistent instability of the shoulder. Displaced fractures of the glenoid fossa can also result in significant posttraumatic arthritis.

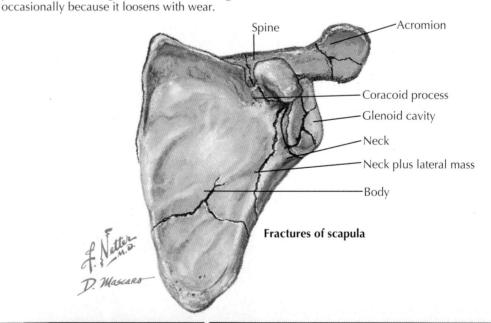

Spine

Acromion

Coracoid process

Glenoid cavity

Neck

Neck plus lateral mass

Body

Fractures of scapula

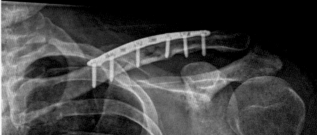

Preoperative (left) and postoperative (right) anteroposterior radiographs of a displaced middle third clavicle fracture with butterfly fragment. The fracture was surgically fixed with a clavicle plate and screws.

Plate 1.35

Upper Limb: PART I

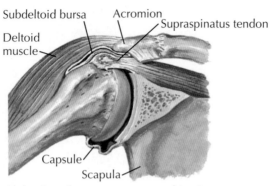

Subdeltoid bursa · Acromion
Deltoid muscle · Supras.pinatus tendon
Capsule · Scapula

Abduction of arm causes repeated impingement of greater tubercle of humerus on acromion, leading to degeneration and inflammation of supraspinatus tendon, secondary inflammation of bursa, and pain on abduction of arm. Calcific deposit in degenerated tendon produces elevation that further aggravates inflammation and pain.

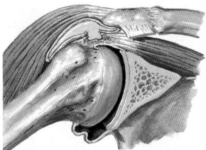

Deposit may rupture spontaneously into bursa and be resorbed, relieving pain and acute inflammation.

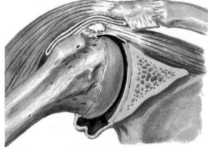

Chronic tendonitis and bursitis with calcific deposit in tendon and minimal inflammation. Chronic deposits do not rupture spontaneously but may be resorbed.

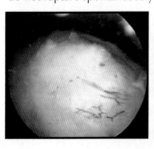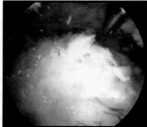

Calcific deposit may rupture spontaneously beneath floor of bursa, with relief of pain and inflammation.

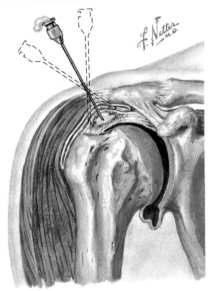

Needle rupture of deposit in acute tendonitis promptly relieves acute symptoms. After administration of local anesthetic, needle introduced at point of greatest tenderness. Several probings may be necessary to reach deposit. This procedure should be done with ultrasonography guidance. Toothpaste-like deposit may ooze from needle. Irrigation of bursa with saline solution using two needles is often done to remove more calcific material. Corticosteroid may be injected for additional relief.

Arthroscopic surgery allows for visualization and location of the calcific deposit within the rotator cuff tendon tissue.

CALCIFIC TENDONITIS

Deposit of calcium mineral within the rotator cuff tendons occurs as a result of a hypoxic state within degenerative tendon tissue. In the phase of deposit formation there are few symptoms. During the phase of deposit absorption the tissues exhibit an acute inflammatory reaction associated with severe pain and a local increase in tissue temperature and, on occasion, local redness and swelling. In an acute phase of absorption, the clinical picture can appear to be an infection, but it is not an infection.

The acute phase can be treated with local cortisone injection to the subacromial bursae with the use of oral antiinflammatory medication. In chronic conditions of persistent pain refractory to nonoperative management, aspiration of the lesion can be done under ultrasound guidance.

The clinical presentation of calcium deposits in the rotator cuff is variable. In some patients, the calcium deposit is seen on radiographs as an incidental finding with a patient reporting a lack of a history of shoulder symptoms or only a remote history of shoulder pain that may have been associated with the deposit. In some patients, an acute episode of pain and inflammation is associated with resorption of the deposit, in which case the symptoms resolve. Other patients have recurrent bouts of acute and severe shoulder pain associated with intervals of no symptoms, and still others have chronic low to moderate pain on a continual basis with some bouts of severe pain. In most cases it is the patient with multiple episodes of severe pain or chronic symptoms whose condition does not respond to nonoperative management and in whom removal of the calcium deposit is indicated.

Arthroscopic surgery can also visualize and locate the calcific deposit within the rotator cuff tendon tissue. Under direct visualization the lesion can be removed with a motorized shaving tool; if the defect is large, repair of the tissue can be performed with arthroscopic technique. At the time of surgery, the deposit can be seen as a bump within the tendon, often surrounded by increased blood vessels. The operative finding is variable, as is the clinical presentation. In most cases requiring surgery, when the calcium deposit is opened, a large amount of calcium debris is extruded under pressure and the material is infiltrated within the tendon substances. The material is granular. Removal of the deposit often results in a defect in the tendon. In many cases with a large calcium deposit, the defect remaining after removal of the deposit is large, and the benefit of arthroscopic removal is the ability to repair the cuff defect at that time. At other times, after opening the deposit, the material found is more the consistency of toothpaste. Other techniques used for removal of calcium deposits in the rotator cuff include the use of high- or low-energy ultrasound and needle aspiration under fluoroscopic control. Open surgery is rarely performed because current minimally invasive techniques are so effective and have lower morbidity than open surgery.

Plate 1.36

Shoulder

CLINICAL PRESENTATION OF FROZEN SHOULDER

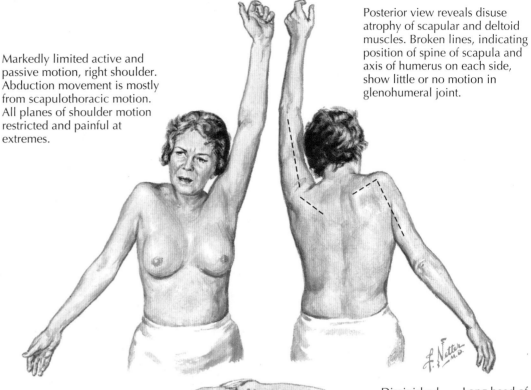

Markedly limited active and passive motion, right shoulder. Abduction movement is mostly from scapulothoracic motion. All planes of shoulder motion restricted and painful at extremes.

Posterior view reveals disuse atrophy of scapular and deltoid muscles. Broken lines, indicating position of spine of scapula and axis of humerus on each side, show little or no motion in glenohumeral joint.

FROZEN SHOULDER

The clinical and anatomic pathology in frozen shoulder is derived from an acute inflammatory synovitis followed by an intracapsular soft tissue fibrosis, resulting in contracture of the capsule. Some have made an analogy of frozen shoulder to Dupuytren contraction in the palmar fascia of the hand. Dupuytren contracture has been associated with myofibroblasts present within the fibrous tissues, and these same cells can be found in the shoulder capsule with frozen shoulder. Frozen shoulder is commonly seen in association with thyroid disorders and diabetes. Patients with these associated systemic diseases often have a more severe and refractory clinical course. When associated with thyroid and diabetic changes, the treatment of frozen shoulder is often more difficult. The recovery phase is longer and protracted, and the recurrence rate and the number of treatment failures are higher with both surgical and nonsurgical treatment.

There is a role for intraarticular therapy with a corticosteroid, particularly in the treatment of early stages of frozen shoulder in which there is acute inflammation of the synovium. As the disease progresses through the second stage with more fibrosis and fewer inflammatory changes, corticosteroid injections appear to have less of a clinical effect. Nonsurgical treatment is focused on passive range-of-motion stretching exercises that should consider all portions of the capsule and affect all arcs of motion to include forward flexion, abduction, and internal and external rotation exercises. In many cases, the patient's shoulder symptoms are accompanied by significant pain; thus the exercise program needs to be performed gently but on a daily basis. Home-based exercise programs instructed by a physical therapist are preferred. Stretching exercises in phase I and phase II are shown later in the discussion on rehabilitation (see Plate 1.62). Home exercises should be done daily and frequently for short periods of time. Typically, each exercise session should include five of the types of stretches shown in the rehabilitation

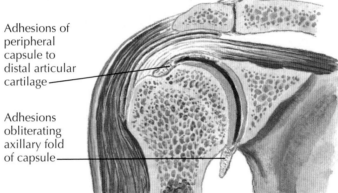

Adhesions of peripheral capsule to distal articular cartilage

Adhesions obliterating axillary fold of capsule

Coronal section of shoulder shows adhesions between capsule and periphery of humeral head.

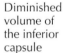

Diminished volume of the inferior capsule

Long head of biceps within the biceps groove

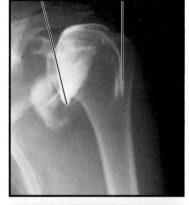

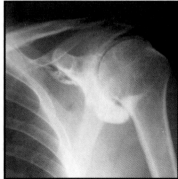

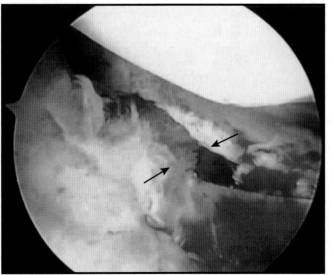

Intraarticular findings of synovitis and loss of capsular volume as well as the arthroscopic releases (*arrows*) performed with arthroscopic surgery

Anteroposterior arthrogram of normal shoulder (*bottom*). Axillary fold and biceps brachii sheath visualized. Volume of capsule normal. Anteroposterior arthrogram of frozen shoulder (*top*). Joint capacity reduced. Axillary fold and biceps brachii sheath not evident.

Plate 1.37

Upper Limb: PART I

RISK FACTORS AND TEST FOR FROZEN SHOULDER

Risk factors

Immobilization after surgery or trauma with cast or sling

Thyroid problems

Diabetes

Long-term bed rest

Passive forward flexion

Degree of rotation from patient with passive forward elevation normally involves both glenohumeral and scapular motion.

Degree of rotation from examiner-assisted passive forward elevation, isolating glenohumeral motion. The terminal elevation can be shown to be entirely from scapulothoracic motion by movement of the arm while palpating the tip of the scapula.

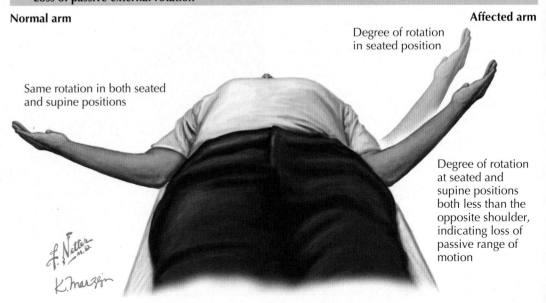

Hand on scapula removes scapular motion from the forward elevation.

Loss of passive external rotation

Normal arm

Affected arm

Degree of rotation in seated position

Same rotation in both seated and supine positions

Degree of rotation at seated and supine positions both less than the opposite shoulder, indicating loss of passive range of motion

FROZEN SHOULDER
(Continued)

discussion, each for 2 minutes for a total of 10 minutes of exercise at regular intervals at least five times per day. Persistence with this regimen accompanied by good pain management will generally result in significant improvement after 6 to 8 weeks in patients with idiopathic adhesive capsulitis. When pain is diminished and range of motion near 80% of normal, a strengthening program can be added to the overall program and the frequency of the stretching program can be diminished and the length of time for each session increased to 15 to 20 minutes three times each day.

In a small percentage of patients with refractory clinical symptoms associated with significant loss of passive arcs of motion, surgical management can be very effective. Idiopathic frozen shoulder (adhesive capsulitis) is most responsive to both nonoperative and surgical management as defined previously. Arthroscopic capsule release involving all portions of the capsule is an effective mechanism to release the contracted tissue and allow for ease of movement and postoperative rehabilitation. Postoperative pain management should include consideration of regional blocks. As with all types of treatment, pain management is important and supports an effective postoperative rehabilitation program.

Examination of the frozen shoulder can demonstrate loss of passive range of motion of the shoulder and is best tested in the supine position. As the examiner tries to further elevate the arm, the examiner's hand realizes loss of GH motion, and the terminal phases of elevation are entirely related primarily to scapular thoracic movement. In addition, loss of passive external rotation can be seen in both the supine and the seated positions. Motion should be tested for both passive and active range of motion. Loss of active range of motion in the setting of normal passive motion is often related to weakness secondary to rotator cuff function (see Plates 1.41, 1.43, and 1.48).

Plate 1.38

Shoulder

BICEPS TENDON TEARS AND SLAP LESIONS: PRESENTATION AND PHYSICAL EXAMINATION

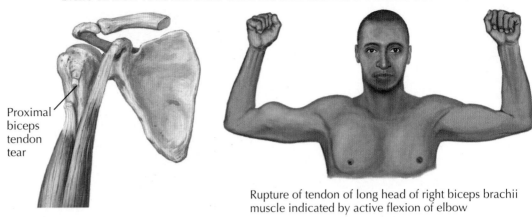

Proximal biceps tendon tear

Rupture of tendon of long head of right biceps brachii muscle indicated by active flexion of elbow

BICEPS TENDON TEARS AND SLAP LESIONS

The classic "Popeye" deformity of the biceps muscle is associated with rupture of the long head of the biceps tendon proximally in the shoulder near its attachment on the superior labrum. When the tendon retracts from its origin, the muscle shortens, resulting in a "bunching up" of the muscle belly in the mid-arm. This is a common condition often associated with rotator cuff tears or impingement syndrome (see Plates 1.41 to 1.43). In many cases, persistent shoulder symptoms after biceps tendon rupture are related to the associated rotator cuff pathologic process rather than symptoms associated with the biceps tendon tear. If shoulder symptoms persist after long head of the biceps tendon rupture, then evaluation of the rotator cuff with magnetic resonance imaging (MRI) or ultrasonography of the shoulder is warranted. In some patients, although uncommon, an isolated tear of the long head of the biceps can result in aching discomfort or cramping of the biceps during forceful elbow flexion or supination of the forearm, both of which are functions of the biceps muscle. Most isolated tears of the long head of the biceps are asymptomatic, and for this reason most are not treated by surgical repair, particularly in the older or more sedentary patient. Isolated acute tears in the younger and active patient in some cases should be considered for surgical repair. When surgically repaired, the torn end of the long head of the biceps tendon is sutured within the biceps groove using a suture anchor or other fixation implant. Alternatively, the tendon can be sutured to local soft tissues such as the PM tendon or the short head of the biceps. This procedure is called a biceps tenodesis. When a tenodesis is performed for management of an acute rupture, the repair is more often performed by open surgery through a small deltopectoral or subpectoral incision. In cases in which a symptomatic partial biceps tear or superior labrum from anterior to posterior (SLAP) tear involving the biceps tendon origin develops from chronic degeneration and is found at the time of arthroscopic surgery, the long head of the biceps tendon can either be released at the site of its origin along the superior labrum and allowed to retract without repair (biceps tenotomy) or a biceps tenodesis can be performed (see Plate 1.39). A biceps tenotomy is usually chosen instead of a tenodesis in an older or more sedentary patient, whereas tenodesis is selected in younger and more active patients who may be at risk for muscle cramping and aching with biceps tenotomy.

Three-part O'Brien test

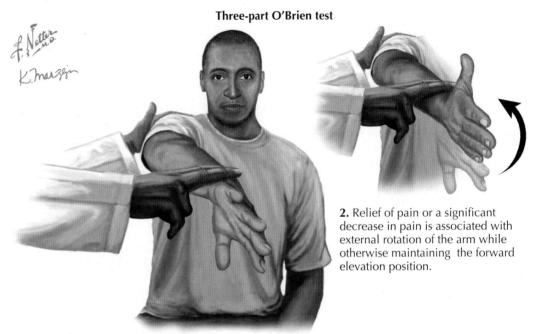

1. Resisted forward elevation with the arm in the sagittal plane with the arm perpendicular to the plane of the body and in 90 degrees of elevation and full internal rotation. If positive, patient will experience pain in the front of the shoulder with downward pressure on the arm.

2. Relief of pain or a significant decrease in pain is associated with external rotation of the arm while otherwise maintaining the forward elevation position.

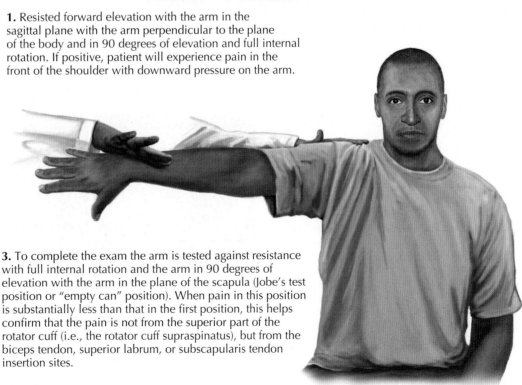

3. To complete the exam the arm is tested against resistance with full internal rotation and the arm in 90 degrees of elevation with the arm in the plane of the scapula (Jobe's test position or "empty can" position). When pain in this position is substantially less than that in the first position, this helps confirm that the pain is not from the superior part of the rotator cuff (i.e., the rotator cuff supraspinatus), but from the biceps tendon, superior labrum, or subscapularis tendon insertion sites.

Plate 1.39

Upper Limb: PART I

BICEPS TENDON TEARS AND SLAP LESIONS: TYPES OF TEARS

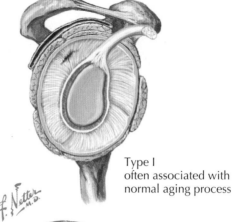

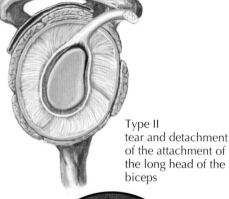

Type I
often associated with
normal aging process

Type II
tear and detachment
of the attachment of
the long head of the
biceps

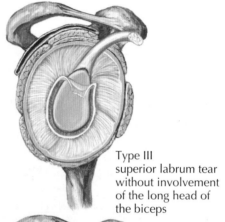

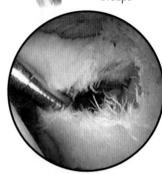

Type III
superior labrum tear
without involvement
of the long head of
the biceps

Arthroscopic view of Type III. Involvement of the superior labrum and biceps tendon but with less severe involvement of the biceps tendon tissue but involvement of the biceps tendon attachment.

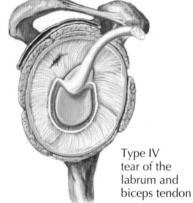

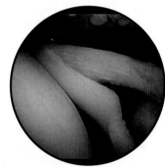

Type IV
tear of the
labrum and
biceps tendon

Arthroscopic view of Type IV. Involvement of the superior labrum along the head of the biceps.

BICEPS TENDON TEARS AND SLAP LESIONS (Continued)

Although a tenotomy will result in a "Popeye" deformity, the patient is most often asymptomatic and the pain that was preoperatively associated with the long head of the biceps tendon is relieved.

The biceps tendon is attached to the superior labrum both anteriorly and posteriorly. Type I SLAP lesions are common and often associated with the normal aging process and as such are not often associated with significant pathology or symptoms. Similarly, when type II lesions are typically seen in the older age population, they are often asymptomatic. Type II SLAP lesions can be symptomatic when they are acute and traumatic, or when chronic and degenerative. They are often seen after a fall onto an outstretched arm or in the overhead-throwing athlete as related to repetitive trauma and may warrant a surgical repair (SLAP repair). Symptomatic chronic, degenerative type II SLAP lesions may not heal well with repair and are therefore more commonly treated with biceps tenodesis. Type III lesions involve a bucket-handle tear of the labrum with mechanical symptoms without biceps tendon involvement and are amenable to surgical treatment specifically to remove that portion of the labrum that is detached (debridement). Type IV SLAP lesions involve both the superior labrum and the long head of the biceps tendon. These lesions are often symptomatic and are generally treated by removal of the labral tissue and with tenodesis of the biceps. Alternatively, the biceps tendon and type IV SLAP lesion can be repaired (SLAP repair) if tendon quality is good and the lesion is relatively small. Less common types of SLAP lesions are associated with tears extending into the anterior inferior labrum (Bankart-type labrum tears) and are associated with GH instability. In these cases, when symptomatic, both lesions are repaired at the time of surgery, most commonly with arthroscopic techniques (Bankart and SLAP repair).

Diagnosis of SLAP lesions is performed with a variety of maneuvers, including the O'Brien test. The O'Brien test is performed with a series of three maneuvers as shown and described in Plate 1.38. A positive test for a SLAP lesion results in pain in the anterior aspect of the shoulder with resisted forward elevation. These symptoms are lessened or relieved with the arm in external rotation and not significantly present with the arm in internal rotation but in the plane of the scapula.

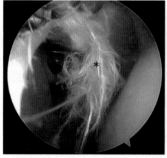

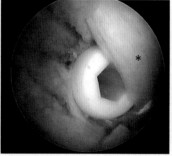

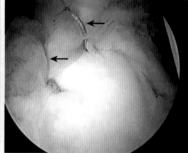

Arthroscopic image of a degenerative partial tear of the long head of the biceps tendon, with the torn tendon marked by the *asterisk*.

The degenerated tearing was arthroscopically treated by releasing the torn tendon from its origin along the superior labrum, removing the damaged tissue and performing a biceps tenodesis, with the healthy tendon (*asterisk*) secured in the biceps groove with an anchor.

Arthroscopic image following repair of a type II SLAP tear. The SLAP tear was fixed with two suture anchors (*arrows*) secured to the glenoid rim posterior to the long head of the biceps tendon.

Plate 1.40

Shoulder

ARTHROSCOPIC SURGERY TO TREAT AC JOINT ARTHRITIS

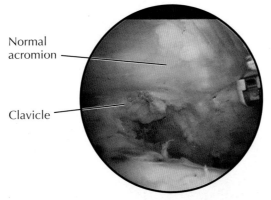

Normal acromion

Clavicle

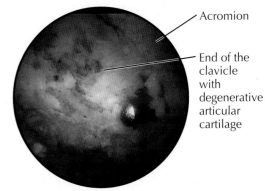

Acromion

End of the clavicle with degenerative articular cartilage

Arthroscopic view of the subacromial space near the AC joint prior to removal of the soft tissues at the AC joint

View of the distal end of the clavicle, after removal of the soft tissue at the undersurface of the joint. There are significant arthritic changes in the joint.

After use of a burr and shaving tool, a space (approximately 1 cm; *double-headed arrow*) is created between the end of the clavicle and the medial portion of the acromion.

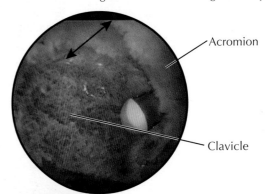

Acromion

Clavicle

ACROMIOCLAVICULAR JOINT ARTHRITIS

The AC joint is formed as the synovial-type joint between the distal end of the clavicle and the acromion. This joint can become arthritic, as can any other joint in the body. When symptomatic, arthritis of the AC joint causes pain over the superior aspect of the shoulder. Occasionally, there is pain that radiates into the area of the trapezius. Pain is often worse with internal rotation, such as placing the arm behind the back. AC joint arthritis is often diagnosed by imaging studies, including AP radiography and MRI of the shoulder. AC joint arthritis can be seen as an isolated lesion or can be associated with rotator cuff and other subacromial pathology. Clinically significant AC joint arthritis is defined as that associated with provocative maneuvers as well as specific tenderness over the AC joint. When associated with significant imaging changes of the arthritic process or cyst or spur formation, the clinical diagnosis of AC joint arthritis is made. Injection of local anesthetic directly into the AC joint will temporarily relieve the pain associated with palpation or the provocative signs and help establish the AC joint as a sole or significant contributor to the shoulder pain. Many patients have AC joint arthritic changes on radiographs and MR images and do not have clinically significant symptoms requiring treatment. It should also be understood that the symptoms and clinical findings of clinically significant AC joint–related pain are very similar to those of the rotator cuff pathologic process and often coexist in the same patient. If clinically significant pain is associated with the AC joint and it is not recognized as a problem separate from concomitant rotator cuff pathologic processes and not treated with the rotator cuff problem, residual pain will occur even if the rotator cuff problem is successfully

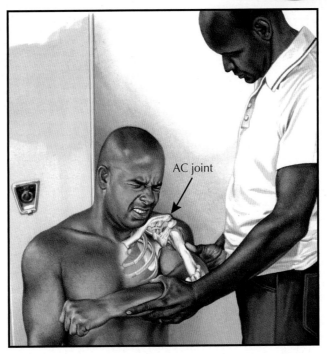

AC joint

The AC joint causes pain over the superior aspect of the shoulder when symptomatic. Tucking in a shirt or cross-body abduction when trying to wash or touch the opposite shoulder also causes pain.

treated. Given the above, the physical examination and use of selective injection tests when it is not clear that the AC joint is involved as a pain generator are critical to making a complete diagnosis of the shoulder problem.

AC joint pain from arthritis can often be treated with antiinflammatory medication, modification of activities, and, on occasion, cortisone injection specifically into the AC joint. When these symptoms remain persistent and significant over a prolonged period, arthroscopic removal of the distal end of the clavicle can be done. This treatment is termed *resection arthroplasty* and is very effective in relief of chronic symptoms associated with AC joint pathology. When done arthroscopically, there is minimal disruption of the AC capsular ligaments and no changes in the corticoclavicular ligaments. This results in a stable shoulder with relief of AC joint–related pain.

Plate 1.41

Upper Limb: PART I

IMPINGEMENT SYNDROME AND THE ROTATOR CUFF: PRESENTATION AND DIAGNOSIS

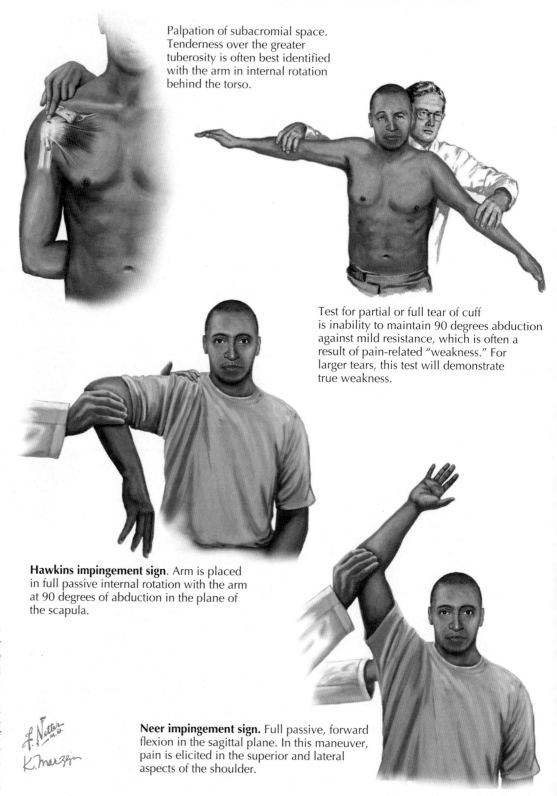

Palpation of subacromial space. Tenderness over the greater tuberosity is often best identified with the arm in internal rotation behind the torso.

Test for partial or full tear of cuff is inability to maintain 90 degrees abduction against mild resistance, which is often a result of pain-related "weakness." For larger tears, this test will demonstrate true weakness.

Hawkins impingement sign. Arm is placed in full passive internal rotation with the arm at 90 degrees of abduction in the plane of the scapula.

Neer impingement sign. Full passive, forward flexion in the sagittal plane. In this maneuver, pain is elicited in the superior and lateral aspects of the shoulder.

IMPINGEMENT SYNDROME AND THE ROTATOR CUFF

Findings associated with pathologic processes involving the rotator cuff relate to tenderness over the rotator cuff, positive impingement signs, and weakness of the rotator cuff demonstrated by the internal and external rotation lag signs. Collectively, these findings are demonstrated in Plates 1.41, 1.43, and 1.48.

The Hawkins and Neer signs are commonly called impingement signs because they are often positive when there is inflammation, degeneration, or tears of the superior and posterior parts of the rotator cuff. The pain associated with these physical examination signs results from contact compression or induced strain on these parts of the rotator cuff under the CA arch or with contact with the glenoid rim. In some cases of shoulder pain it is not clear to the examiner if the pain is originating from a pathologic process in the subacromial space (e.g., bursitis, partial rotator cuff tear, or full tear) when the impingement signs are equivocal. In these cases, the examiner can perform an impingement test with the injection of 10 mL of lidocaine or similar local anesthetic into the subacromial space under sterile conditions. The method of injection is shown on Plate 1.61. Several minutes after the injection the examiner should repeat the impingement signs of the physical examination. A positive impingement test is defined as a significant improvement in the pain associated with these physical findings that was present before the injection (usually 50%–100% relief).

Chronic rotator cuff symptoms may be progressive and symptomatic. The acromion along with the coracoid and AC ligament form the CA arch. In many cases these chronic symptoms are associated with narrowing of the subacromial space or subcoracoid space. The subacromial space is defined as the space between the undersurface of the acromion and the rotator cuff that contains a bursa that may become compromised in size by bone spurs that form under the acromion, often within the CA ligament. This mechanical narrowing of the space below the CA arch can be associated with an acquired bone spur that can cause mechanical irritation of the underlying rotator cuff. It is not certain if the

Plate 1.42   Shoulder

IMPINGEMENT SYNDROME AND THE ROTATOR CUFF: RADIOLOGIC AND ARTHROSCOPIC IMAGING

Burred lateral acromion

Burred medial acromion showing bone spur

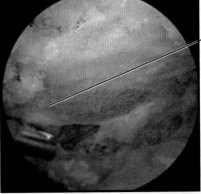

Completely burred acromion with bone spur removed and the acromion now flat

Arthroscopic view showing the under-surface of the acromion with partial removal of the spur on the lateral portion of the acromion

Arthroscopic view showing the final completion of the acromioplasty with the acromion being made smooth and flat throughout

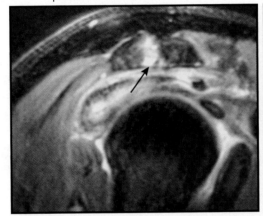

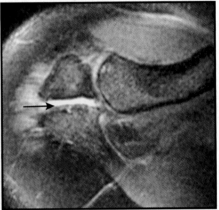

Sagittal and coronal MRI of an unfused segment (*arrow*) (meso os acromiale is most common type)

IMPINGEMENT SYNDROME AND THE ROTATOR CUFF (Continued)

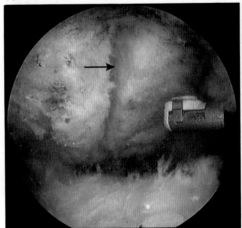

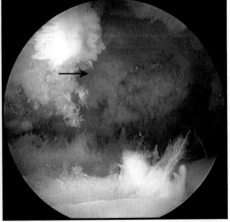

Arthroscopic view of a meso os acromiale

Arthroscopic view of treatment by removal of the anterior segment by arthroscopic technique (*arrows*) in an older, less active patient. Open reduction and internal fixation may be preferred in a younger, more active patient.

spur forms first and then causes mechanical irritation of the rotator cuff, resulting in partial-thickness or full-thickness rotator cuff tears or if the tear results in weakness of the rotator cuff, resulting in the formation of a spur. In either case, the spur can be part of the pain associated with the impingement. In many cases subacromial impingement is not the cause or source of the rotator cuff pathology. The rotator cuff pathology is often intrinsic to degeneration of the tendon or because of repetitive or single-event trauma.

Subacromial impingement and symptoms may also occur from failure of the ossification centers of the acromion to fuse in early adult life, resulting in a developmental anomaly called an os acromiale. These lesions are associated with a much higher likelihood of having a rotator cuff tear. In cases with this lesion, the tears are often larger and occur in a younger patient population than tears that typically occur as a result of tendon degeneration. The most common of these types of os acromiale is associated with lack of fusion between the anterior half and posterior half of the acromion, resulting in two separate bones called a meso os acromiale. These lesions should not be confused with an acute fracture or a nonunion of an acute fracture.

The lesions can be asymptomatic. In some cases, a radiolucent line is seen on imaging, but the bone is not mobile and is associated with a stable fibrous tissue interface. The findings are bilateral in about 60% of cases. In some cases, a bone segment is mobile and often tilted downward. The anterior half of the acromion can cause mechanical irritation of the cuff and is associated with a large tear; this more often occurs in younger patients than the age group with degenerative

or attritional tears. The os acromiale lesions are often best seen on the axillary radiograph or with axial CT or MRI. The arthroscopic near complete removal of a lesion is generally reserved for the less active individual. Open reduction and internal fixation with screw fixation and, on occasion, tension band wiring are often done to treat this problem in someone who performs heavier physical activities or heavier labor or who participates in certain sporting activities.

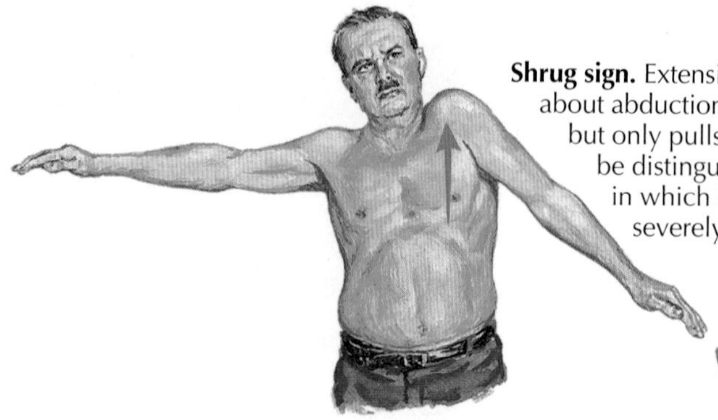

Plate 1.43

Upper Limb: PART I

Shrug sign. Extensive rupture of left cuff. To bring about abduction, trapezius muscle contracts strongly but only pulls scapula upward (*arrow*). This should be distinguished from a frozen shoulder (Plate 1.36), in which both active and passive range of motion are severely limited.

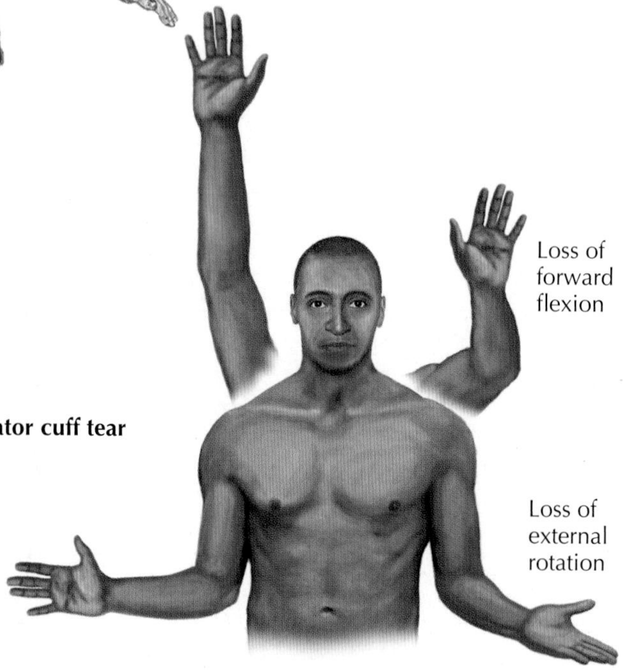

ROTATOR CUFF TEARS: PHYSICAL EXAMINATION

The rotator cuff tendons surround the humeral head and provide rotational control and strength to the shoulder. Along with the large deltoid muscle, these muscles are primarily responsible for elevation of the shoulder. When there are significant tears of the rotator cuff, there is loss of elevation of the shoulder and weakness. There is often tenderness and subacromial crepitation with rotational motion of the arm. External rotation weakness is demonstrated by the external rotation lag sign and demonstrates involvement of the supraspinatus and infraspinatus tendons and, on occasion, the teres minor tendon. These tendons are primarily responsible for external rotation strength. Tears involving these three tendons can cause a positive external rotation lag sign. The level of weakness as seen by the amount of internal rotation drift from the point of full passive external rotation is associated with the size of the tear and the number of tendons involved. In some cases there can be weakness of external rotation secondary to nerve injury (see Plate 1.58). The supraspinatus and infraspinatus muscles are innervated by the SSN. When there is injury to this nerve, often because of a compressive lesion at the suprascapular notch or the spinoglenoid notch, the muscle will be weak and is best tested by resistance in external rotation or by the external rotation lag sign.

Large and massive rotator cuff tears often involving two or more of the rotator cuff tendons will typically result in the patient's inability to either raise the arm or maintain an elevated position of the arm against moderate resistance. The shrug sign is defined as the inability to elevate the arm associated with compensatory elevation of the scapula. In some cases there is an inability to raise the arm, but this is not associated with elevation of the scapula. This can resemble paralysis of the shoulder, but in these cases the nerves to the muscles are normal, and thus this is termed *pseudoparalysis*. This loss of elevation is generally associated with superior escape of the shoulder due to deficiency of the CA arch (see Plate 1.55). All these signs of loss of elevation are physical examination findings associated with rotator cuff weakness and are associated with different parts of the rotator cuff and other associated shoulder pathologic processes, such as deficiency of the CA arch. For the diagnosis to be related to a large rotator cuff tear when the shrug sign or other signs of rotator cuff weakness are present, there should be full or near-full passive range of motion of the shoulder and the apparent weakness should not related to significant pain. In some cases of large and massive tears, the patient can achieve full active elevation yet have weakness that can be demonstrated by the inability to hold the arm at 90 degrees of elevation against mild to moderate resistance. Smaller tears, particularly those without severe pain, can demonstrate normal range of motion and

Left arm rotator cuff tear

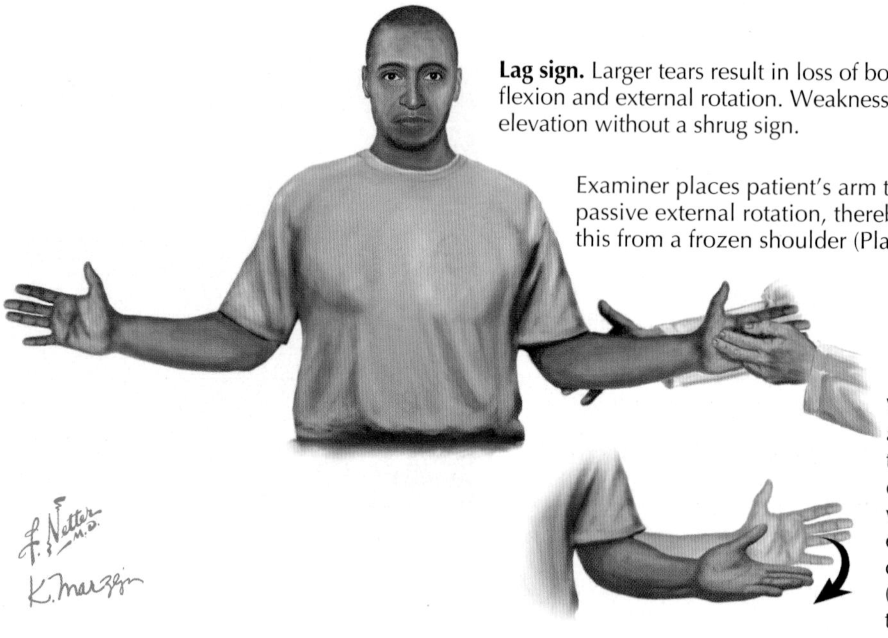

Loss of forward flexion

Loss of external rotation

Lag sign. Larger tears result in loss of both active forward flexion and external rotation. Weakness of forward flexion elevation without a shrug sign.

Examiner places patient's arm to obtain full passive external rotation, thereby distinguishing this from a frozen shoulder (Plate 1.36).

When released, arm drifts inward toward abdomen, demonstrating weakness of the external rotators of the cuff (infraspinatus teres minor).

remarkably good strength with these tests; negative tests are not an indication for lack of a full-thickness tear often in the 1- to 2-cm range. Patients with smaller tears will often demonstrate weakness with the internal and external rotation strength testing or lag signs tested with the arm by the side of the body. Sometimes the validity of these tests is in question as they relate to testing the strength of the shoulder because of pain associated with stiffness due to a frozen shoulder or subacromial pain due to inflammation of the bursae or other soft tissues of the shoulder. If this is the case, injection of a local anesthetic to either the GH joint and/or to the subacromial space will often relieve the pain. This both confirms the location of the pain and pathologic process to the shoulder (i.e., cervical spine or other non–shoulder-related referred pain to the shoulder) and allows for reexamination for shoulder strength in a setting of minimal or much reduced shoulder pain.

Plate 1.44

Shoulder

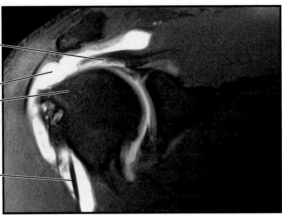

Supra-
spinatus

Infra-
spinatus

Teres
minor

Subscap-
ularis

Coronal oblique view of T1-weighted image (*left*) showing increase in signal in the distal portion of the supraspinatus tendon, which shows further increase in signal (white area) on fat saturation sequence image (*right*).

T1 sagittal oblique view demon-strates significant atrophy of the supraspinatus muscle belly along with some increase in fatty material within the muscle demonstrated by the areas of increased signal within the muscle.

Rotator cuff tendon
Subacromial contrast
Glenohumeral joint contrast

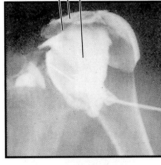

Communication between shoulder joint and subdeltoid bursa on arthrogram is patho-gnomonic of cuff tear.

Supra-
spinatus
tendon

Fluid
contrast
material

Greater
tuberosity
tendon
insertion
site

Long
head
of the
biceps
tendon

Coronal MRI view of the supraspinatus tendon with a tendon tear and retraction of the tendon to the midhu-meral head. There is significant effusion of the joint, and the joint outlines the tendon defect. In this particular case, the muscle tissue is very healthy as this is an acute tear less than 6 weeks old and no muscle atrophy is seen.

Supraspinatus normal muscle filling the entire supra-spinous fossa (in contrast to a more chronic tear shown above)

Subscapularis

Infraspinatus

Teres minor (no muscle atrophy)

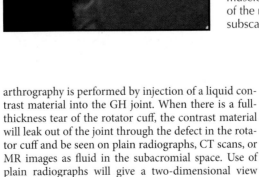

Sagittal MRI view showing a very large and biconvex muscle with a homogeneous muscle signal within all of the rotator cuff muscles (supraspinatus and infraspinatus subscapularis and teres minor muscles).

IMAGING OF SUPRASPINATUS AND INFRASPINATUS ROTATOR CUFF TEARS

The rotator cuff tendons surround the humeral head and are attached to the lesser tuberosity (subscapularis) and the greater tuberosity (supraspinatus and infraspi-natus tendons and teres minor). Between the two tuberosities is the bicipital groove through which is the long head of the biceps tendon (see Plate 1.5).

Rotator cuff tears can be either partial or full thick-ness. Partial-thickness tears involve only a superficial surface (bursal or articular surface) of the tendon and may extend into the tendon substance but are not through-and-through defects. A full-thickness defect involves the full thickness of the tendon and may in-volve more than one tendon.

Tendon tear type is defined as either partial thick-ness or full thickness and is also defined by the size in centimeters of involvement and the tendons involved (e.g., supraspinatus, infraspinatus). When a large ten-don tear is present, often involving more than one tendon such as the supraspinatus and infraspinatus, there is retraction of the tendon from its insertion site. When a tear is present for a substantial period, the muscle tissue in the area of the involved tendons un-dergoes muscular atrophy and fatty infiltration. These changes are often seen using MRI and are important prognostic factors with respect to the ability of the tendon to be repaired or the potential for healing of the repaired tendon. Larger tears of the superior and pos-terior rotator cuff result in loss of both active forward flexion and external rotation.

Imaging of the rotator cuff can include ultrasonogra-phy, MRI, and CT arthrogram. Ultrasonography pro-vides a simple and cost-effective means of assessing the presence of a both partial- and full-thickness tears of the rotator cuff. The efficacy of ultrasonography is im-proved with dynamic assessment and recording of the images and should be done by an experienced radiolo-gist. Many healthcare systems have not developed the same expertise with the use of ultrasound compared with CT arthrography or MRI with or without the use of contrast enhancement of the images. Contrast

arthrography is performed by injection of a liquid con-trast material into the GH joint. When there is a full-thickness tear of the rotator cuff, the contrast material will leak out of the joint through the defect in the rota-tor cuff and be seen on plain radiographs, CT scans, or MR images as fluid in the subacromial space. Use of plain radiographs will give a two-dimensional view of the shoulder, but when taken in multiple planes, ra-diographs can give a clearer definition of the size and

location of the tear. Much more information is available with thin-slice tomographic imaging available with CT and MRI. In addition, an assessment of the muscle at-rophy and amount of fatty infiltration of the muscle can be seen with CT and MRI. For most clinicians, MRI is preferred as the study providing the most information related to cuff tear size, location of the tear, degree of tendon retraction, and the changes in the muscle asso-ciated with the location of the tear.

Plate 1.45

Upper Limb: PART I

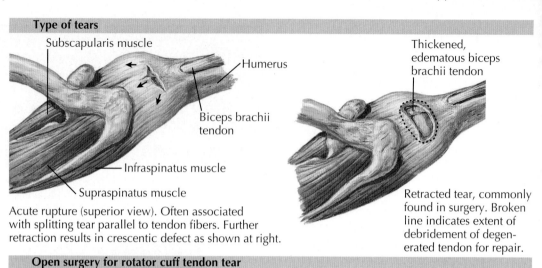

Type of tears

Subscapularis muscle

Humerus

Biceps brachii tendon

Infraspinatus muscle

Supraspinatus muscle

Acute rupture (superior view). Often associated with splitting tear parallel to tendon fibers. Further retraction results in crescentic defect as shown at right.

Thickened, edematous biceps brachii tendon

Retracted tear, commonly found in surgery. Broken line indicates extent of debridement of degenerated tendon for repair.

Surgical Management of Supraspinatus and Infraspinatus Rotator Cuff Tears

Most rotator cuff tears occur by avulsion of the tendon from the tuberosity. In some cases there is a remnant of tissue that remains on the tuberosity. This tissue is often very degenerative and of poor quality and cannot be used to repair the tendon. This tissue, if it is present at the time of surgery, is removed to create a fresh bone bed for the reattachment of the rotator cuff tendon. The principles of surgical repair are the same if the surgery is performed by traditional open surgery or arthroscopic surgery. In most cases, primary repair (first-time surgery) is performed by arthroscopic technique because it is less invasive by not having to make a major incision or detach any portion of the deltoid muscle. As a result, the surgery is less painful, there is less tissue damage, and therefore no risk for damage to the deltoid or need to repair the deltoid and there is less risk of infection or postoperative shoulder stiffness. The view of the damage and tissues is better with arthroscopic surgery. Open surgery in most cases is now reserved for more complex rotator cuff reconstruction in patients with massive chronic tears who may benefit from muscle transfer surgery or augmentation with tissue grafts.

The principles of primary rotator cuff repair include mobilization of the tendon to remove scar tissue and any contracture of the capsule so that the tendon can be pulled laterally from its retracted position to the prepared bed of the tuberosity. Sutures are passed through the tendon, and suture anchors in the bone allow for suturing of the tendon to the bone. Alternatively, tunnels are made through the bone through which the sutures in the tendon are passed and then tied over a bone bridge. When suture anchors are used, they are placed directly into the tuberosity bone and the sutures are then passed through the tendon. In either case, when the sutures are tied, the tendon edge is placed in direct approximation to the tuberosity. An anatomic repair places the tendon back to the bone to cover the entire original footprint of the tendon to bone. In many cases there are splits in the tendon in the mediolateral direction such that sutures are also placed in the sides of the tear, thus effecting a tendon-to-tendon repair.

Open surgery for rotator cuff tendon tear

Rotator cuff

The open rotator cuff repair view demonstrates a large tear of the supraspinatus and infraspinatus tendons.

Greater tuberosity

Arthroscopic surgery for rotator cuff tendon tear

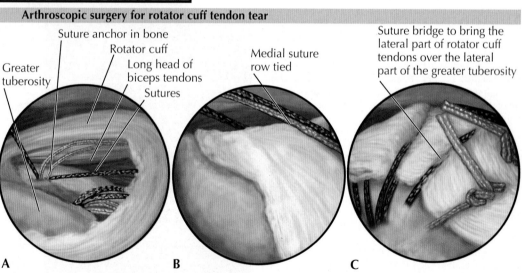

Suture anchor in bone

Rotator cuff

Greater tuberosity

Long head of biceps tendons

Sutures

Medial suture row tied

Suture bridge to bring the lateral part of rotator cuff tendons over the lateral part of the greater tuberosity

A

B

C

In this technique, sutures are placed in the medial portion of the greater tuberosity and then passed through the lateral edge of the rotator cuff tendon approximately 1.5 cm from the tendon edge (**A**). When these sutures are tied, the tendon comes to the medial border of the greater tuberosity (**B**). The suture ends are then pulled over the greater tuberosity to help compress the lateral edge of the greater tuberosity (**C**).

Protection of the repair after surgery avoids active motion of the shoulder, specifically any lifting, reaching, pushing, or pulling for 6 to 12 weeks, depending on the size of the tear and the quality of the tissues and repair. During this time, there is protection of the shoulder in a sling or pillow brace to place the shoulder in approximately 20 degrees of abduction. This position takes some tension off the repair site. Postoperative shoulder stiffness (frozen shoulder) is minimized by close postoperative evaluation of shoulder motion by the surgeon or other healthcare provider over the first 2 months after surgery. Starting with passive range-of-motion exercises during the first 6 to 8 weeks from surgery, therapy is individualized based on the size of the tear, quality of the tissues and repair, and amount of stiffness that occurred over the first few weeks after surgery.

Plate 1.46

Shoulder

SUPERIOR CAPSULAR RECONSTRUCTION AND BALLOON ARTHROPLASTY

Superior capsular reconstruction

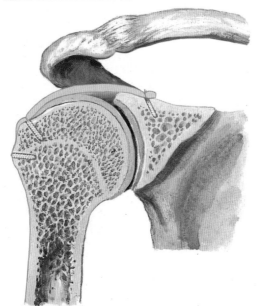

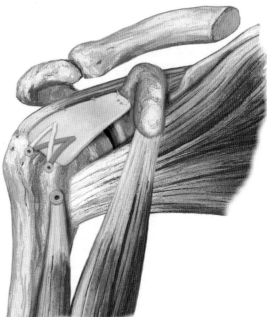

SURGICAL MANAGEMENT OF IRREPARABLE SUPRASPINATUS AND INFRASPINATUS CUFF TEAR

SUPERIOR CAPSULAR RECONSTRUCTION

Treatment of irreparable rotator cuff tear with advanced fatty infiltration and atrophy in rotator cuff musculature remains challenging. When nonoperative management fails and pain is the main symptom, an arthroscopic debridement with biceps tenodesis has proven effective but durability of this procedure in unpredictable. Teruhisa Mihata first defined the role of superior capsular complex in GH stability in a cadaveric model and showed reduction in superior migration of the humeral head by attachment of a graft from the glenoid to humeral head. He published his clinical experience with superior capsular reconstruction (SCR) in 2012 using a tensor fascia lata autograft and showed good pain and functional improvement. In recent years SCR has gained popularity in North America using a cadaveric dermal allograft to minimize donor site morbidity and reduce operative time. A graft shaped to the shape of the defect is fashioned to bridge between the rim of the glenoid and rotator cuff footprint using several suture anchors, and the SCR graft is also repaired to the native tendon posteriorly in a side-to-side fashion. Although early results in small series have been positive, including good pain control and preserved function after SCR, it appears that the type of graft is an important predictor of the outcome. The tensor fascia lata graft has shown superior performance in restoring GH stability over the dermal allograft, and its outcome has been stable in midterm follow-up. There is limited high-quality evidence on the long-term outcome, cost-benefit analysis, and longevity of this surgery.

BALLOON ARTHROPLASTY

The superior translation of the humeral head is the hallmark of massive rotator cuff tear. The biodegradable subacromial balloon spacer is a new technology for treatment of irreparable rotator cuff tear. The subacromial balloon is inserted percutaneously through a small lateral incision to fill the subacromial space and restore GH stability. Before insertion of the balloon, a limited arthroscopic subacromial decompression is performed, and it is recommended to address any concomitant pathology of the long head of the biceps tendon. Early experience shows that the balloon degrades in 9 to 12 months, whereas pain relief and improved patient-reported outcome have persisted beyond 1 year, which is attributed to the restoration of joint mechanics and scarring of the capsular structures. The midterm results of balloon arthroplasty in Europe have been promising in small series. Although indications and the long-term outcome of this procedure are not well established, early experience suggests that patients with limited overhead range of motion or advanced cuff tear arthropathy may not be good candidates for this procedure.

Superior capsular reconstruction using a dermal allograft for irreparable posterosuperior rotator cuff tear. In order to restore the force couples across the glenohumeral joint, a rectangular-shaped allograft is attached to the rim of the glenoid and footprint of the rotator cuff to prevent the humeral head from migrating superiorly.

The dermal allograft is attached to the greater tuberosity using a double row suture anchor repair and is attached to remnants of the posterior rotator cuff tendon in a side-to-side fashion.

Balloon arthroplasty

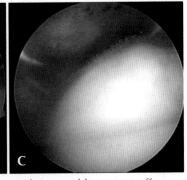

Subacromial balloon that acts as a cushion to restore stability of the glenohumeral joint

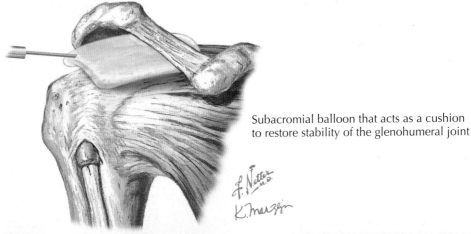

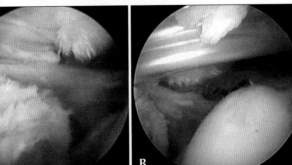

Arthroscopic images of application of subacromial balloon in a patient with irreparable rotator cuff tear, minimal arthritis, and preserved forward elevation. **A,** Irreparable rotator cuff tear with minimal arthritis and a torn long head of the biceps tendon after a limited subacromial decompression. **B,** Insertion of folded biodegradable balloon in the subacromial space. **C,** Inflation of the balloon in the subacromial space by injection of normal saline to create a cushioning effect for the humeral head.

Plate 1.47

Upper Limb: PART I

SURGICAL MANAGEMENT OF IRREPARABLE SUPRASPINATUS AND INFRASPINATUS CUFF TEAR (Continued)

LATISSIMUS TRANSFER

The LD transfer was initially described by L'Episcopo in patients with obstetric brachial plexus palsy. The main purpose of LD transfer is to restore external rotation and vertical stability of the humeral head. The modern application of LD transfer to irreparable posterosuperior rotator cuff tear was described by Christian Gerber. Surgery is done through a double incision technique. The first incision is performed in the axilla to release and harvest the LD tendon from its insertion on the humerus. The second incision is made superiorly through the deltoid to identify the rotator cuff tear, prepare the greater tuberosity, and attach the harvested and transferred LD tendon to the greater tuberosity footprint. The LD transfer technique has been modified recently to be performed arthroscopically assisted using a single open incision and in an all-arthroscopic fashion. The LD transfer is indicated in young patients with irreparable posterosuperior rotator cuff tear who have preserved shoulder height elevation; it is contraindicated in patients with superior escape, subscapularis tendon tear, and deltoid dysfunction. Mid- to long-term follow-up of patients shows that LD transfer improves pain and function in three out of four patients, and the majority can perform their activities of daily living with minimal limitation. The gain in external rotation and abduction strength is limited, and more data are needed on the long-term effect of LD transfer on long-term progression of arthritis.

TRAPEZIUS TRANSFER

The lower trapezius tendon (LTT) transfer was initially described for the paralytic shoulder and has emerged as an effective treatment for irreparable rotator cuff tear in a young patient with profound external rotation weakness. The LTT attaches to the inferomedial edge of the scapular spine and can be harvested through a transverse incision. It is important to completely detach the tendinous portion from the scapula and separate the lower and middle trapezius tendon for maximum excursion. The extension of the harvested tendon to the shoulder is accomplished by sewing an Achilles allograft to the tendon. Bassam Elhassan has popularized the application of LTT transfer for irreparable rotator cuff tear. The original series was done open through an acromial osteotomy. Although this provided great exposure and access to the entire cuff insertion, there is concern for nonunion of the osteotomy and deltoid dysfunction. Recently the LTT transfer has been modified to an arthroscopically assisted technique to facilitate the passage and fixation of the allograft in the shoulder obviating the need for acromial osteotomy. The short to midterm outcome of LTT transfer for irreparable rotator cuff tear has been promising, and most patients report an improvement in pain and external rotation. Gain in range of motion was most consistent in patients who had more than 60 degrees of forward elevation before surgery.

LATISSIMUS DORSI AND LOWER TRAPEZIUS TENDON TRANSFERS

Latissimus dorsi tendon transfer

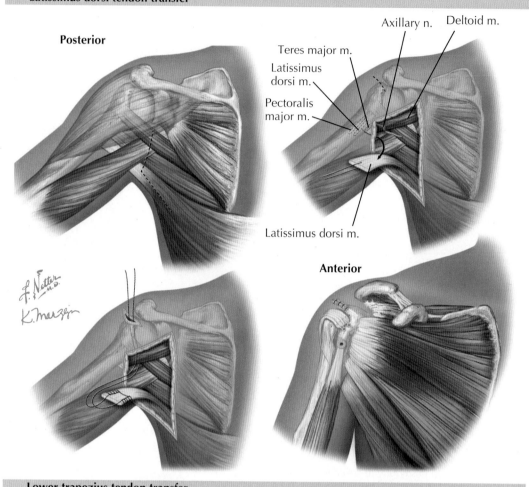

Posterior

Axillary n.   Deltoid m.
Teres major m.
Latissimus dorsi m.
Pectoralis major m.
Latissimus dorsi m.

Anterior

Lower trapezius tendon transfer

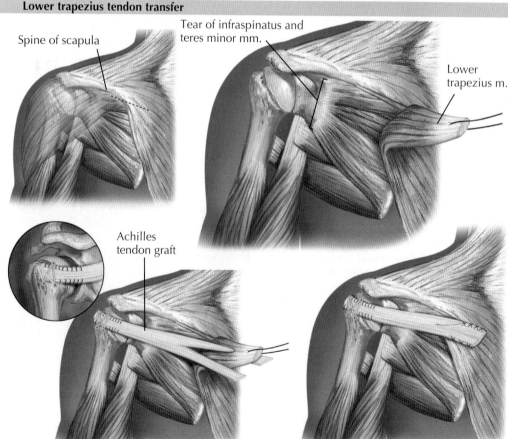

Spine of scapula

Tear of infraspinatus and teres minor mm.

Lower trapezius m.

Achilles tendon graft

Plate 1.48   Shoulder

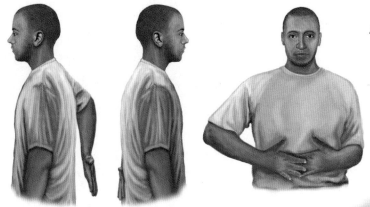

- Trapezius
- Coracoid
- Subscapularis
- Long head of biceps tendon

Coronal MRI showing the normal left subscapularis muscle belly passing under the coracoid and then attaching to the lesser tuberosity

MANAGEMENT OF SUBSCAPULARIS ROTATOR CUFF TEARS

Subscapularis tears can be isolated to the subscapularis tendon or can be associated with tears involving the superior and posterior portions of the rotator cuff. MRI can show the subscapularis muscle belly passing under the coracoid and then attaching to the lesser tuberosity. With the location of the subscapularis muscle being posterior to the chest wall, its most significant function is internal rotation, seen with the arm closest to the body. Therefore the function of the subscapularis muscle and its associated tendon is most responsible for the internal rotation function of the shoulder, particularly internal rotation strength near the center of the body. This important function specific to the subscapularis results in defining the most sensitive physical examination tests for weakness associated with this part of the rotator cuff. The other large internal rotator muscles (i.e., PM, LD, and pectoralis minor) also provide internal rotation strength to the shoulder but provide most of the strength to the shoulder when the arm is away from the body. For these reasons, the best method of testing for subscapularis function is a test of internal rotation strength close to the trunk rather than away from the body. The abdominal compression test or internal rotation lag sign are the two best methods for testing subscapularis function. Most subscapularis tendon tears will be missed on physical examination if these specific subscapularis tests are not performed. Internal rotation strength, tested in various degrees of abduction and external rotation, is not as reliable an indication of subscapularis muscle weakness because other internal rotators of the shoulder are so strong in that arm position and these tests are less specific than the belly press or internal rotation lag sign.

The abdominal compression test demonstrates the inability to internally rotate the arm with the hand against the abdomen with or without resistance to internal rotation. When performing this test, it is critical to be sure that the patient keeps the palm of the hand completely against the abdomen. Elevation of the palm off the abdomen to achieve some internal rotation of the shoulder is a sign of weakness of the subscapularis. In addition, demonstrated weakness in a true positive abdominal compression test (positive means weakness and inability to fully perform the test) must be accompanied by the examiner demonstrating the ability to passively achieve full internal rotation by the examiner passively lifting the elbow and achieving full passive internal rotation. This is necessary to rule out loss of motion secondary to shoulder stiffness, which will give a false-positive result of the abdominal compression test.

Another test for subscapularis function is the lift-off or internal rotation lag sign. This test is more difficult for many patients to do because of shoulder pain, and it requires good passive range of motion and normal elbow function. For these reasons, this test is not always performed in patients with larger rotator cuff tears. This test is more sensitive to define minor weakness of the rotator cuff associated with smaller or

Excessive passive external rotation of left side indicating detachment of the subscapularis tendon

Positive lift-off test (left shoulder) or internal rotation lag sign

Examiner able to passively internally rotate arm, demonstrating that the patient's inability to do this is a result of weakness, not loss of passive range of motion.

Abdominal compression test

Consistent with loss of subscapularis tendon attachment to the left shoulder to the lesser tuberosity. Patient unable to internally rotate the arm and place the elbow parallel to the torso.

partial tears, and in these cases most patients can perform the abdominal compression test. A positive lift-off or internal rotation lag sign is defined by the patient's inability to lift the hand off the buttock without extension of the elbow.

In addition to a loss of active internal rotation, there can be increase in passive external rotation with large or near full tears of the subscapularis tendon, because of loss of the continuity of the subscapularis muscle and tendon to the lesser tuberosity. In this case increased passive external rotation is easily seen when the patient is placed in the supine position and each shoulder is passively externally rotated and compared.

Acute traumatic full-thickness subscapularis tears are best treated by early diagnosis, which is best done by physical examination. With subscapularis tendon tears there is often damage to the long head of the biceps. This subscapularis tendon tear is associated with a dislocation in the long head of the biceps tendon from the biceps groove. Repairs can be done by either open or arthroscopic suture technique. The principles and methods of repair are the same as those described for supraspinatus and infraspinatus tears. Long head of the biceps damage or dislocation is treated by release of the long head of the biceps or tenodesis of the tendon, as described in the discussion of pathologic processes of the biceps.

Plate 1.49

Upper Limb: PART I

PECTORALIS TRANSFER AND LATISSIMUS TRANSFER

Pectoralis transfer

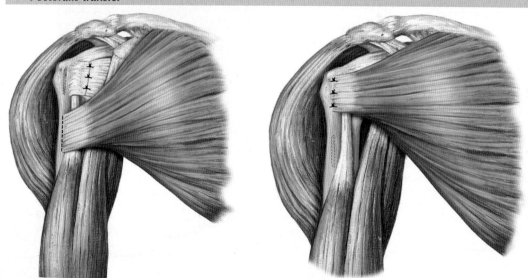

Pectoralis major transfer for irreparable subscapularis tendon tear showing transfer of both sternal and clavicular head over the lesser tuberosity

Latissimus transfer

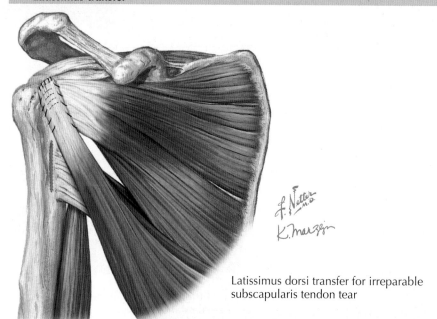

Latissimus dorsi transfer for irreparable subscapularis tendon tear

MANAGEMENT OF IRREPARABLE SUBSCAPULARIS TEARS

PECTORALIS TRANSFER

Historically, the PM transfer has been the main treatment option for irreparable subscapularis tear. Studies have shown no difference in the outcome whether the sternal or clavicular head of the PM is transferred. Also, it has been suggested in biomechanical studies that subcoracoid PM transfer underneath the conjoint tendon will better replicate the line of pull of the subscapularis and may result in better outcome. The PM transfer results in good outcome with reduced pain and increased range of motion, especially in internal rotation in the majority of patients. It has been shown that patients with massive rotator cuff tear, those with anterior humeral head subluxation, and those who had the PM transfer after shoulder replacement had less favorable outcomes.

LATISSIMUS TRANSFER

The LD transfer is an alternative to PM transfer for irreparable subscapularis tendon tear. This technique has gained more acceptance because of the similarity between the line of pull of the LD and subscapularis as both are muscles in the posterior chest wall, whereas the PM originates from the anterior chest wall. This surgery can be done open or arthroscopically assisted, and there is no clinically significant difference in the outcome of the two techniques. A recent meta-analysis showed both LD and PM can provide good pain relief, but overall LD might result in superior outcome. These results are based on small case series, and multicenter studies with mid- to long-term follow-up are necessary to learn about the outcome of this procedure.

Preoperative (**A**) and postoperative (**B**) radiographs of a patient with cuff tear arthropathy who underwent reverse total shoulder arthroplasty with a monoblock screw-on baseplate with lateralized center of rotation glenosphere and a short-stem inlay, partially coated stem.

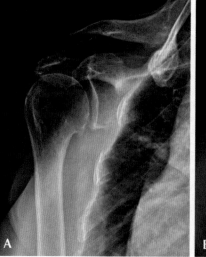

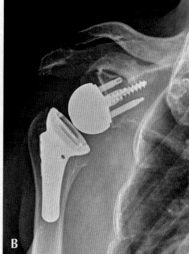

Plate 1.50

Shoulder

PALPATION ANTERIOR AND POSTERIOR JOINT LINES

Tenderness at anterior joint line

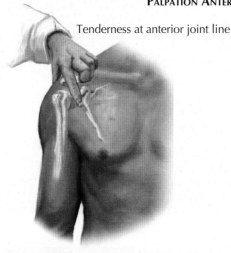

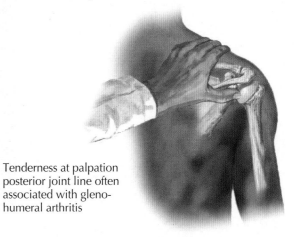

Tenderness at palpation posterior joint line often associated with glenohumeral arthritis

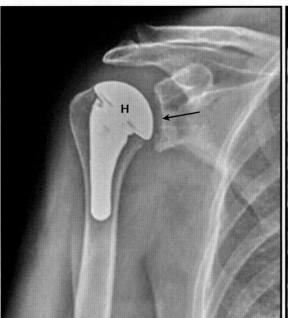

Center of glenoid

Posterior glenoid wear

Severe posterior subluxation of humeral head (more than 50% of humeral head)

Center of the humeral head

Axillary radiograph

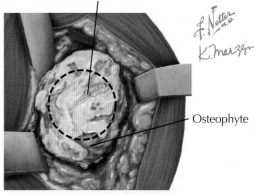

Irregular and very enlarged humeral head resulting from peripheral osteophyte, no cartilage (circled area indicates normal humeral head size)

Osteophyte

Loss of the uniformly white articular cartilage on the surface of the humeral head and proliferation of bone (osteophyte) along the periphery of the humeral head. Severe arthritic changes of the humeral head have more peripheral osteophyte formation.

OSTEOARTHRITIS OF THE GLENOHUMERAL JOINT

Osteoarthritis of the shoulder is considered a degenerative condition of the articular cartilage. It may be associated with inflammatory changes of the joint, but the damage to the cartilage is not primarily based on an inflammatory pathologic process as it is for rheumatoid arthritis (RA). The rotator cuff tendons are almost always intact in patients with osteoarthritis, and there is a proliferative osteophyte formation around the periphery of the humeral head, making it much larger than normal. The joint enlargement and flattening of the humeral head result in loss of motion. There is loss of the uniformly white articular cartilage on the surface of the humeral head, and there is proliferation of bone (osteophyte) along the periphery of the humeral head. The head becomes flattened and larger, sometimes resembling a mushroom. In most cases of osteoarthritis, the humeral head is well centered within the glenoid in AP radiographs. This is defined as the center of the humeral head being close to the midline of the center of the glenoid. Another method of assessing this alignment is a smooth and continuous scapulohumeral line at the inferior part of the humeral neck (Maloney line). This is a result of an intact rotator cuff. A continuous Maloney line is not seen when the rotator cuff is damaged, as seen on the AP radiographs in rotator cuff tear arthropathy (see Plates 1.56 and 1.57). In many patients with osteoarthritis, there is asymmetric bone loss of the posterior part of the glenoid, resulting in increased retroversion of the glenoid. The Modified Walch Classification defines the full spectrum of osteoarthritis pathology.

The clinical findings of advanced osteoarthritis are significant loss of passive (stiffness) and active

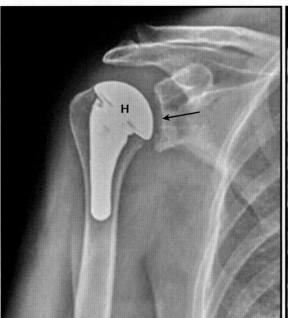

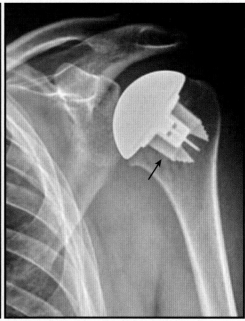

Short-stem humeral anatomic prosthetic (H). The stem is limited to the region of the humeral metaphysis and proximal junction of the metaphysis. The *arrow* demonstrates the location of the back side of the plastic glenoid component.

Stemless (canal-sparing) humeral component. The humeral stem *(arrow)* is limited to the region of the humeral metaphysis, avoiding placement of the stem into the humeral canal.

Plate 1.51

Upper Limb: PART I

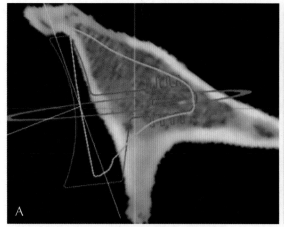

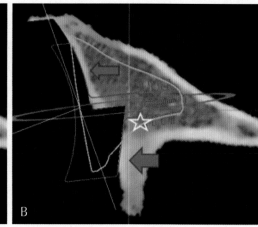

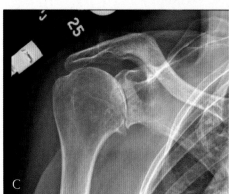

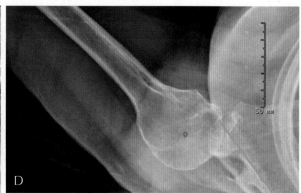

OSTEOARTHRITIS OF THE GLENOHUMERAL JOINT (Continued)

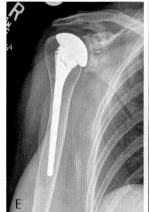

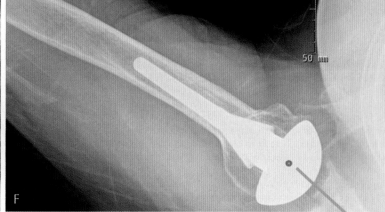

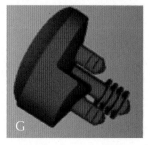

(pain-related) GH motion. Significant pain in the shoulder is typically along the anterior and posterior joint line with deep palpation. Advanced-stage osteoarthritis is often treated by total shoulder arthroplasty. Total shoulder arthroplasty involves osteotomy (removal) of the humeral head at the anatomic neck (see Plates 1.1 and 1.2) and insertion of a stem down the medullary canal to which is attached an anatomically sized and positioned prosthetic humeral head. Patients with better bone quality (most patients) and osteoarthritis can be treated with shorter stems, with some stems limited to the metaphysis. In addition, there is the preparation of the glenoid bone surface to correct pathologic version and insertion of a plastic glenoid component. After total shoulder arthroplasty with an intact rotator cuff without severe glenoid bone loss, there is restoration of the normal anatomic relationships between the humeral head center and glenoid center line on both the AP and axillary radiographs. In patients with posterior bone loss, a posterior augmented glenoid component can correct the increased posterior bone loss and recenter the humeral head.

Nonoperative treatment for early and midstage arthritis would include modification activities, oral antiinflammatory medication, and, occasionally, corticosteroid injection (see Plate 1.61). Viscosupplementation with high-molecular-weight hyaluronic acid injected into the joint over a series of one to five injections spaced 1 week apart has been used as an effective nonoperative treatment for knee and shoulder osteoarthritis.

A and B, Preoperative 3D planning: axial CT image of the glenoid demonstrating a biconcave glenoid surface with posterior glenoid bone loss described as a Walch B2 glenoid morphology. The light blue outline of the glenoid vault model demonstrating the premorbid joint line within the pathologic glenoid. The pink outline of the posterior augmented stepped glenoid component. C and E, Pre- and postoperative anterior posterior radiographs of a patient with osteoarthritis of the shoulder. D and F, Pre- and postoperative axillary radiographs of a patient with osteoarthritis and a Walch B2 glenoid showing correction of the posterior humeral head subluxation using the augmented stepped (G) glenoid component.

Plate 1.52

Shoulder

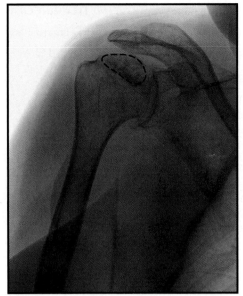

Preoperative anteroposterior radiograph. Dotted line represents area of avascular necrosis.

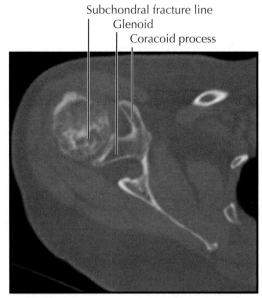

Subchondral fracture line
Glenoid
Coracoid process

CT scan

AVASCULAR NECROSIS OF THE HUMERAL HEAD

AVN of the humeral head is caused by loss of blood flow to a portion of the humeral head. This can be associated with trauma, as seen in multiple-part fracture-dislocations. AVN can also be seen in a wide variety of systemic diseases associated with sickle cell anemia, caisson disease (deep sea diver decompression sickness), mucopolysaccharidoses, or the use of systematically administered corticosteroids, particularly when used at high dosage.

Early AVN has almost no symptoms of pain, weakness, or stiffness. In most cases AVN is due to a single insult to the bone, although in some patients with systemic disease the vascular loss may result in multiple infarcts to the bone and, as such, the areas of AVN can become larger over time. In all these cases the symptoms occur secondary to humeral head deformity associated with humeral head collapse, subchondral fracture, or secondary damage to the cartilage surface due to joint incongruity. When a late pathologic process and symptoms occur, joint replacement is often needed. In many of these cases, patients are young and active, and long-term survivorship of the prosthetic components is shorter than in patients who are older and less active. For these reasons, early screening of the joints at risk is recommended in patients with known risk factors and when one joint is diagnosed with AVN. Multiple joint involvement is common in patients with systemic causes for AVN. In most cases, the weight-bearing joints will become symptomatic first, followed by the non–weight-bearing joints. A skeletal survey or a bone scan to screen for AVN in other asymptomatic joints is the most cost-effective means for detecting early AVN. MRI is the most sensitive test for AVN but may be less practical for screening owing to cost and time needed for each scan.

AVN in the humeral head is characterized by a segmental loss of blood supply and is seen on radiography and MRI as an area of sclerosis with well-demarcated margins. In more advanced stages, the humeral segment involved undergoes collapse, initially seen as a crescent sign below the subchondral surface. A crescent sign represents a sheer fracture between the subchondral bone and the avascular segment of cancellous bone below the articular surface. Later collapse of the

Supraspinatus muscle
Glenoid
Irregularity of subchondral bone plate
AVN
Fracture line
Suprascapular nerve
Suprascapular notch

humeral head will result in nonspherical head and, later, arthritic changes, which are most severe on the humeral side.

In later stages of the disease, secondary damage occurs to the glenoid surface when articulated with a deformed humeral head over a long period of time. In patients with significant articular deformity and chronic and refractory pain, joint replacement either as hemiarthroplasty or total shoulder arthroplasty is

Intact scapulo-humeral line (Maloney line) represented by a centered humeral head (HH) in the glenoid
Glenoid compound; metal wire in center of plastic compound
AC joint
Clavicle
HH
Humeral stem in medullary canal

Postoperative anteroposterior radiograph

performed. When both sides of the joint are significantly involved, total shoulder arthroplasty is preferred to treat both sides of the joint.

Some surgeons have advocated surgical decompression of the avascular segment in early stages of AVN by drilling small holes into the bone from the distal aspect of the bone proximally into the lesion. This is generally done by percutaneous methods using fluoroscopic image control.

Plate 1.53

Upper Limb: PART I

RADIOGRAPHIC PRESENTATIONS AND TREATMENT OPTIONS OF RHEUMATOID ARTHRITIS OF GLENOHUMERAL JOINT

Radiographic presentations of rheumatoid arthritis of glenohumeral joint

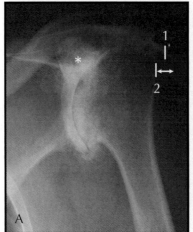
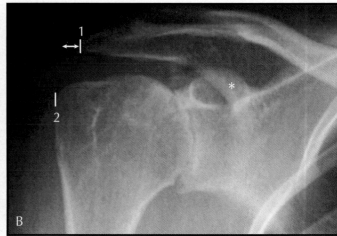

Glenoid bone loss is often centered within glenoid fossa resulting in the medial migration of the humeral head (* = coracoid). The two lines represent (**1**) lateral acromion and (**2**) lateral part of greater tuberosity. In the more normal shoulder in RA (**B**), line 2 is lateral to line 1. In the more severe RA shoulder (**A**) with medial glenoid bone loss, line 2 is medial to line 1.

RHEUMATOID ARTHRITIS OF THE GLENOHUMERAL JOINT

RA is an inflammatory disease based within the joint lining (synovium). This inflammatory disease can be very destructive to the articular cartilage and bone but also affects the surrounding soft tissues. Shoulder RA specifically can cause severe thinning and then tearing of the rotator cuff and biceps tendon as well as progressive destruction of the articular cartilage on both sides of the joint.

Unlike osteoarthritis, RA is a nonproliferative arthritic condition and there is minimal new bone formation, resulting in minimal osteophyte formation. This feature is important in distinguishing between the two most common causes of shoulder arthritis. There can be progressive bone loss with osteopenia and demineralization of the humeral head. This is similar to patients with rotator cuff arthritis. Patients with osteoarthritis have hard bone that becomes whiter on radiography related to new bone formation. Glenoid bone loss is often centered within the glenoid fossa in RA, resulting in medial migration of the humeral head. Osteoarthritis shows more eccentric glenoid wear primarily on the posterior glenoid. In many cases of RA, there is superior migration of the humeral head seen on radiographic views that is associated with destructive changes of the rotator cuff. In these cases, glenoid bone loss can occur in the superior part of the glenoid fossa. RA, rotator cuff tear arthritis, and crystal-induced arthritis (hydroxyapatite deposition disease, "Milwaukee shoulder") produce large rotator cuff tears and superior migration of the humeral head, which, in turn, can result in asymmetric superior glenoid bone loss. All these findings are best seen on routine radiographs. CT is also helpful in demonstrating these bone changes. The synovitis and joint effusion and the rotator cuff damage are best seen with MRI.

The humeral head can show lack of proliferative osteophyte formation but severe erosive changes of the articular surface. A treatment option for younger patients is a conservative humeral replacement maintaining most of the humeral bone stock using a

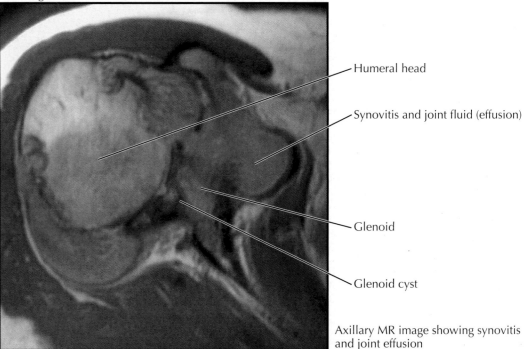

- Humeral head
- Synovitis and joint fluid (effusion)
- Glenoid
- Glenoid cyst

Axillary MR image showing synovitis and joint effusion

Treatment option: anatomic total shoulder arthroplasty

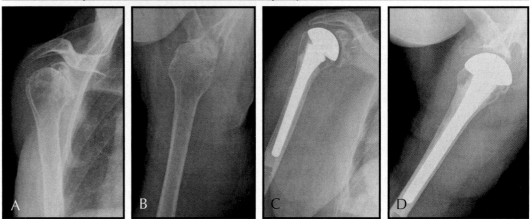

When the rotator is intact, a more traditional treatment is an anatomic total shoulder arthroplasty. A cemented stemmed total shoulder arthroplasty is shown in AP (**C**) and axillary (**D**) views.

Plate 1.54

Shoulder

CONSERVATIVE HUMERAL HEAD SURFACE REPLACEMENT

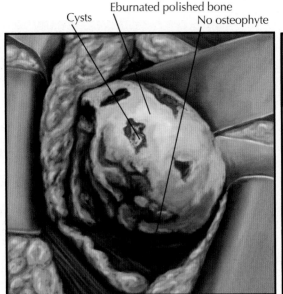

Cysts
Eburnated polished bone
No osteophyte

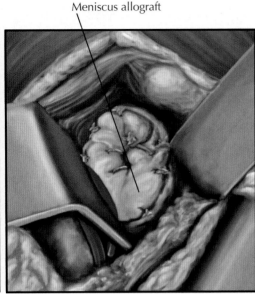

Meniscus allograft

Humeral head shows lack of proliferative osteophyte formation but severe erosive changes of the articular surface.

Avoidance of a glenoid prosthetic plastic component was achieved by use of meniscal allograft sutured to the cartilage-deficient glenoid surface.

RHEUMATOID ARTHRITIS OF THE GLENOHUMERAL JOINT (Continued)

surface-only arthroplasty (no stem). Avoidance of a glenoid prosthetic plastic component is preferred in these patients. This remains a controversial method of treatment because the results are not as consistent or predictable as those for traditional complete prosthetic joint replacement (total shoulder arthroplasty). Traditional complete joint replacement can have its own difficulties with long-term survivorship, and for very young patients, a more conservative joint replacement avoiding the humeral stem and plastic glenoid prosthetic component can result in good clinical outcome and therefore remains a surgical treatment option for the young active patient. This is indicated primarily when the rotator cuff is intact and well functioning, and a centered humeral head is seen on the preoperative AP radiographs.

More traditional treatment of RA when the rotator cuff is intact is anatomic total shoulder arthroplasty. If the rotator cuff is intact, the patient may be treated with an uncemented or cemented stemmed total shoulder arthroplasty depending on bone quality. When the rotator cuff is damaged and there is associated superior migration of the humeral head, hemiarthroplasty is preferred over total shoulder replacement. Most patients with severe RA needing shoulder replacement are best treated with a reverse total shoulder arthroplasty because the rotator cuff is deficient or not functional. Reverse shoulder arthroplasty avoids the superior migration of the humeral head associated with anatomic total shoulder replacement. This results in contact with only the superior part of the glenoid component and thus a continuous eccentric loading of the glenoid component and associated early loosening of the glenoid component. Many of the newer disease-modifying biologic drugs block the factors that result in the inflammatory mechanism that lead to severe joint destruction. For this reason the need for shoulder replacement in patients with RA has markedly decreased in the past 10 to 15 years.

A conservative humeral surface replacement without a humeral stem in the shape of the humerus maintains most of the humeral bone stock using only a surface replacement.

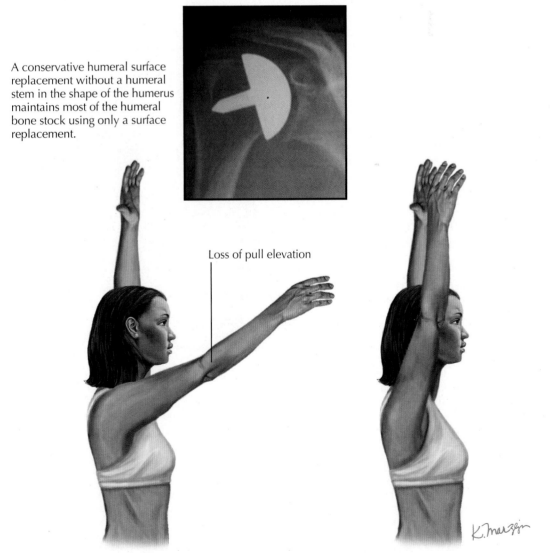

Loss of pull elevation

Conservative humeral surface replacement can result in good clinical outcome as seen on the preoperative versus 1-year postoperative examination.

Plate 1.55

Upper Limb: PART I

PHYSICAL FINDINGS AND APPEARANCE

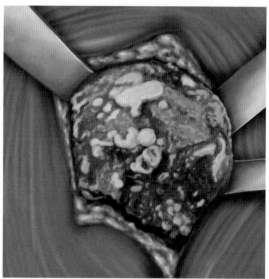

Rotator cuff tear arthropathy. Severe erosive arthritis, little or no rotator cuff tissue surrounding the humeral head.

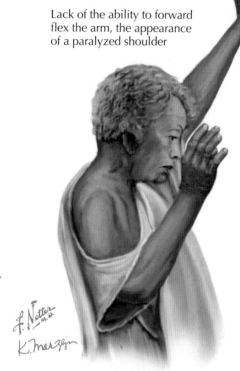

Lack of the ability to forward flex the arm, the appearance of a paralyzed shoulder

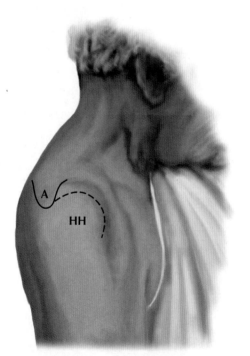

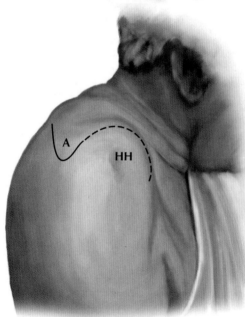

ROTATOR CUFF–DEFICIENT ARTHRITIS (ROTATOR CUFF TEAR ARTHROPATHY)

CUFF TEAR ARTHROPATHY WITH A CONTAINED AND STABLE HUMERAL HEAD

In some cases of arthritis there is severe damage to the rotator cuff along with arthritic changes of the articular surfaces of the joint. This can occur in severe cases of RA, in cases of crystalline arthropathy, or in patients with large chronic rotator cuff tears. These diseases result in severe erosive arthritis and superior migration of the humeral head. This often is associated with erosion and bone loss along the superior portion of the glenoid (see Plate 1.57). When these patients come to surgery, there is often little or no rotator cuff tissue surrounding the humeral head.

Patients with less severe rotator cuff–deficient arthritis have superior migration of the humeral head, yet the humeral head is still stable and contained within an intact CA arch. When the humeral head is contained within the CA arch and glenoid surface, along with sufficient remaining rotator cuff tissue to maintain a stable fulcrum for rotation of the humeral head within the intact CA arch, a humeral head hemiarthroplasty can be performed with a satisfactory clinical result. In

Physical findings consistent with superior escape of the humeral head and pseudoparalytic shoulder. With the arm in the resting position, there is relatively normal contour to the anterior aspect of the shoulder with the humeral head (HH) below the acromion (A). With attempted active elevation of the shoulder, there is a superior shift of the humeral head and a prominence of the humeral head anteriorly above the acromion (A).

patients with a contained and stable humeral head, the physical examination will generally demonstrate the ability to elevate the arm to at least 90 degrees, and the humeral head remains contained under the CA arch. The clinical findings of superior escape and pseudoparalysis of the shoulder are not found in these patients. The shoulder examination is more consistent with the

middle image on Plate 1.43 than the upper image on Plate 1.43 or the examination seen on Plate 1.55.

Although hemiarthroplasty can be performed in this subset of patients with rotator cuff–deficient arthritis, the results can be variable. In most cases, reverse total shoulder arthroplasty is the preferred treatment in the older and less active patient.

Plate 1.56   Shoulder

ROTATOR CUFF–DEFICIENT ARTHRITIS (ROTATOR CUFF TEAR ARTHROPATHY): RADIOGRAPHIC FINDINGS

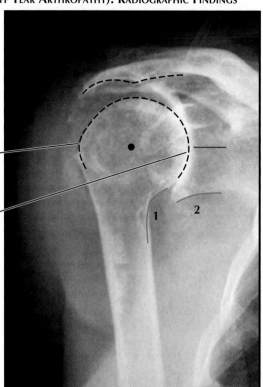

Rounding off of the humeral head, and loss of rotator cuff

The humeral head is contained within the coracoacromial arch and the glenoid surface. Humeral hemiarthroplasty can be performed with a satisfactory clinical result.

- - - = erosion of undersurface of acromion

• = center of rotation of humeral head

ROTATOR CUFF–DEFICIENT ARTHRITIS (ROTATOR CUFF TEAR ARTHROPATHY) (Continued)

SEVERE ROTATOR CUFF–DEFICIENT ARTHRITIS NEEDING REVERSE TOTAL SHOULDER REPLACEMENT

When rotator cuff–deficient arthritis is associated with loss of the containment mechanism of the humeral head within the CA arch, the patient does not have a fulcrum to rotate the humeral head; this result is termed *pseudoparalysis of the shoulder*. When these conditions occur in the older and less active patient, the best treatment is reverse shoulder arthroplasty. Physical findings, consistent with superior escape of the humeral head and pseudoparalytic shoulder, include a relatively normal contour to the anterior aspect of the shoulder with the arm in the resting position. With attempted active elevation of the shoulder, there is a superior shift of the humeral head and a prominence of the humeral head anteriorly. In the most severe cases the superior migration of the humeral head outside of the CA arch is seen at rest with the arm by the side of the body. Pseudoparalysis is associated with lack of the ability to forward flex the arm as well as weakness of active external rotation (loss of the superior and posterior parts of

Loss of joint space and subacromial space

Humeral head prosthesis, without glenoid component hemiarthroplasty

Colinear intact Maloney line and the center of rotation of the humeral head are now aligned with center line of glenoid (red line).

1 = humeral neck
2 = glenoid neck
———— = center line of glenoid
• = center of rotation of humeral head

the rotator cuff) and/or loss of active internal rotation. Classic radiographic findings of rotator cuff tear arthropathy are marked degenerative changes and collapse of the humeral head, superior migration of the humeral head, and associated severe rotator cuff deficiency and subchondral cyst formation in the humeral head.

Reverse total shoulder arthroplasty means that the components are designed to be opposite to the normal

anatomy. The convex surface is on the glenoid side, and the concave surface is on the humeral side. This causes a semiconstrained joint, resulting in a fixed center of rotation, thereby substituting for the function of the rotator cuff. When there is loss of function of the CA arch to contain the superiorly migrated humeral head and there is superior escape of the humeral head and resultant pseudoparalysis of the shoulder, a hemiarthroplasty will not provide any improvement of

Plate 1.57

Upper Limb: PART I

ROTATOR CUFF–DEFICIENT ARTHRITIS (ROTATOR CUFF TEAR ARTHROPATHY): RADIOGRAPHIC FINDINGS (CONTINUED)

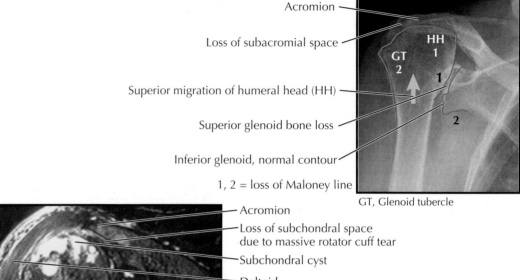

Acromion

Loss of subacromial space

Superior migration of humeral head (HH)

Superior glenoid bone loss

Inferior glenoid, normal contour

1, 2 = loss of Maloney line

GT, Glenoid tubercle

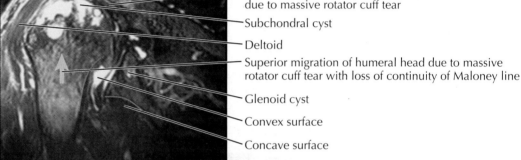

Acromion

Loss of subchondral space due to massive rotator cuff tear

Subchondral cyst

Deltoid

Superior migration of humeral head due to massive rotator cuff tear with loss of continuity of Maloney line

Glenoid cyst

Convex surface

Concave surface

ROTATOR CUFF–DEFICIENT ARTHRITIS (ROTATOR CUFF TEAR ARTHROPATHY) (Continued)

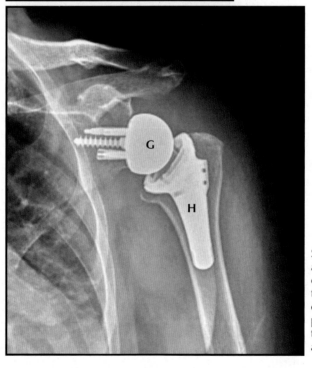

Short-stem reverse total shoulder arthroplasty. The humeral component (H) contains the concave plastic surface, and the glenoid component (G) contains the convex metal surface. This reverse prosthetic articulation is typically used to treat patients with rotator cuff tear arthropathy.

function. The reverse arthroplasty enforces a fixed fulcrum for rotation of the humeral component around the glenoid component and therefore partially substitutes for the containment function of the rotator cuff with the center of the humeral head within the glenoid. With a reverse total shoulder replacement the center of rotation is shifted from the center of the humeral head in the normal shoulder anatomy toward the center of the spherical glenoid component. This results in a medial shift in the center of rotation. A medial shift in the center of rotation results in an increase in the moment arm of the deltoid, thereby improving its mechanical advantage and ability to elevate the arm. In addition, medialization of the center of rotation of the glenoid bone and its surface contact with the glenoid component minimizes the moment arm for the forces around the glenoid component that would occur if the center of rotation was at the location of the normal shoulder. The amount of medial shift of the center of rotation varies greatly between types of reverse arthroplasty. The reverse total shoulder replacement does dramatically improve the patient's ability to elevate the arm as a result of these mechanical features. The best outcomes of the reverse total shoulder occur in patients with some posterior rotator cuff function before surgery (e.g., an intact teres minor tendon). Patients with some external rotation function will often achieve near full elevation of the shoulder after reverse total shoulder replacement. Those patients without any external rotation function before surgery will generally get less improvement with reverse replacement but generally will get shoulder-level elevation. Some patients without any external rotation function may benefit from a muscle (lower trapezius) transfer. This muscle transfer can be done at the time of the replacement surgery or after the surgery. LD transfer is best performed at the time of joint replacement.

Plate 1.58

Shoulder

SUPRASCAPULAR NERVE

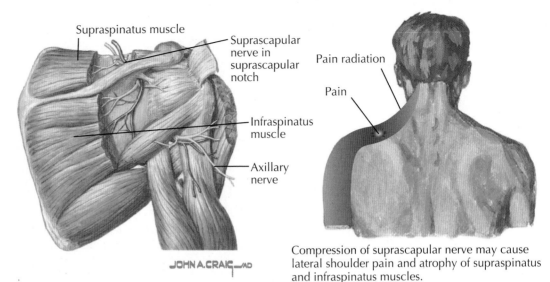

Supraspinatus muscle

Suprascapular nerve in suprascapular notch

Infraspinatus muscle

Axillary nerve

JOHN A.CRAIG—AD

Pain radiation

Pain

Compression of suprascapular nerve may cause lateral shoulder pain and atrophy of supraspinatus and infraspinatus muscles.

NEUROLOGIC CONDITIONS OF THE SHOULDER

The long thoracic nerve innervates the serratus anterior muscle. The serratus anterior muscle has its origin in the anterior chest wall and then inserts along the medial border of the scapula with most of its fibers attaching to the distal third of the scapular body (see Plate 1.13).

When there is a lesion of the long thoracic nerve and weakness of the serratus anterior muscle, there is winging of the scapula. When severe, there is limitation of active elevation of the shoulder because of an unstable scapula that is not able to appropriately rotate laterally and maintain its position along the chest wall. In this case, by using overactive rhomboid function and trapezius function the patient is trying to compensate for loss of the function of the serratus anterior muscle. When this lesion occurs as a result of a viral insult or closed trauma, then spontaneous recovery often occurs over a period of several months to a year. When recovery is either incomplete or results in significant long-term disability, PM muscle transfer to the tip of the scapula is a well-defined and effective treatment.

Charcot arthropathy of the shoulder can be associated with severe destructive lesions of both the humeral head and glenoid and is often evident on radiographs as multiple-joint bony debris. In some cases this is associated with a cervical syrinx, resulting in loss of proprioception and proprioceptive fibers to the shoulder girdle. When there is loss of sense of joint position, normal activities and pain associated with injury are not perceived by the patient, resulting in severe destructive damage to the joint. Often patients have much less pain and better function than what would be expected by the severity of the joint damage. Because of the underlying cause of the shoulder damage, joint replacement or any type of surgical reconstruction has a high rate of complications, including prosthetic dislocation, periprosthetic fractures, and loosening of the prosthetic components.

SSN lesions can be associated with entrapment of the suprascapular notch or spinal glenoid notch. They can also be associated with ganglion cyst formation that can

Ganglion cyst

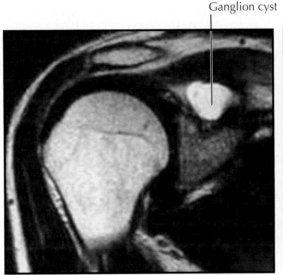

MR image showing ganglion cyst causing compressive neuropathy of suprascapular nerve

Humeral head   Ganglion cyst

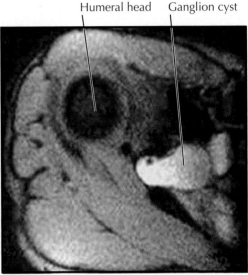

MR image of suprascapular nerve compression by a large ganglion cyst

Arthroscopic view of an intact ganglion cyst

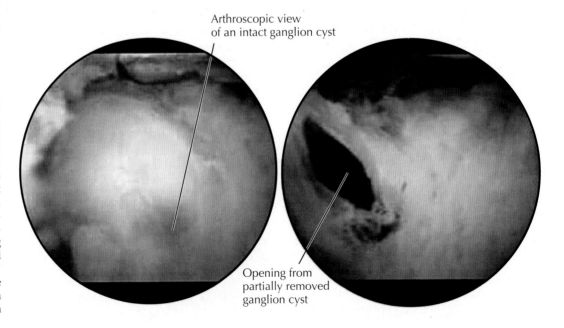

Opening from partially removed ganglion cyst

Plate 1.59

Upper Limb: PART I

Long thoracic nerve

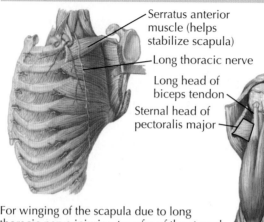

Serratus anterior muscle (helps stabilize scapula)

Long thoracic nerve

Long head of biceps tendon

Sternal head of pectoralis major

Winging of scapula

Normal

Path of tendon transfer

For winging of the scapula due to long thoracic nerve injuries, transfer of the sternal head of the pectoralis major tendon to the inferomedial border of the scapula is a common surgical treatment. The transferred tendon replaces the function of the dysfunctional serratus muscles in retracting the scapula as the arm elevates to avoid winging of the scapula. The sternal head is removed from its insertion on the humerus just lateral to the long head of the biceps tendon. The clavicular head is left intact or released and repaired. The released sternal head is then passed along the chest wall and fixed to the inferior medial border of the scapula with heavy sutures.

NEUROLOGIC CONDITIONS OF THE SHOULDER (Continued)

cause compression of the nerve. SSN compression will result in weakness of external rotation and an external rotation lag sign (see Plate 1.43). Atrophy of the musculature of the supraspinous fossa and infraspinous fossa should be evaluated. Ganglion cyst formation can be associated with a superior labral tear (Plate 1.58). The ganglion cyst forms as a synovial fluid-filled sac. When this ganglion encroaches on the suprascapular notch or spinoglenoid notch, there is an SSN compressive neuropathy.

These lesions can be treated by aspiration under image guidance. When treated by needle aspiration the ganglion can recur because the SLAP lesion is not repaired. Arthroscopic repair of the SLAP lesion can result in spontaneous resolution of the ganglion cyst. Alternatively, the SLAP lesion can be repaired arthroscopically with excision of the ganglion cyst. The clinical appearance for suprascapular neuropathy is severe atrophy of the supraspinatus or infraspinatus musculature. Isolated atrophy of the infraspinatus muscle is associated with entrapment of the infraspinatus branch of the SSN at the spinoglenoid notch.

Lesions of the spinal accessory nerve involve weakness or paralysis isolated to the trapezius muscle. Spinal accessory nerve lesions can also be associated with viral syndromes. They can also be seen as an iatrogenic lesion associated with cervical node biopsy. The shoulder demonstrates drooping of the scapula, noted when one shoulder is not level to the other, the neck contour is distorted, and the rhomboid muscles are prominently seen because the middle trapezius is atrophied. This lesion also causes winging of the scapula with predominant involvement of the upper half of the scapula. It can be distinguished from the long thoracic nerve palsy with serratus anterior muscle weakness that affects predominately the lower pole of the scapula. Chronic lesions that are associated with incomplete or lack of recovery can be treated with transfer of the levator scapulae and rhomboid musculature (Eden-Lange procedure). This is an effective muscle transfer as a salvage procedure for this nerve and muscle lesion.

Spinal accessory nerve

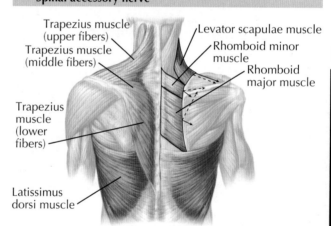

Trapezius muscle (upper fibers)

Trapezius muscle (middle fibers)

Trapezius muscle (lower fibers)

Latissimus dorsi muscle

Levator scapulae muscle

Rhomboid minor muscle

Rhomboid major muscle

Winging of the scapula due to spinal accessory nerve injuries or trapezial dysfunction can be surgically treated with the Eden-Lange (solid arrows) or triple transfer (dotted arrows) when nonoperative management has failed. Both transfers involve transferring the levator scapulae, rhomboid minor, and rhomboid major from their medial scapular insertions to more lateral scapular insertions to replace the dysfunctional trapezius muscle. The triple transfer inserts the tendons on the scapular spine to re-create the trapezial insertions rather than the scapular body as described with the Eden-Lange transfer.

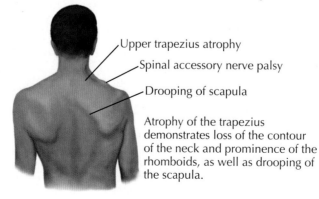

Upper trapezius atrophy

Spinal accessory nerve palsy

Drooping of scapula

Atrophy of the trapezius demonstrates loss of the contour of the neck and prominence of the rhomboids, as well as drooping of the scapula.

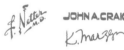

Charcot arthropathy

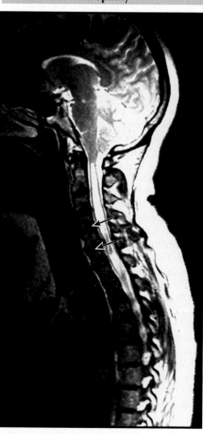

MR image showing cervical syrinx (arrows) resulting in loss of proprioception and proprioceptive fibers to the shoulder girdle, which can cause a Charcot arthropathy of the shoulder

Plate 1.60

Shoulder

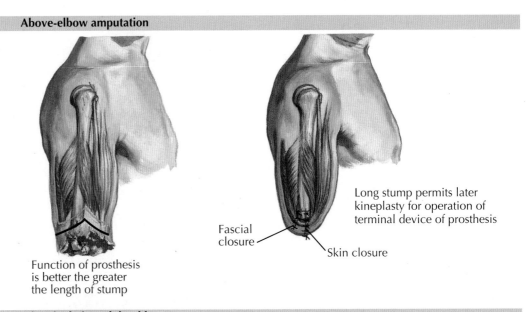

Above-elbow amputation

Long stump permits later kineplasty for operation of terminal device of prosthesis

Fascial closure

Skin closure

Function of prosthesis is better the greater the length of stump

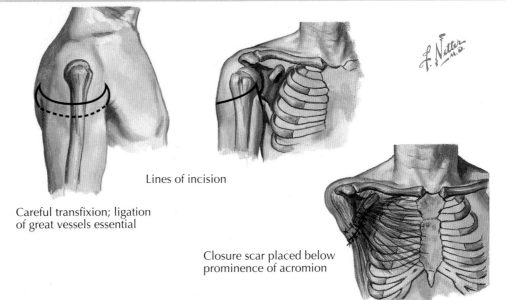

Disarticulation of shoulder

Lines of incision

Careful transfixion; ligation of great vessels essential

Closure scar placed below prominence of acromion

AMPUTATION OF UPPER ARM AND SHOULDER

ABOVE-ELBOW AMPUTATION

An amputation above the elbow should be designed to preserve as much length of the residual limb as possible. To function successfully, an artificial upper limb must have a long lever arm, and as much of the humerus as possible should be saved to provide this lever (Plate 1.60, *top*). Even a very short humerus stump should be retained, if possible, because disarticulation of the shoulder greatly diminishes the powering of the artificial limb.

Occasionally, a kineplasty technique is used to enable the patient to operate the terminal device of an upper limb prosthesis. In this procedure, a tunnel is made beneath the biceps brachii muscle and the entire tunnel is covered with skin, creating a loop of muscle. The cables for the operation of a terminal device of an upper limb prosthesis are attached to this muscle loop.

FOREQUARTER AMPUTATION

This radical procedure is usually reserved for the treatment of aggressive, malignant tumors. In contrast to the disarticulation of the shoulder joint, a forequarter amputation removes all the bone architecture and muscles of the upper limb (Plate 1.60, *bottom*). It is a devastating amputation that provides no residual base to support an artificial limb. Consequently, it is usually very difficult to obtain a satisfactory fit of the prosthesis.

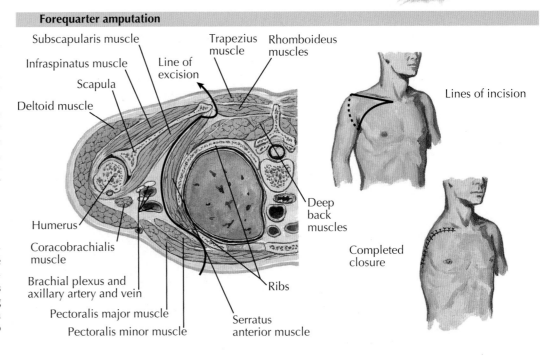

Forequarter amputation

Subscapularis muscle

Infraspinatus muscle

Scapula

Deltoid muscle

Trapezius muscle

Rhomboideus muscles

Line of excision

Humerus

Coracobrachialis muscle

Brachial plexus and axillary artery and vein

Pectoralis major muscle

Pectoralis minor muscle

Deep back muscles

Ribs

Serratus anterior muscle

Lines of incision

Completed closure

Plate 1.61

Upper Limb: PART I

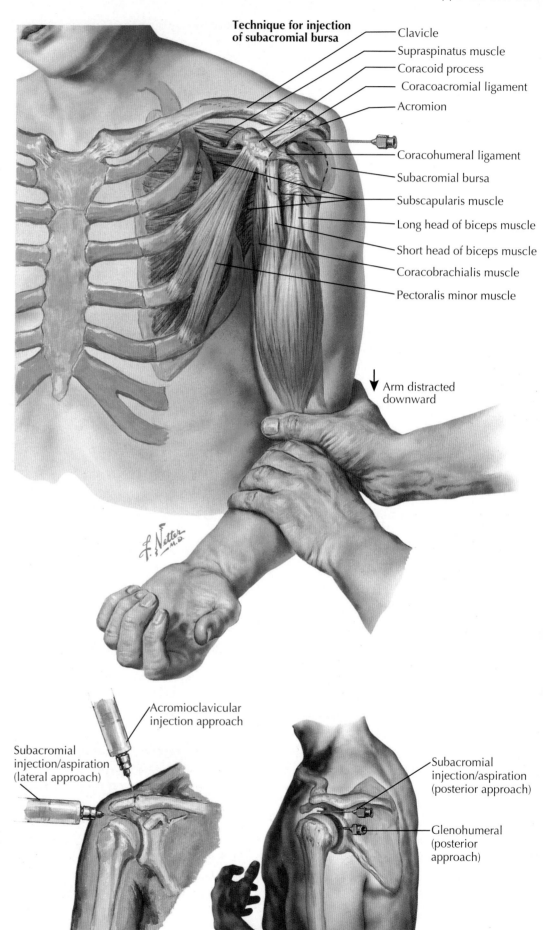

Technique for injection of subacromial bursa

Clavicle
Supraspinatus muscle
Coracoid process
Coracoacromial ligament
Acromion
Coracohumeral ligament
Subacromial bursa
Subscapularis muscle
Long head of biceps muscle
Short head of biceps muscle
Coracobrachialis muscle
Pectoralis minor muscle

Arm distracted downward

Acromioclavicular injection approach

Subacromial injection/aspiration (lateral approach)

Subacromial injection/aspiration (posterior approach)

Glenohumeral (posterior approach)

SHOULDER INJECTIONS

Injections to the shoulder can be performed either for diagnostic purposes or for aspiration of joint fluid. This can be done for evaluation of possible infection or crystalline arthritis.

Injections for therapeutic reasons are often used to place a corticosteroid into the joints or subacromial space. Knowing the basic anatomy and surface landmarks of the shoulder for the subacromial space, GH joint, and AC joint is critically important for safe and effective joint aspiration or injection. Injections should be performed under aseptic conditions with thorough preparation of the skin and using sterile technique. Local anesthetic can be given at the time of injection and is often helpful in localizing the shoulder pain, particularly if the injection is precisely given into a specific compartment and followed by reexamination of the shoulder soon after the injection. In most cases, these injections are given in the office setting using ultrasound guidance.

Plate 1.62

Shoulder

BASIC, PASSIVE, AND ACTIVE-ASSISTED RANGE-OF-MOTION EXERCISES

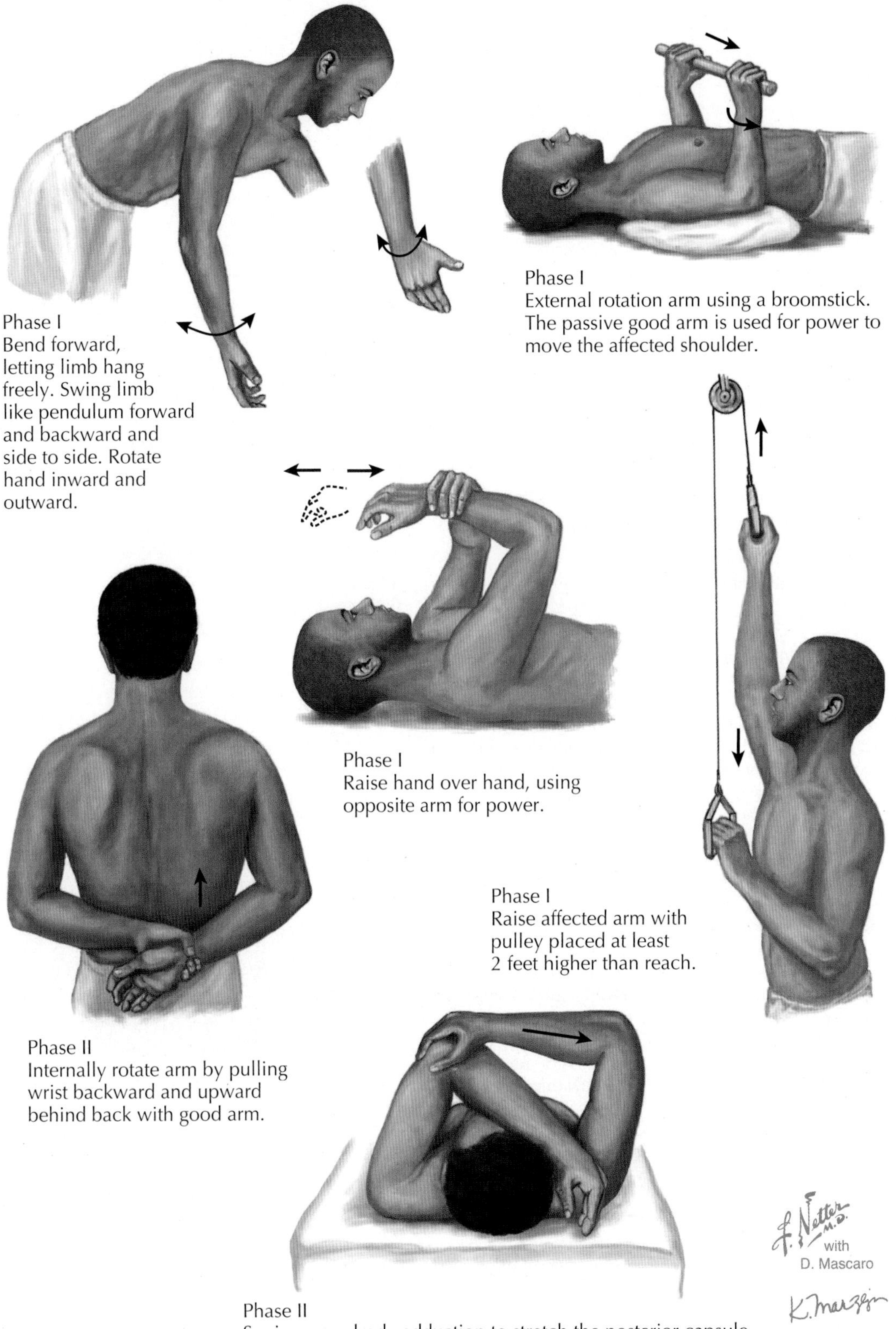

Phase I
Bend forward, letting limb hang freely. Swing limb like pendulum forward and backward and side to side. Rotate hand inward and outward.

Phase I
External rotation arm using a broomstick. The passive good arm is used for power to move the affected shoulder.

Phase I
Raise hand over hand, using opposite arm for power.

Phase I
Raise affected arm with pulley placed at least 2 feet higher than reach.

Phase II
Internally rotate arm by pulling wrist backward and upward behind back with good arm.

with
D. Mascaro

Phase II
Supine cross-body adduction to stretch the posterior capsule

EXERCISES FOR RANGE OF MOTION AND STRENGTHENING OF SHOULDER

BASIC, PASSIVE, AND ACTIVE-ASSISTED RANGE-OF-MOTION EXERCISES

The rehabilitation exercises shown in this section are applicable to both nonoperative and postoperative treatment for all the shoulder conditions discussed in this book. The specific exercises used, their progression, and their coordination with other treatment modalities are specific to the diagnosis, the severity of the pathologic process, and many other patient and surgical factors. A detailed discussion for each of these conditions is beyond the scope of this book.

In general principles, the exercise program should start with the easiest exercises to perform and can be progressed when the early-phase exercises can be done easily and with comfort. The keys in rehabilitation of the shoulder are pain management and avoiding injury during the exercises. Pain management may include one or more of the following: application of ice or heat; use of nonsteroidal antiinflammatory agents, nonnarcotic medication, corticosteroid injections, or bracing; nerve blocks; or surgery. The first priority is to regain most of the passive range of motion before concentrating on strengthening. Strengthening should include both the shoulder and scapula as well as the trunk musculature. Strengthening of the scapula should begin when phase I strengthening of the GH musculature starts. Scapula-strengthening exercises include shoulder shrugs and rowing-type exercises (shoulder protraction and retraction). Coordination of scapula strengthening with GH strengthening is necessary for successful progression to the overhead exercises of phase II. In general, the progression of strengthening of the GH muscles should be first strengthening the rotator cuff in nonimpingement arcs of motion (phase I) to obtain good strength in rotation by the side as well as good scapula strength before beginning active elevation strengthening. Before starting resisted elevation with weights, the patient should have full active elevation without a weight. If this is not achieved, continue phase I strengthening and perform scapula strengthening. Use of gatching and closed-chain active elevation strengthening can be an intermediate step to gaining strength and coordinated muscle function before active strengthening in a seated or standing position. When performing gatching or closed-chain supine elevation, it is important to achieve full active elevation without resistance before starting phase II strengthening.

Most effective rehabilitation programs require daily home-based effort by the patient. In most circumstances the exercises should be spread out over the day and not be concentrated into an intense once-a-day regimen. This basic principle of early shoulder rehabilitation is particularly important in the early or acute stages of rehabilitation when the shoulder is at its worst with respect to pain, motion, or strength. The worse the problems, the more frequent and gentle the exercises should be performed, but with short periods of exercise to avoid overuse and time to recover before the next interval of exercise.

Plate 1.63

Upper Limb: PART I

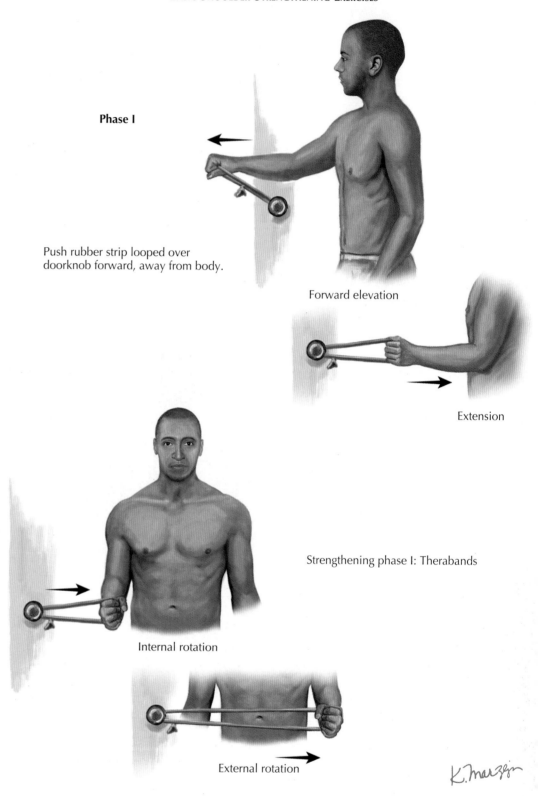

BASIC SHOULDER-STRENGTHENING EXERCISES

Phase I

Push rubber strip looped over doorknob forward, away from body.

Forward elevation

Extension

Strengthening phase I: Therabands

Internal rotation

External rotation

K. marzen

EXERCISES FOR RANGE OF MOTION AND STRENGTHENING OF SHOULDER (Continued)

The initial program should focus on the most key and deficient problems for that diagnosis. For example, the primary problem with early severe frozen shoulder is pain and loss of passive range of motion. This should result in the need to achieve effective pharmacologic pain management and to focus on passive range-of-motion exercises to achieve improvements in passive range of motion and improvement in pain before considering adding strengthening exercises to the program. The more painful the shoulder, the gentler the exercises, which are done for a shorter duration but frequently during the day. As the shoulder improves, the exercise periods can be more consolidated for longer duration and then progressed with respect to intensity.

Patient education and participation are critical to success for either nonoperative rehabilitation or postoperative rehabilitation. Clear and precise communication among the physician, patient, and therapist is as important to a successful outcome as is the precision and expertise by which all the other treatment is performed, including surgery.

Pendulum exercises are performed with the patient leaning forward with the opposite arm supported on a stable structure such as a table and the waist bent at approximately 90 degrees. The affected extremity is allowed to dangle in front of the patient's body, and small circular motions are made either clockwise or counterclockwise, allowing for general passive range of motion of the GH joint.

Supine passive forward elevation is done in the supine position using the unaffected extremity to move the affected arm passively or with active-assisted elevation (some muscle activity of the affected shoulder). This is generally done in the plane of the scapula. The plane of the scapula is midway between the true coronal plane (parallel to the plane of the body [pure abduction] and the sagittal plane, which is perpendicular to the plane of the body [pure forward flexion]). The plane of the scapula lies 30 to 40 degrees anterior to the coronal plane. The plane of the scapula for motion exercises places the rotator cuff and other muscles of the shoulder in the most physiologic and natural position with

respect to the scapula body. For all passive exercises, when the arm reaches its maximum level of gentle passive arc, there is a gentle stretch given to increase the arc of motion. Repetitive movements are done during one session a few times each day.

Active-assisted forward flexion can also be done using an assistive device such as an exercise wand in the standing position. Passive external rotation is done using a device such as a cane or exercise wand. Cross-body

adduction stretches the posterior capsule, and normal posterior capsule length is important to achieve full forward elevation or full internal rotation.

BASIC SHOULDER-STRENGTHENING EXERCISES

Progressive resistant strengthening exercises can be performed in phases. Phase I involves the use of an

Plate 1.64

Shoulder

BASIC SHOULDER-STRENGTHENING EXERCISES (CONTINUED)

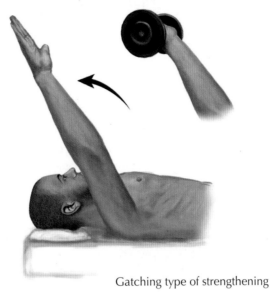

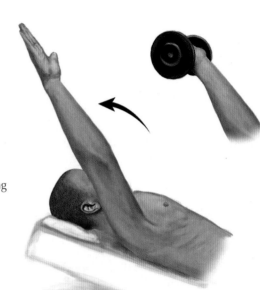

Gatching type of strengthening

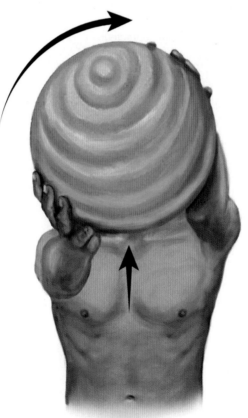

Closed-chain active-assisted
strengthening in forward elevation

EXERCISES FOR RANGE OF MOTION AND STRENGTHENING OF SHOULDER (Continued)

elastic band for external rotation with the arm by its side to avoid impingement or overstressing of the rotator cuff tendons. The concept of progression of strengthening from phase I to phase II is to first strengthen the rotator cuff by doing rotational exercises in the least difficult or pain-provocative arm and body position. After achievement of better rotator cuff strength and shoulder function with the phase I exercises performed with the arm by the side, then the shoulder should be better able to tolerate the more difficult exercises for phase II strengthening.

Phase I strengthening can be done either using both hands with an elastic band or with the elastic band to a stationary object, such as a doorknob, with a pillow under the arm to provide slight abduction and then external rotation away from the body. It is best to use a stationary object so that the better or stronger shoulder does not overpower the weaker shoulder. Internal rotation can likewise be performed with the arm in slight abduction and internal rotation toward the abdomen. Extension is performed in a similar matter with the elbow by the side pulling the band. Forward flexion is shown with the elastic band with the arm moving in the forward position generally below shoulder level. Many of these same exercises can be performed with alternative techniques using handheld 1- to 5-lb weights.

For patients with severe weakness of forward elevation, graduated exercises are performed starting initially in the supine position without a weighted extremity. This is called the gatching technique. The arm is actively elevated with the patient in the supine position.

When this can be easily achieved with multiple repetitions, a small 1- to 2-lb handheld weight is used again until this can be done easily and repetitively. When this is accomplished, the patient is then elevated with the torso at 30 to 40 degrees without a weighted extremity. This is again tested repetitively until this can be done with ease, after which a small 1- to 2-lb handheld weight is added. This is repetitively accomplished until the patient can gradually bring the arm up actively in a seated position.

An alternative way to graduate to the full active elevation without assistance is the use of closed-chain active-assistance strengthening in forward flexion. This can be done with an exercise wand or preferably with a lightweight exercise ball. The patient places both arms on the ball and with assistance squeezes the ball and raises the arm above the head. The weak side is on the upper portion of the ball and is assisted by the strong arm, which is on the lower part of the ball. As the weak shoulder becomes stronger, the patient moves his or her hands to an equal and opposite side of the ball and when very strong can use the affected arm on the underside of the ball as an assistant to the normal side. These exercises are useful as an intermediate step to achieve full active elevation and progressive resistive exercises and forward flexion above shoulder level.

Plate 1.65

Upper Limb: PART I

COMMON SURGICAL APPROACHES TO THE SHOULDER

The deltopectoral approach is most commonly used for major reconstruction of the shoulder for treatment of complex fractures of the proximal humerus or glenoid. It is the most common approach for joint replacement for all indications. The incision is generally 10 to 15 cm in length and is located over the anterior aspect of the shoulder and is centered over the tip of the coracoid. For major reconstructive procedures, the incision is angled from the lateral third of the clavicle toward the insertion site of the deltoid muscle and follows the cephalic vein. The deep part of the approach separates the natural plane between the deltoid and PM muscles, usually bringing the cephalic vein with the deltoid muscle as it is retracted laterally. Entry into the GH joint is through the subscapularis tendon. This can be done by splitting the tendon and muscle fibers from lateral to medial without detachments of the insertion site. This provides exposure of limited procedures. Most of the indications for this approach have been replaced by arthroscopic procedures. Larger reconstructive procedures such as a joint replacement are generally performed by midtendon incision, as shown on Plate 1.65, with a similar incision in the underlying capsule. Alternatively, the subscapularis tendon can be sharply removed from the lesser tuberosity and then sewn back to the position using sutures in the bone. Recent advances have shown better healing and clinical results when the tendon is removed with a thin piece of its bony insertion and then reattached with suture to achieve bone-to-bone healing, which is generally more reliable than tendon-to-bone healing or tendon-to-tendon healing, particularly in older patients who have age-related tendon degeneration.

Most repair and reconstructive procedures are done by arthroscopic techniques. In general, several small 3- to 4-mm incisions (portals) are made for a repair or reconstructive procedure and can be placed in superior, anterior, and posterior aspects of the shoulder. In most reconstructive procedures, multiple portals are used at the same time. At least one portal at any one time is always used for the arthroscope to view the surgical procedure while at least one other is used to pass instruments or devices to modify the tissue and to repair or insert an implant. In general, procedures that are performed within the GH joint use portals in the posterior and anterior joint line for ligament reconstruction; the superior portals are often used for SLAP repairs, and the superior and lateral portals are often used for rotator cuff repairs.

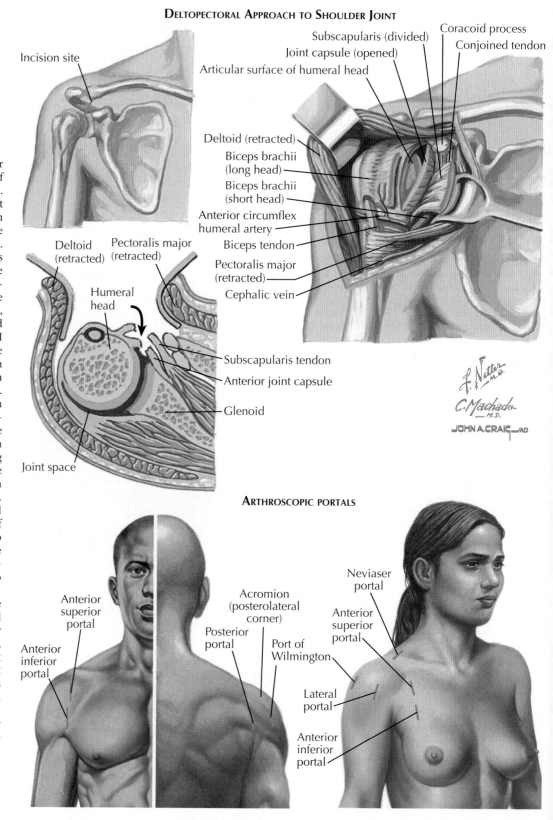

DELTOPECTORAL APPROACH TO SHOULDER JOINT

Incision site

Subscapularis (divided)
Coracoid process
Joint capsule (opened)
Conjoined tendon
Articular surface of humeral head

Deltoid (retracted)
Biceps brachii (long head)
Biceps brachii (short head)
Anterior circumflex humeral artery
Biceps tendon
Pectoralis major (retracted)
Cephalic vein

Deltoid (retracted)
Pectoralis major (retracted)
Humeral head

Subscapularis tendon
Anterior joint capsule
Glenoid

Joint space

ARTHROSCOPIC PORTALS

Anterior superior portal
Anterior inferior portal

Acromion (posterolateral corner)
Posterior portal
Port of Wilmington

Neviaser portal
Anterior superior portal
Lateral portal
Anterior inferior portal

UPPER ARM AND ELBOW

Plate 2.1

Upper Limb: PART I

TOPOGRAPHIC ANATOMY OF UPPER ARM AND ELBOW

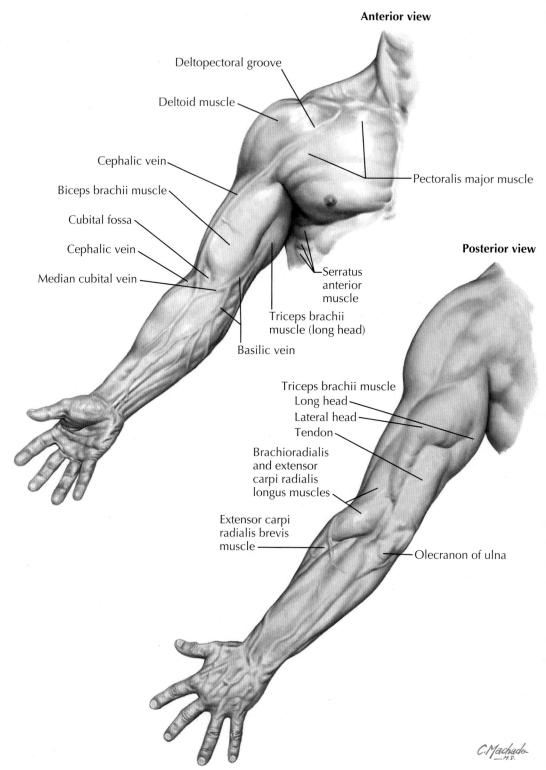

Anterior view

Deltopectoral groove

Deltoid muscle

Cephalic vein

Biceps brachii muscle

Cubital fossa

Cephalic vein

Median cubital vein

Pectoralis major muscle

Serratus anterior muscle

Triceps brachii muscle (long head)

Basilic vein

Posterior view

Triceps brachii muscle
Long head
Lateral head
Tendon

Brachioradialis and extensor carpi radialis longus muscles

Extensor carpi radialis brevis muscle

Olecranon of ulna

BONY ANATOMY AND LANDMARKS

Anteriorly, the contour of the biceps muscle is seen starting in the upper arm and extending distally into the *cubital fossa,* which is the inverted triangular depression on the anterior aspect of the elbow. The flexion crease along the anterior elbow is in line with the medial and lateral epicondyles and is 1 to 2 cm proximal to the joint line when the elbow is extended. The superficial cephalic and basilic veins are the most prominent superficial major contributions of the anterior venous system and communicate by way of the median cephalic and median basilic veins to form a pattern resembling an "M" over the cubital fossa. Laterally, the tip of the olecranon, the lateral epicondyle, and the radial head form a palpable triangle called the *posterolateral soft spot* that can show evidence of an effusion from the elbow joint and serves as an important landmark for joint aspiration and for elbow arthroscopy. The *proximal extensor forearm musculature* originates from the lateral epicondyle and forms the lateral margin of the cubital fossa and the lateral contour of the forearm and comprises the brachioradialis and the extensor carpi radialis longus and brevis muscles. The *proximal flexor pronator musculature* forms the contour of the medial anterior forearm extending from the medial epicondyle and includes the pronator teres, flexor carpi radialis, palmaris longus, and flexor carpi ulnaris. The relationship of these muscles can be approximated by placing the opposing thumb and the index, long, and ring fingers over the anterior medial forearm. Posteriorly, the contour of the triceps muscle is seen in the upper arm extending to the tip of the olecranon. More distally, the proximal forearm is contoured dorsally by the lateral

extensor musculature, consisting of the anconeus, extensor carpi ulnaris, extensor digitorum quinti, and extensor digitorum communis.

The main bone of the upper arm is the *humerus*. It is a long bone composed of a shaft and two articular extremities. The proximal humerus, which includes the humeral head, greater and lesser tuberosity, and surgical neck, is discussed in detail in Section 1, Shoulder. The

body, or shaft, of the humerus begins just below the surgical neck. It is somewhat rounded above and prismatic in its lower portion. Above and medially, the coracobrachialis muscle is received near the middle of the shaft; about opposite laterally is the prominent *deltoid tuberosity.* This is continued upward in a V-shaped roughening for the insertion of the deltoid muscle. Just below the deltoid tuberosity, a groove for the radial

Plate 2.2

Upper Arm and Elbow

ANTERIOR AND POSTERIOR VIEWS OF HUMERUS

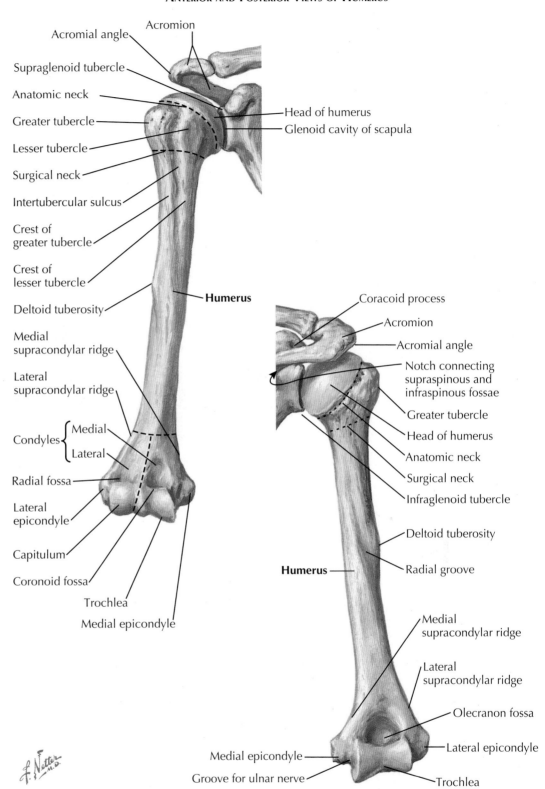

Acromial angle
Acromion
Supraglenoid tubercle
Anatomic neck
Greater tubercle
Lesser tubercle
Surgical neck
Intertubercular sulcus
Crest of greater tubercle
Crest of lesser tubercle
Deltoid tuberosity
Head of humerus
Glenoid cavity of scapula
Humerus
Medial supracondylar ridge
Lateral supracondylar ridge
Condyles { Medial / Lateral }
Radial fossa
Lateral epicondyle
Capitulum
Coronoid fossa
Trochlea
Medial epicondyle

Coracoid process
Acromion
Acromial angle
Notch connecting supraspinous and infraspinous fossae
Greater tubercle
Head of humerus
Anatomic neck
Surgical neck
Infraglenoid tubercle
Deltoid tuberosity
Humerus
Radial groove
Medial supracondylar ridge
Lateral supracondylar ridge
Olecranon fossa
Lateral epicondyle
Medial epicondyle
Groove for ulnar nerve
Trochlea

BONY ANATOMY AND LANDMARKS (Continued)

nerve indents the bone posteriorly, spiraling lateralward as it descends. Sharp lateral and medial supracondylar ridges spring from the respective borders inferiorly and continue into the lateral and medial epicondyles of the humerus. The inferior extremity of the bone is flattened anteroposteriorly and mediolaterally, and it is widened by the medial and lateral epicondyles. The lateral epicondyle is not conspicuous, but the medial epicondyle forms a marked medial projection above the elbow. Projecting somewhat backward, it is grooved behind for the ulnar nerve.

The *articular surfaces* for the radius, ulna, capitellum, and trochlea are directed somewhat forward; consequently, the inferior extremity of the humerus appears to curve anteriorly. The *capitellum* is roughly globular. Smaller than the trochlea, it articulates with the cupped upper surface of the radius. Above it is a shallow fossa, the *radial fossa,* for the reception of the edge of that bone during full flexion of the elbow. The *trochlea* is shaped like a spool, with a deep depression between two well-marked margins. The depression is slightly spiral and receives the central ridge of the trochlear notch of the ulna. The medial rim of the trochlea is the more prominent; the lateral rim is only a small elevation separating the trochlea from the capitellum. Above the trochlea is the *coronoid fossa* for the reception of the coronoid process of the ulna in front and the *olecranon fossa* for the olecranon behind.

The humerus ossifies from eight centers of ossification: one for the shaft and seven for the processes—head, greater and lesser tuberosities, trochlea, capitellum, lateral epicondyle, and medial epicondyle. The

shaft appears near the middle of the bone in the eighth week of fetal life and then extends toward its extremities. At birth, the humerus is ossified in nearly its whole length; only its extremities remain cartilaginous. Shortly after birth, ossification begins in the head of the bone, followed by the appearance of the centers in the greater and lesser tuberosities at 3 to 5 years of age, respectively. By age 6, all these

centers have merged into one large epiphysis. In the distal humerus, secondary centers appear for the capitellum at age 2, for the trochlea at age 9 or 10, and in the lateral epicondyle at ages 13 to 14. These centers unite and fuse with the shaft at about age 13 in females and age 15 in males. The separate center for the medial epicondyle appears at ages 6 to 8 and fuses with the shaft at ages 14 to 16.

Plate 2.3   Upper Limb: PART I

BONES OF ELBOW

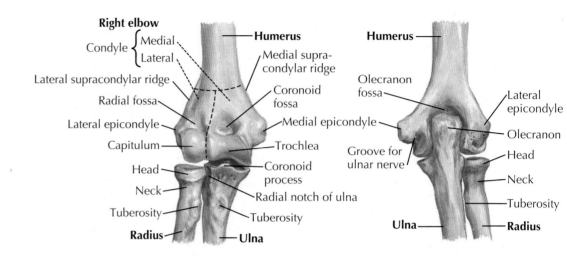

Right elbow

Condyle { Medial / Lateral
Lateral supracondylar ridge
Radial fossa
Lateral epicondyle
Capitulum
Head
Neck
Tuberosity
Radius

Humerus
Medial supra-condylar ridge
Coronoid fossa
Medial epicondyle
Trochlea
Coronoid process
Radial notch of ulna
Tuberosity
Ulna

Humerus
Olecranon fossa
Groove for ulnar nerve
Ulna
Lateral epicondyle
Olecranon
Head
Neck
Tuberosity
Radius

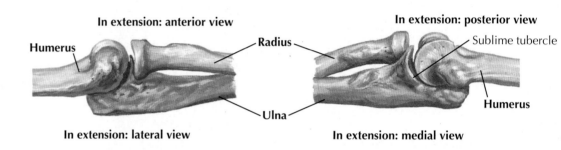

In extension: anterior view

Humerus

In extension: lateral view

In extension: posterior view

Radius
Sublime tubercle
Humerus
Ulna

In extension: medial view

ELBOW JOINT

The elbow joint, composed of the humeroradial, humeroulnar, and proximal radioulnar articulations within a common capsule, necessarily involves the proximal portions of the radius and ulna as well as the distal part of the humerus. The humeroulnar articulation acts as a hinge and allows flexion and extension of the elbow, whereas rotational movements occur through the humeroradial and proximal radioulnar articulations. Therefore the elbow is not considered a simple hinge joint, but rather a trochoginglymoid joint that possesses two degrees of freedom or motion: flexion-extension and pronation-supination. The center of rotation of the elbow runs through the center of the articular surface of the distal humerus formed by the trochlea and the capitellum, lying just anterior to the anterior cortex of the distal humerus on the lateral view. The carrying angle of the elbow, formed by the humerus and ulna with the hand and forearm fully supinated and the elbow fully extended, has been reported to range from 11 to 14 degrees of valgus in men and from 13 to 16 degrees of valgus in women. The carrying angle is typically about a degree greater on the dominant compared with the nondominant side. Valgus (cubitus valgus) or varus (cubitus varus) malalignment is diagnosed when the carrying angle is greater than or less than these normal values, respectively.

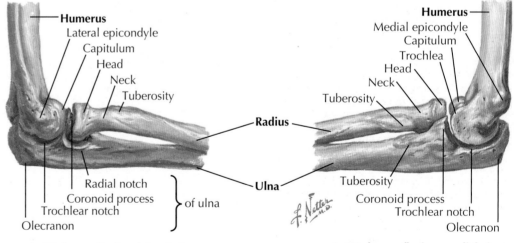

Humerus
Lateral epicondyle
Capitulum
Head
Neck
Tuberosity
Radial notch
Coronoid process } of ulna
Trochlear notch
Olecranon

In 90-degree flexion: lateral view

Humerus
Medial epicondyle
Capitulum
Trochlea
Head
Neck
Tuberosity
Radius
Tuberosity
Coronoid process
Trochlear notch
Olecranon
Ulna

In 90-degree flexion: medial view

In the region of the elbow joint, the special parts of the radius are the head, neck, and tuberosity. The radial head is round; it is a thick disk, articular both on its circumference and over its cupped upper free surface. The latter surface articulates with the capitellum of the humerus. The articular circumference of the head is broader medially for contact with the radial notch of the ulna, forming a 240-degree arc for articulation with the ulna, and narrower where it is held by the annular ligament. The neck of the radius is the constriction below the head, and the tuberosity is an oval prominence just distal to the neck. Its posterior portion is roughened for the reception of the biceps brachii tendon; its anterior part is smooth and is in contact with the bicipitoradial bursa.

Plate 2.4

Upper Arm and Elbow

ELBOW: RADIOGRAPHS

Anteroposterior radiograph

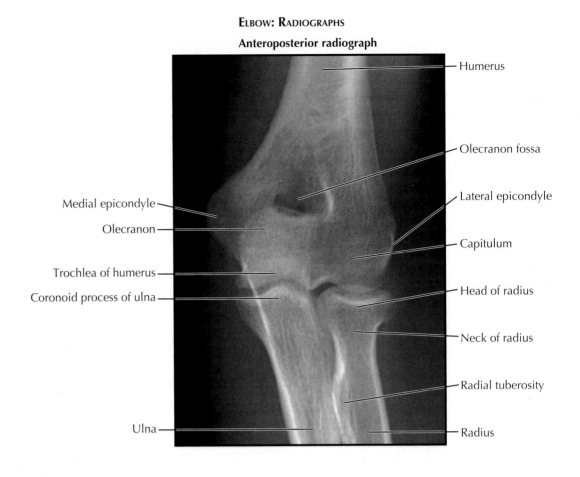

Humerus

Olecranon fossa

Lateral epicondyle

Capitulum

Head of radius

Neck of radius

Radial tuberosity

Radius

Medial epicondyle

Olecranon

Trochlea of humerus

Coronoid process of ulna

Ulna

Lateral radiograph

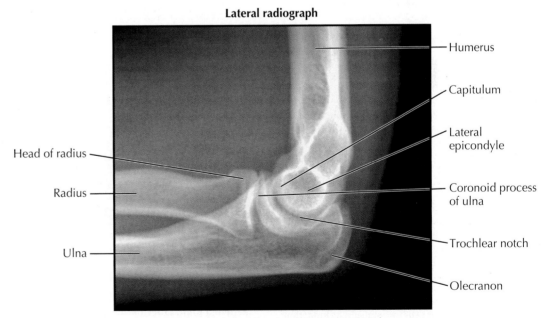

Humerus

Capitulum

Lateral epicondyle

Coronoid process of ulna

Trochlear notch

Olecranon

Head of radius

Radius

Ulna

ELBOW JOINT (Continued)

The proximal end of the ulna has a more complex architecture. Its heavy proximal extremity exhibits the opened jaws of the trochlear notch, olecranon, coronoid process, and radial notch.

The *trochlear notch* is a concavity that describes about one-third of a circle and is divided by a longitudinal ridge into medial and lateral parts. The waist of the notch is constricted, and a roughness across the waist separates the part deriving from the olecranon from the part formed by the coronoid process. The trochlear notch receives the trochlea of the humerus. In extreme flexion, the coronoid process of the ulna enters the coronoid fossa of the humerus; in extreme extension, the olecranon enters the olecranon fossa.

The *olecranon* contributes part of the trochlear notch and forms the posterior projection of the elbow. Its blunt end receives the tendon of the triceps brachii muscle and is attached to the capsule of the elbow joint along the bounding margin of the trochlear notch. Between these attachments, the bone is smooth for the subtendinous bursa of the triceps brachii muscle.

The *coronoid process* is a strong, triangular projection of the anterior surface of the ulna; it also forms the anterior part of the trochlear notch. The anterior surface of the coronoid process is rough for the insertion of the tendon of the brachialis muscle. The junction of this surface with the shaft is the location of the tuberosity of the ulna, which receives the oblique cord of the radius.

The *radial notch of the ulna,* a shallow concavity on the lateral aspect of the coronoid process, receives the circumferential articular surface of the head of the radius. Its prominent edges give attachment to the ends of the annular ligament of the radius.

OSSIFICATION

The radius is ossified by means of a center of ossification that appears in the shaft (which is bony at birth) at the eighth week of intrauterine life. Ossification for the radial head begins at 4 or 5 years, and this portion fuses with the shaft at 14 to 16 years.

Ossification of the ulna begins near the middle of the shaft at the eighth week of intrauterine life, and the shaft is bony at birth.

Plate 2.5

Upper Limb: PART I

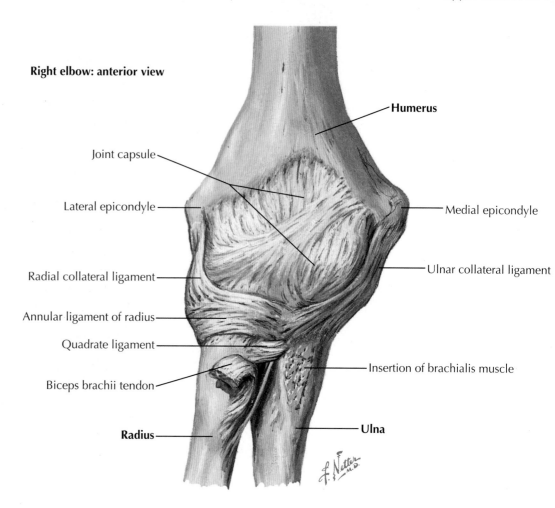

Right elbow: anterior view

Humerus

Joint capsule

Lateral epicondyle

Medial epicondyle

Ulnar collateral ligament

Radial collateral ligament

Annular ligament of radius

Quadrate ligament

Insertion of brachialis muscle

Biceps brachii tendon

Ulna

Radius

ELBOW LIGAMENTS

LIGAMENTS AND CAPSULE

As discussed previously, the elbow is not just a simple hinge joint, but instead possesses two degrees of freedom or motion: flexion-extension and pronation-supination. However, with the primary range of motion occurring in the flexion-extension direction, there are reciprocally convex and concave articular surfaces along the distal humerus, radius, and ulna; a capsule, loose on the sides toward which movement takes place; strong collateral ligaments; and a grouping of muscle masses at the borders where they are not in the direction of movement.

The *articular surfaces* are the spool-shaped trochlea and the rounded capitellum of the humerus proximally and the trochlear notch of the ulna and the cupped upper surface of the humeral head of the radius distally. The capitellum of the humerus is directed forward and downward, with the articular surfaces most completely in contact when the elbow is flexed to a 90-degree angle. Contact is weak between the humerus and the radius, and both the stability of the joint and its limitation of motion to flexion and extension are due to the ridged and grooved relationship of the humerus and the ulna.

The *articular capsule* is weak in front and behind but strengthened at the sides by the ulnar and radial collateral ligaments. In front, it is attached on the humerus from the medial to the lateral epicondyles along the superior borders of the coronoid and radial fossae. Distally, it is attached to the anterior border of the coronoid process of the ulna and to the annular ligament of the radius; it is continuous on either side with the collateral ligaments. The posterior portion of the capsule is

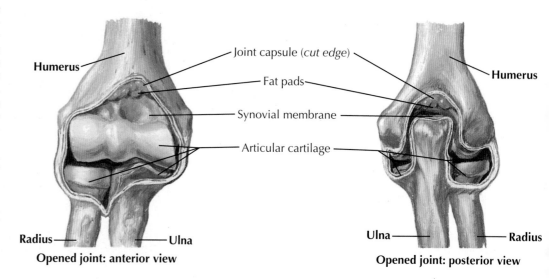

Humerus

Joint capsule (*cut edge*)

Fat pads

Humerus

Synovial membrane

Articular cartilage

Radius

Ulna

Opened joint: anterior view

Ulna

Radius

Opened joint: posterior view

membranous. Its attachments are the margins of the olecranon and the edges of the olecranon fossa, the lateral epicondyle, the annular ligament, and the posterior border of the radial notch of the ulna.

The *collateral ligaments* are strong, triangular thickenings of the articular capsule, attached by their apices to the medial and lateral epicondyles of the humerus. Their broader distal attachments are to the forearm bones and the annular ligament of the radius. These

ligaments place strict limitations on side-to-side displacements of the joint.

The *ulnar collateral ligament* has thickened borders, with the *anterior band* reaching the medial edge of the coronoid process and the *posterior band* attaching to the corresponding edge of the olecranon. The thinner *intermediate portion* ends below, in transverse fibers stretched between the coronoid process and the olecranon.

Plate 2.6

Upper Arm and Elbow

In 90-degree flexion: lateral view

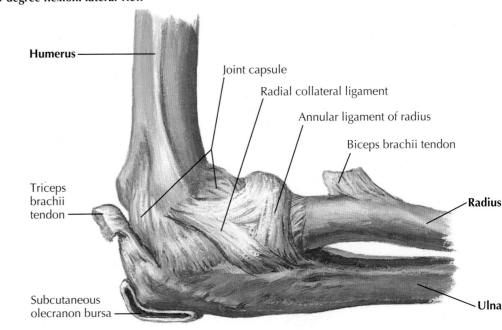

Humerus

Joint capsule

Radial collateral ligament

Annular ligament of radius

Biceps brachii tendon

Triceps brachii tendon

Radius

Subcutaneous olecranon bursa

Ulna

In 90-degree flexion: medial view

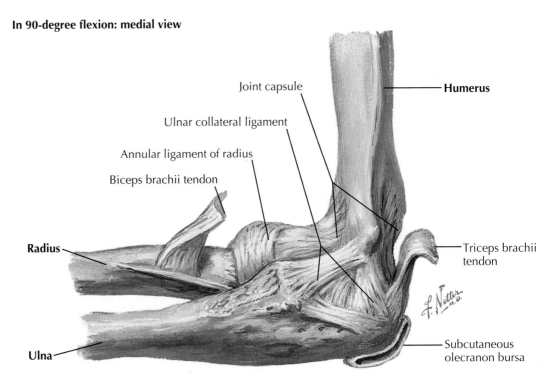

Joint capsule

Ulnar collateral ligament

Annular ligament of radius

Biceps brachii tendon

Humerus

Radius

Triceps brachii tendon

Ulna

Subcutaneous olecranon bursa

ELBOW LIGAMENTS (Continued)

The *radial collateral ligament,* a narrower, less distinct thickening, is stretched between the underside of the lateral epicondyle above and the annular ligament and the margins of the radial notch of the ulna below.

The *synovial membrane* of the elbow joint lines the capsule and is reflected onto the borders of the radial and coronoid fossae of the humerus in front and the olecranon fossa behind. Below, it continues into the proximal radioulnar articulation.

MOVEMENTS

The hinge action at the elbow joint is not exactly in the line of the long axis of the humerus. In extension, the forearm deviates from a straight line with the arm, forming the carrying angle of the forearm, which is obliterated when the hand is pronated. As discussed previously, the carrying angle has been reported to range from 11 to 14 degrees of valgus in men and from 13 to 16 degrees of valgus in women. Because of a slight spiral orientation of the ridge of the trochlear notch and of the groove of the trochlea, flexion does not bring the forearm bones medial to the humerus. The habitual ease with which the hand is carried to the mouth in elbow flexion is due to the slight medial rotation of the humerus and the semipronated position of the hand.

PROXIMAL RADIOULNAR ARTICULATION

The head of the radius rotates in a ring formed by the radial notch of the ulna and the annular ligament of the radius. The *annular ligament of the radius* is a strong, curved band attaching to the anterior and posterior margins of the radial notch of the ulna. It serves as a restraining ligament, which prevents withdrawal of the head of the radius from its socket. The annular ligament receives the radial collateral ligament and blends with the capsule of the elbow joint. Below, a lax band, called the *quadrate ligament,* passes from the lower border of the radial notch of the ulna to the adjacent medial surface of the neck of the radius.

The *synovial membrane* of this joint is continuous with that of the elbow joint. A reflection of the membrane below the annular ligament forms a loose sac around the neck of the radius, which accommodates to the rotation of the head of the radius.

Plate 2.7   Upper Limb: PART I

MUSCLE ORIGINS AND INSERTIONS OF UPPER ARM AND ELBOW

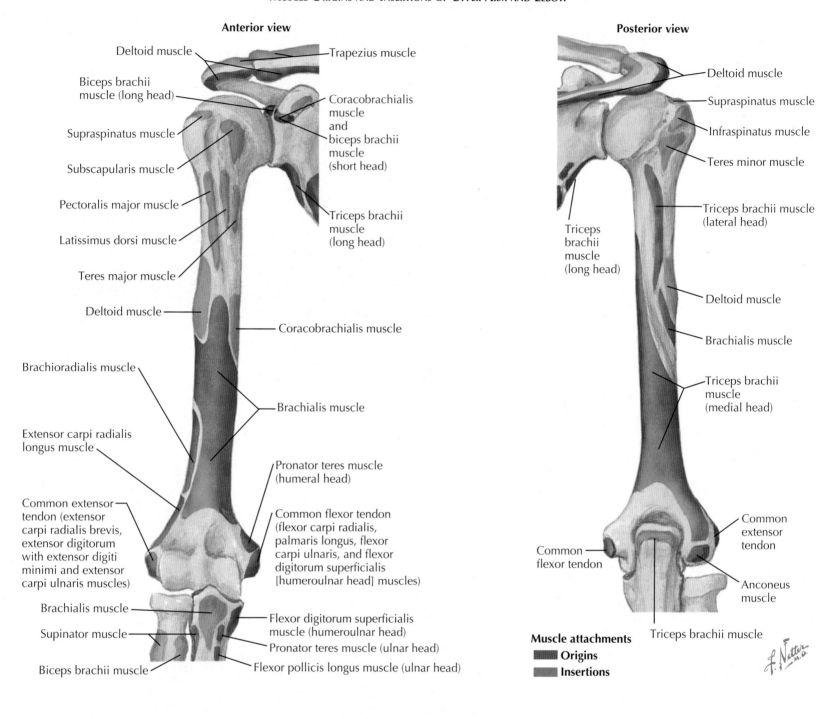

Anterior view

Deltoid muscle

Biceps brachii muscle (long head)

Supraspinatus muscle

Subscapularis muscle

Pectoralis major muscle

Latissimus dorsi muscle

Teres major muscle

Deltoid muscle

Brachioradialis muscle

Extensor carpi radialis longus muscle

Common extensor tendon (extensor carpi radialis brevis, extensor digitorum with extensor digiti minimi and extensor carpi ulnaris muscles)

Brachialis muscle

Supinator muscle

Biceps brachii muscle

Trapezius muscle

Coracobrachialis muscle and biceps brachii muscle (short head)

Triceps brachii muscle (long head)

Coracobrachialis muscle

Brachialis muscle

Pronator teres muscle (humeral head)

Common flexor tendon (flexor carpi radialis, palmaris longus, flexor carpi ulnaris, and flexor digitorum superficialis [humeroulnar head] muscles)

Flexor digitorum superficialis muscle (humeroulnar head)

Pronator teres muscle (ulnar head)

Flexor pollicis longus muscle (ulnar head)

Posterior view

Deltoid muscle

Supraspinatus muscle

Infraspinatus muscle

Teres minor muscle

Triceps brachii muscle (lateral head)

Triceps brachii muscle (long head)

Deltoid muscle

Brachialis muscle

Triceps brachii muscle (medial head)

Common extensor tendon

Common flexor tendon

Anconeus muscle

Triceps brachii muscle

Muscle attachments
■ Origins
■ Insertions

MUSCLES OF UPPER ARM AND ELBOW

The upper arm, or brachium, is the region between the shoulder joint and the elbow. The arm muscles are few, and they are served by certain terminal branches of the brachial plexus and portions of the great vascular channels of the limb (see Plates 2.7 to 2.11).

BRACHIAL FASCIA

A strong tubular investment of the deeper parts of the arm, the brachial fascia is continuous above with the pectoral and axillary fasciae and with the fascial covering of the deltoid and latissimus dorsi muscles. Below, the brachial fascia is attached to the epicondyles of the humerus and to the olecranon and then is continuous with the antebrachial fascia. It is perforated for the passage of the basilic vein, for the medial antebrachial cutaneous nerve, and for many lesser nerves and vessels.

Two *intermuscular septa* are prolonged upward from the epicondylar attachments of the brachial fascia. These blend with the periosteum of the humerus along its supracondylar ridges and borders and fuse peripherally with the brachial fascia to form the anterior and posterior compartments of the arm. Above, the *lateral intermuscular septum* ends at the insertion of the deltoid muscle; the *medial intermuscular septum* ends in continuity with the fascia of the coracobrachialis muscle. The medial intermuscular septum has an additional, weaker anterior lamina, and the anterior and posterior laminae

together with the brachial fascia form the neurovascular compartment of the arm (see Plate 2.10).

MUSCLES

The muscles of the arm are separated both positionally and functionally by the humerus and the intermuscular septa into an anterior and a posterior group or compartments (see Plates 2.8 and 2.9). The anterior group comprises the coracobrachialis, biceps brachii, and brachialis muscles. The posterior group includes the triceps brachii and anconeus muscles. Important neurovascular structures in the anterior compartment include the musculocutaneous nerve, median nerve, ulnar nerve (proximally), radial nerve (distally), and brachial artery. Important neurovascular structures in the posterior

Plate 2.8

Upper Arm and Elbow

MUSCLES OF THE UPPER ARMS: ANTERIOR VIEWS

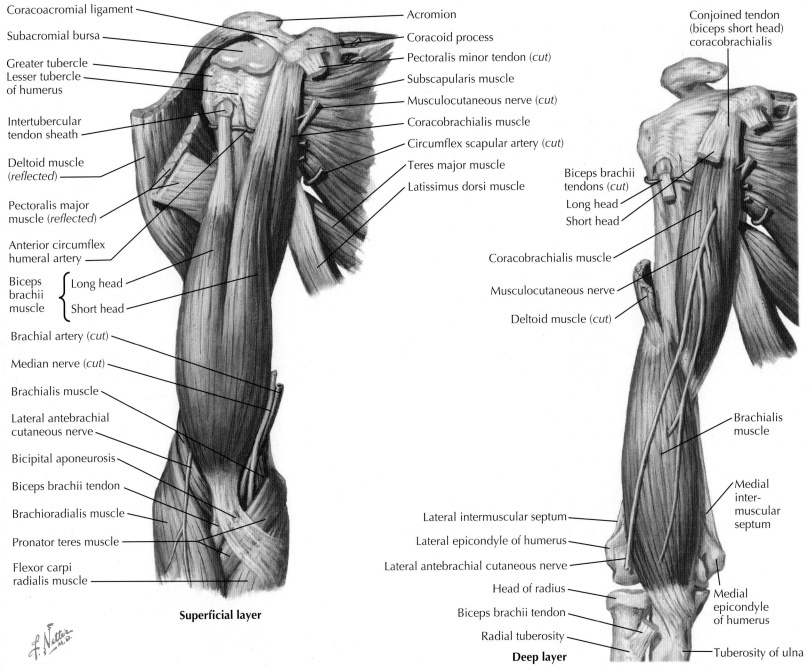

Coracoacromial ligament

Subacromial bursa

Greater tubercle
Lesser tubercle
of humerus

Intertubercular
tendon sheath

Deltoid muscle
(*reflected*)

Pectoralis major
muscle (*reflected*)

Anterior circumflex
humeral artery

Biceps
brachii
muscle { Long head
Short head

Brachial artery (*cut*)

Median nerve (*cut*)

Brachialis muscle

Lateral antebrachial
cutaneous nerve

Bicipital aponeurosis

Biceps brachii tendon

Brachioradialis muscle

Pronator teres muscle

Flexor carpi
radialis muscle

Acromion

Coracoid process

Pectoralis minor tendon (*cut*)

Subscapularis muscle

Musculocutaneous nerve (*cut*)

Coracobrachialis muscle

Circumflex scapular artery (*cut*)

Teres major muscle

Latissimus dorsi muscle

Superficial layer

Conjoined tendon
(biceps short head)
coracobrachialis

Biceps brachii
tendons (*cut*)
Long head
Short head

Coracobrachialis muscle

Musculocutaneous nerve

Deltoid muscle (*cut*)

Lateral intermuscular septum

Lateral epicondyle of humerus

Lateral antebrachial cutaneous nerve

Head of radius

Biceps brachii tendon

Radial tuberosity

Brachialis
muscle

Medial
inter-
muscular
septum

Medial
epicondyle
of humerus

Tuberosity of ulna

Deep layer

MUSCLES OF UPPER ARM AND ELBOW (Continued)

compartment include the ulnar nerve (distally), radial nerve (proximally), and radial recurrent arteries. The median nerve, ulnar nerve, and brachial artery run along the medial aspect of the upper arm, and the radial nerve runs laterally. The musculocutaneous nerve travels more in the midline, between the biceps brachii and brachialis muscles. Key origin and insertion points of the muscles of the arm are pictured in Plate 2.7.

Coracobrachialis Muscle

A short, band-like muscle of the upper arm, the coracobrachialis, arises from the tip of the coracoid process

and acts to flex and adduct the arm. The short head of the biceps brachii muscle originates from the lateral side of the coracoid process and runs side by side with the coracobrachialis to form the conjoined tendon. The coracobrachialis inserts by a flat tendon into the medial surface of the humerus just proximal to its mid-length. The musculocutaneous nerve supplies the coracobrachialis muscle and passes diagonally through the muscle at its mid-length.

Biceps Brachii Muscle

The biceps brachii is a long, fusiform muscle of the anterior aspect of the arm. Its *long head* arises as a rounded tendon from the supraglenoid tubercle of the scapula, crosses the head of the humerus within the capsule of the shoulder joint, and emerges from that capsule to travel down the bicipital groove of the

proximal humerus, between the greater and lesser tuberosities. It is covered by the intertubercular synovial sheath. The *short head* of the biceps brachii muscle arises by a thick, flattened tendon from the tip of the coracoid process, in common with the coracobrachialis muscle and, unlike the long head, never has an intraarticular course.

The two bellies of the biceps brachii muscle unite at about the middle of the arm to form the most prominent muscle of the anterior compartment. The tendon of insertion is a strong, vertical cord palpable down the center of the cubital fossa. Here, its deeper part turns its anterior surface lateralward to end on the tuberosity of the radius, separated from the anterior part of the tuberosity by the small *bicipitoradial bursa*. The variable *interosseous cubital bursa* may separate the tendon from the ulna and its covering muscles. The musculocutaneous

Plate 2.9

Upper Limb: PART I

Muscles of the Upper Arms: Posterior Views

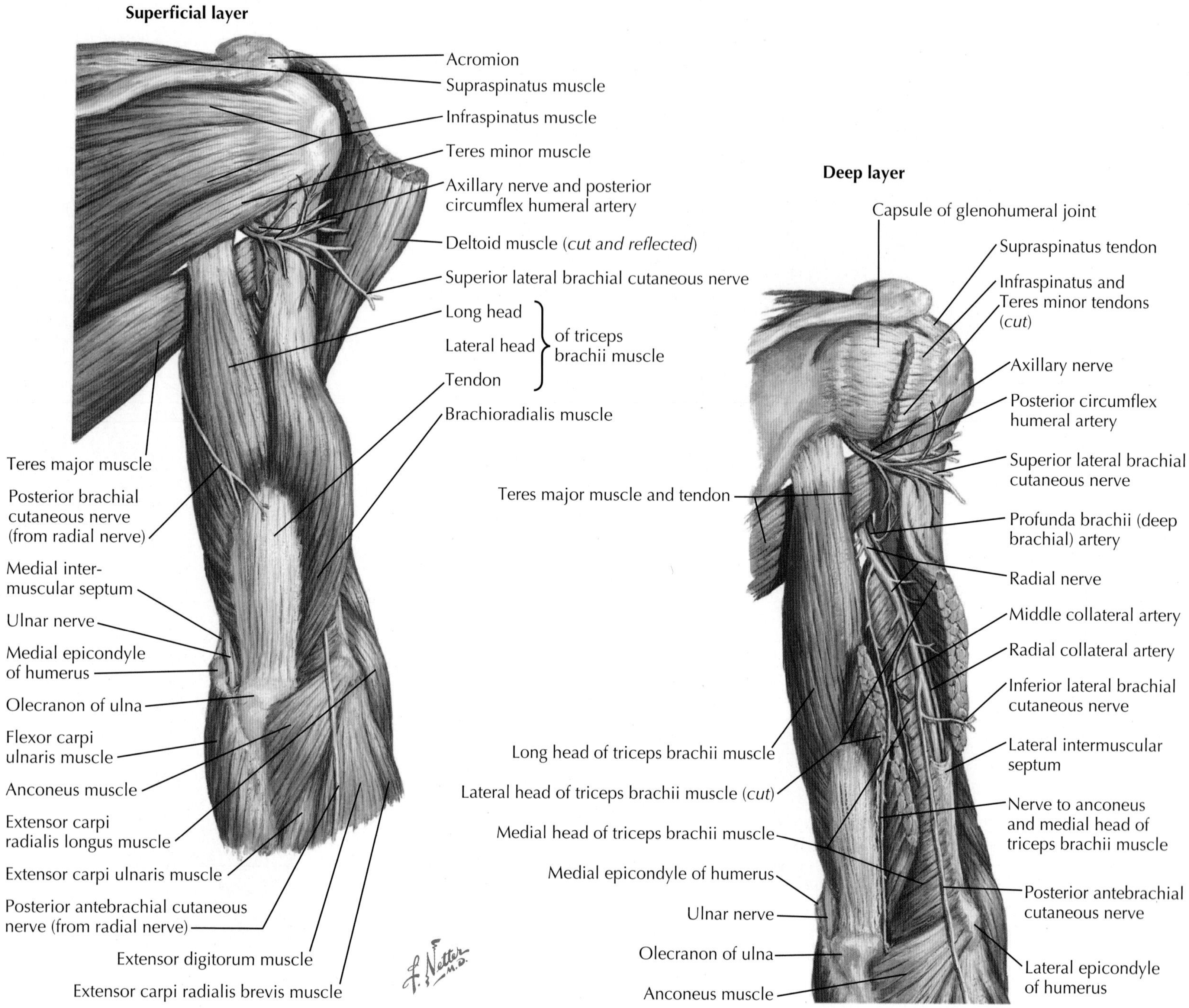

Superficial layer

Acromion
Supraspinatus muscle
Infraspinatus muscle
Teres minor muscle
Axillary nerve and posterior circumflex humeral artery
Deltoid muscle (*cut and reflected*)
Superior lateral brachial cutaneous nerve
Long head
Lateral head } of triceps brachii muscle
Tendon
Brachioradialis muscle

Teres major muscle
Posterior brachial cutaneous nerve (from radial nerve)
Medial inter-muscular septum
Ulnar nerve
Medial epicondyle of humerus
Olecranon of ulna
Flexor carpi ulnaris muscle
Anconeus muscle
Extensor carpi radialis longus muscle
Extensor carpi ulnaris muscle
Posterior antebrachial cutaneous nerve (from radial nerve)
Extensor digitorum muscle
Extensor carpi radialis brevis muscle

Deep layer

Capsule of glenohumeral joint
Supraspinatus tendon
Infraspinatus and Teres minor tendons (*cut*)
Axillary nerve
Posterior circumflex humeral artery
Superior lateral brachial cutaneous nerve
Teres major muscle and tendon
Profunda brachii (deep brachial) artery
Radial nerve
Middle collateral artery
Radial collateral artery
Inferior lateral brachial cutaneous nerve
Lateral intermuscular septum
Long head of triceps brachii muscle
Lateral head of triceps brachii muscle (*cut*)
Medial head of triceps brachii muscle
Nerve to anconeus and medial head of triceps brachii muscle
Medial epicondyle of humerus
Ulnar nerve
Posterior antebrachial cutaneous nerve
Olecranon of ulna
Anconeus muscle
Lateral epicondyle of humerus

f. Netter M.D.

Muscles of Upper Arm and Elbow (Continued)

nerve supplies both heads of the biceps brachii, whose function is unique in that it acts across both the shoulder and elbow joints. At the shoulder, the muscle assists in forward flexion, joint stabilization (long head), and adduction (short head). At the elbow, its main actions are to flex the elbow and supinate the forearm. The biceps acts as an elbow flexor particularly when the forearm is supinated and is a strong supinator with the elbow at least partially flexed and with the forearm in a more pronated position.

The *bicipital aponeurosis,* or lacertus fibrosus, formed from the more anterior and medial tendon fibers of the muscle, arises at the bend of the elbow and passes obliquely over the brachial artery and median nerve to blend with the antebrachial fascia over the flexor group of the forearm (see Plate 2.8). The pull of the bicipital aponeurosis is largely exerted on the ulna.

Brachialis Muscle

This muscle arises from the lower half of the anterior surface of the humerus and the two intermuscular septa and lies deep to the biceps. Its upper extent has two pointed processes positioned on either side of the insertion of the deltoid muscle (Plate 2.8). The muscular fibers converge to a thick tendon, which adheres to the capsule of the elbow joint and inserts on the tuberosity of the ulna and on the anterior surface of its coronoid process. Its major attachment is to the coronoid process about 2 mm distal from the articular margin. This muscle bulges beyond the biceps brachii muscle on either side,

and anterior to its medial border lie the brachial vessels and the median nerve. The medial half of this muscle is supplied by the musculocutaneous nerve, whereas the lateral portion is supplied by the radial nerve. The muscle's main action is to flex the elbow. The brachialis has the largest cross-sectional area of any of the muscles that flex the elbow, but it has a poor mechanic advantage owing to its close proximity to the axis of rotation. This natural internervous plane within the muscle allows it to be split during a routine anterolateral surgical approach to the humerus to come down on the anterior surface of the humerus, typically for fixation of a humeral shaft fracture.

Triceps Brachii Muscle

This large muscle with three heads occupies the entire dorsum of the arm. Each head of the triceps (long, lateral, medial) originates distal to the other, with a progressively larger area of origin. The *long head* arises

Plate 2.10

Upper Arm and Elbow

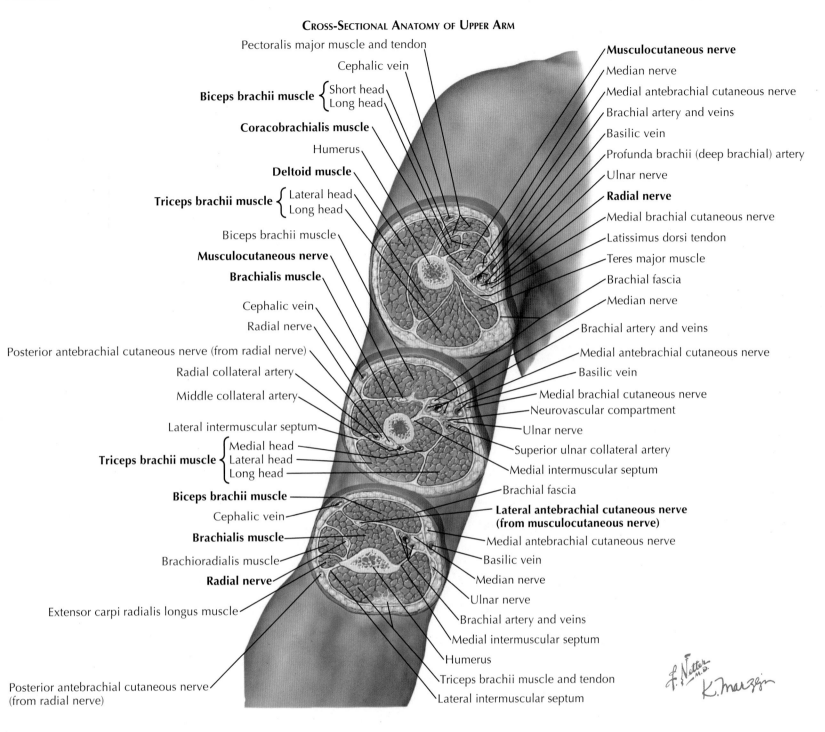

CROSS-SECTIONAL ANATOMY OF UPPER ARM

Pectoralis major muscle and tendon

Cephalic vein

Biceps brachii muscle { Short head / Long head

Coracobrachialis muscle

Humerus

Deltoid muscle

Triceps brachii muscle { Lateral head / Long head

Biceps brachii muscle

Musculocutaneous nerve

Brachialis muscle

Cephalic vein

Radial nerve

Posterior antebrachial cutaneous nerve (from radial nerve)

Radial collateral artery

Middle collateral artery

Lateral intermuscular septum

Triceps brachii muscle { Medial head / Lateral head / Long head

Biceps brachii muscle

Cephalic vein

Brachialis muscle

Brachioradialis muscle

Radial nerve

Extensor carpi radialis longus muscle

Posterior antebrachial cutaneous nerve (from radial nerve)

Musculocutaneous nerve

Median nerve

Medial antebrachial cutaneous nerve

Brachial artery and veins

Basilic vein

Profunda brachii (deep brachial) artery

Ulnar nerve

Radial nerve

Medial brachial cutaneous nerve

Latissimus dorsi tendon

Teres major muscle

Brachial fascia

Median nerve

Brachial artery and veins

Medial antebrachial cutaneous nerve

Basilic vein

Medial brachial cutaneous nerve

Neurovascular compartment

Ulnar nerve

Superior ulnar collateral artery

Medial intermuscular septum

Brachial fascia

Lateral antebrachial cutaneous nerve (from musculocutaneous nerve)

Medial antebrachial cutaneous nerve

Basilic vein

Median nerve

Ulnar nerve

Brachial artery and veins

Medial intermuscular septum

Humerus

Triceps brachii muscle and tendon

Lateral intermuscular septum

MUSCLES OF UPPER ARM AND ELBOW (Continued)

by a strong tendon from the infraglenoid tubercle of the scapula. Its belly descends between the teres major and teres minor muscles and joins the lateral and medial heads of the triceps in a common insertion on the olecranon. The long head is a defining border of the triangular space (lateral border), which contains the circumflex scapular artery; the quadrangular space (medial border), which contains the axillary nerve and the posterior humeral circumflex artery; and triangular interval (medial border), which contains the radial nerve and the profunda brachii artery. The *lateral head* takes origin from the posterior surface and lateral

border of the humerus above and lateral to the radial groove and from the lateral intermuscular septum. Crossing the groove and concealing the radial nerve and deep brachial vessels, its fibers join in the common tendon insertion on the olecranon. The lateral head is the lateral border of both the quadrangular space and triangular interval. The *medial head* arises from the humerus entirely medial and below the radial groove from as high as the insertion of the teres major muscle to as low as the olecranon fossa of the humerus (see Plate 2.9). It also takes origin from the entire length of the medial intermuscular septum and from the lateral septum below the radial nerve groove. The medial head is deep to the other heads and is hidden by them. The tendon of the muscle appears as a flat band covering its distal two-fifths. It inserts on the posterior part of the

olecranon and into the deep fascia of the forearm on either side of it.

All three heads of the triceps brachii are innervated by the radial nerve and have a primary action of elbow extension. The long and lateral heads are innervated by branches of the radial nerve that arise proximal to the radial groove, whereas the branch to the medial head originates distal to the radial groove and also innervates the anconeus. A radial nerve injury at the midshaft of the humerus therefore usually does not disrupt function of the more proximally innervated long and lateral heads of the triceps. The humeral shaft can be surgically approached posteriorly by splitting the triceps muscle to come down onto the posterior cortex or by elevating the muscle along its lateral border and reflecting all three heads of the muscle medially. This approach may

Plate 2.11

Upper Limb: PART I

CROSS-SECTIONAL ANATOMY OF ELBOW

Coronal view

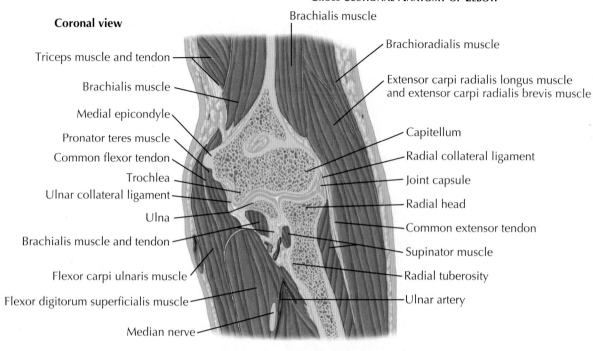

Trices muscle and tendon

Brachialis muscle

Medial epicondyle

Pronator teres muscle

Common flexor tendon

Trochlea

Ulnar collateral ligament

Ulna

Brachialis muscle and tendon

Flexor carpi ulnaris muscle

Flexor digitorum superficialis muscle

Median nerve

Brachialis muscle

Brachioradialis muscle

Extensor carpi radialis longus muscle and extensor carpi radialis brevis muscle

Capitellum

Radial collateral ligament

Joint capsule

Radial head

Common extensor tendon

Supinator muscle

Radial tuberosity

Ulnar artery

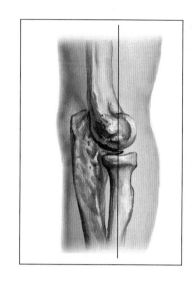

Axial view

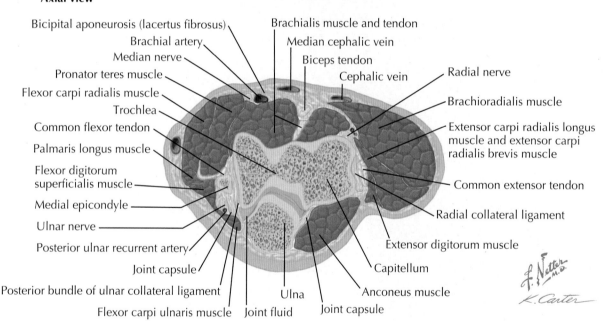

Bicipital aponeurosis (lacertus fibrosus)

Brachial artery

Median nerve

Pronator teres muscle

Flexor carpi radialis muscle

Trochlea

Common flexor tendon

Palmaris longus muscle

Flexor digitorum superficialis muscle

Medial epicondyle

Ulnar nerve

Posterior ulnar recurrent artery

Joint capsule

Posterior bundle of ulnar collateral ligament

Flexor carpi ulnaris muscle   Joint fluid   Joint capsule

Ulna

Brachialis muscle and tendon

Median cephalic vein

Biceps tendon

Cephalic vein

Radial nerve

Brachioradialis muscle

Extensor carpi radialis longus muscle and extensor carpi radialis brevis muscle

Common extensor tendon

Radial collateral ligament

Extensor digitorum muscle

Capitellum

Anconeus muscle

J. Netter M.D.
K. Carter

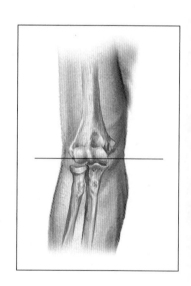

MUSCLES OF UPPER ARM AND ELBOW (Continued)

afford more exposure than an anterolateral approach in more distal fractures of the humeral shaft.

Anconeus Muscle

This is a small, triangular muscle that arises from a broad site on the posterior aspect of the lateral epicondyle of the humerus (see Plate 2.9). Its fibers diverge from this origin and insert into the side of the olecranon and the adjacent one-fourth of the posterior surface of the ulna. The muscle is deep to the dorsal antebrachial fascia and extends across the elbow and the superior radioulnar joints. It is innervated by the terminal branch of the radial nerve that also innervates the medial head of the triceps. The function of this muscle has been the subject of some debate and includes assisting in elbow extension and stabilizing the elbow joint. Joint stabilization may be its primary role. The anconeus serves as a key landmark in the lateral or Kocher approach to the elbow, in which the interval between the extensor carpi ulnaris anteriorly and the anconeus posteriorly is utilized to approach the lateral or posterolateral aspect of the elbow.

Muscle Actions

The principal movements produced by the muscles of the arm are flexion and extension of the forearm at the elbow. The brachialis and biceps brachii muscles are the principal flexors. In this action, the brachialis muscle is always active; the biceps brachii muscle becomes active against resistance and is most effective when flexion of the forearm is combined with supination. It is a powerful supinator of the forearm and one of the primary muscles for producing this movement. Extension of the forearm is produced by the triceps brachii muscle and assisted by the anconeus muscle. The medial head of the triceps brachii muscle is usually active, and the lateral and long heads are recruited for extra powers.

Certain heads of these muscles are active at the shoulder joint. The long head of the biceps brachii muscle flexes the arm at the shoulder, and its tendon aids in stabilization of the joint. The long head of the triceps brachii muscle assists in extension and adduction of the arm.

Plate 2.12

Upper Arm and Elbow

CUTANEOUS NERVES AND SUPERFICIAL VEINS OF UPPER ARM AND ELBOW

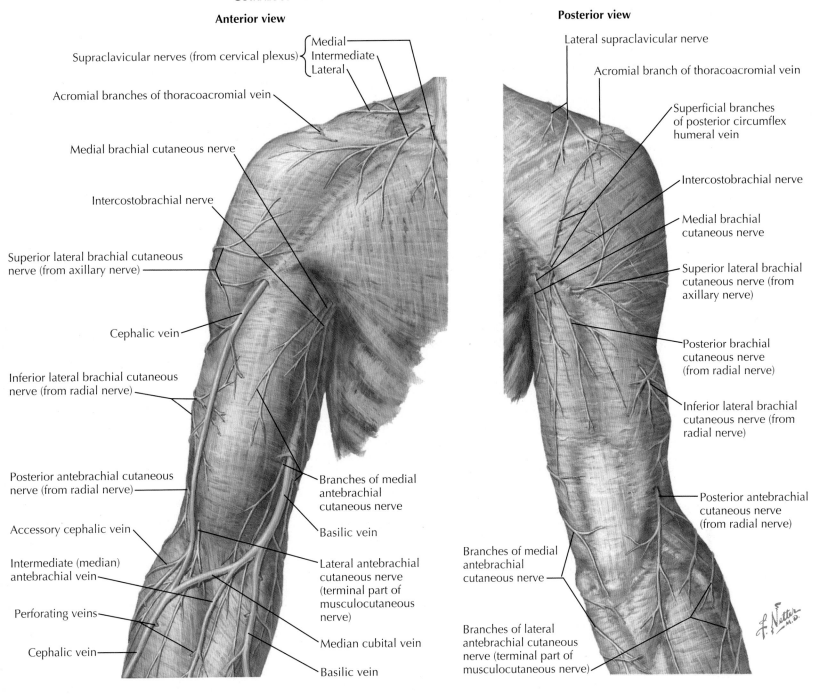

Anterior view

Supraclavicular nerves (from cervical plexus)
{ Medial
Intermediate
Lateral }

Acromial branches of thoracoacromial vein

Medial brachial cutaneous nerve

Intercostobrachial nerve

Superior lateral brachial cutaneous nerve (from axillary nerve)

Cephalic vein

Inferior lateral brachial cutaneous nerve (from radial nerve)

Posterior antebrachial cutaneous nerve (from radial nerve)

Accessory cephalic vein

Intermediate (median) antebrachial vein

Perforating veins

Cephalic vein

Branches of medial antebrachial cutaneous nerve

Basilic vein

Lateral antebrachial cutaneous nerve (terminal part of musculocutaneous nerve)

Median cubital vein

Basilic vein

Posterior view

Lateral supraclavicular nerve

Acromial branch of thoracoacromial vein

Superficial branches of posterior circumflex humeral vein

Intercostobrachial nerve

Medial brachial cutaneous nerve

Superior lateral brachial cutaneous nerve (from axillary nerve)

Posterior brachial cutaneous nerve (from radial nerve)

Inferior lateral brachial cutaneous nerve (from radial nerve)

Posterior antebrachial cutaneous nerve (from radial nerve)

Branches of medial antebrachial cutaneous nerve

Branches of lateral antebrachial cutaneous nerve (terminal part of musculocutaneous nerve)

CUTANEOUS NERVES

The cutaneous nerves of the upper limb and elbow are for the most part derived from the brachial plexus, although the uppermost nerves to the shoulder are derived from the cervical plexus. Some of the cutaneous nerves arise directly from the medial, lateral, or posterior cord of the brachial plexus, whereas others are terminal branches of the peripheral nerves of the upper extremity.

SHOULDER

The *supraclavicular nerves* (C3, C4) become superficial at the posterior border of the sternocleidomastoid muscle within the posterior triangle of the neck. They pierce the superficial layer of the cervical fascia and the platysma muscle, radiating in three lines: (1) the medial supraclavicular nerves cross over the clavicle anteriorly to cover the shoulder more medially, (2) the intermediate supraclavicular nerves also run anteriorly and go toward the acromion laterally, and (3) the lateral or posterior supraclavicular nerves cross over the scapula to cover the shoulder posteriorly.

UPPER ARM

The *superior lateral brachial cutaneous nerve* (C5, C6) is the termination of the lower branch of the axillary nerve of the brachial plexus. Leaving the axillary nerve, it turns superficially around the posterior border of the lower third of the deltoid muscle to pierce the brachial fascia. Its cutaneous distribution is the lower half of the deltoid muscle and the long head of the triceps brachii

in the most proximal aspect of the upper arm, both anteriorly and posteriorly.

The *inferior lateral brachial cutaneous nerve* (C5, C6) is derived from the posterior antebrachial cutaneous nerve shortly after this nerve branches from the radial nerve. The inferior lateral brachial cutaneous nerve becomes superficial in line with the lateral intermuscular septum a little below the insertion of the deltoid muscle. It accompanies the lower part of the cephalic vein and distributes in the lower lateral surface of the arm, below the area covered by the superior lateral brachial cutaneous nerve and extending both anteriorly and posteriorly.

The *posterior brachial cutaneous nerve* arises within the axilla as a branch of the radial nerve (C5 to C8). Traversing the medial side of the long head of the triceps brachii muscle, the nerve penetrates the brachial

Plate 2.13

Upper Limb: PART I

CUTANEOUS INNERVATION OF THE UPPER LIMB

Anterior (palmar) view

Posterior (dorsal) view

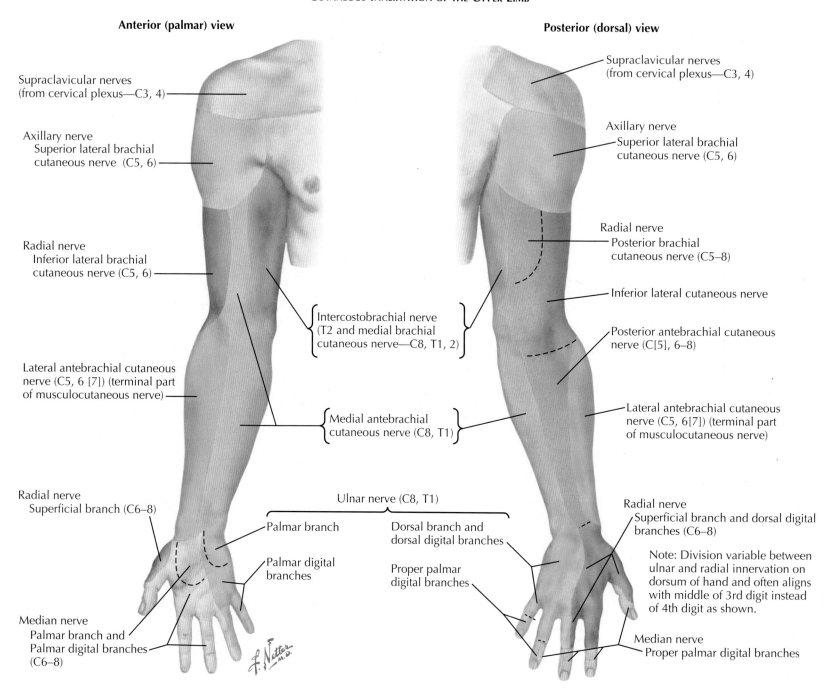

Supraclavicular nerves
(from cervical plexus—C3, 4)

Axillary nerve
Superior lateral brachial
cutaneous nerve (C5, 6)

Radial nerve
Inferior lateral brachial
cutaneous nerve (C5, 6)

Lateral antebrachial cutaneous
nerve (C5, 6 [7]) (terminal part
of musculocutaneous nerve)

Radial nerve
Superficial branch (C6–8)

Median nerve
Palmar branch and
Palmar digital branches
(C6–8)

Intercostobrachial nerve
(T2 and medial brachial
cutaneous nerve—C8, T1, 2)

Medial antebrachial
cutaneous nerve (C8, T1)

Ulnar nerve (C8, T1)
Palmar branch
Palmar digital
branches
Dorsal branch and
dorsal digital branches
Proper palmar
digital branches

Supraclavicular nerves
(from cervical plexus—C3, 4)

Axillary nerve
Superior lateral brachial
cutaneous nerve (C5, 6)

Radial nerve
Posterior brachial
cutaneous nerve (C5–8)

Inferior lateral cutaneous nerve

Posterior antebrachial cutaneous
nerve (C[5], 6–8)

Lateral antebrachial cutaneous
nerve (C5, 6[7]) (terminal part
of musculocutaneous nerve)

Radial nerve
Superficial branch and dorsal digital
branches (C6–8)

Note: Division variable between
ulnar and radial innervation on
dorsum of hand and often aligns
with middle of 3rd digit instead
of 4th digit as shown.

Median nerve
Proper palmar digital branches

CUTANEOUS NERVES (Continued)

fascia to distribute in the middle third of the back of the arm, below the area covered by the superior lateral brachial cutaneous nerve and lateral to the distribution of the medial brachial cutaneous nerve and the intercostobrachial nerve.

The *medial brachial cutaneous nerve* (C8, T1) arises from the medial cord of the brachial plexus in the lower axilla. It descends along the medial side of the brachial artery to the middle of the arm, where it pierces the brachial fascia and supplies the skin of the posteromedial surface of the lower third of the arm as far as the olecranon.

The *intercostobrachial nerve* is the larger part of the lateral cutaneous branch of the second thoracic nerve (T2). In the second intercostal space at the axillary line,

it pierces the serratus anterior muscle to enter the axilla. Here, it usually anastomoses with the medial brachial cutaneous nerve and then pierces the brachial fascia just beyond the posterior axillary fold. Its cutaneous distribution is along the medial and posterior surfaces of the arm from the axilla to the elbow.

The *medial antebrachial cutaneous nerve* arises from the medial cord of the brachial plexus. A small branch pierces the axillary fascia and supplies the skin over the medial anterior area of the arm.

ELBOW

Cutaneous innervation about the elbow can be more variable and includes coverage by the inferior lateral brachial cutaneous nerve laterally and posteriorly, the medial brachial cutaneous nerve medially and

posteriorly, and the medial antebrachial cutaneous nerve anteriorly. As the elbow continues into the proximal forearm, coverage is taken over by the antebrachial cutaneous nerves (medial, lateral, posterior). The *medial antebrachial cutaneous nerve* (C8, T1) is a continuation of the medial cord of the brachial plexus after the medial brachial cutaneous nerve, whereas the *lateral antebrachial cutaneous nerve* (C5, C6) is the terminal branch of the musculocutaneous nerve, running next to the cephalic vein. The *posterior antebrachial cutaneous nerve* (C5 to C8) is another cutaneous branch of the radial nerve after the posterior brachial cutaneous nerve has branched off more proximally. All three of the antebrachial cutaneous nerves continue along distally to provide cutaneous innervation for the entire forearm, down to the level of the wrist.

Plate 2.14

Upper Arm and Elbow

MUSCULOCUTANEOUS NERVE

PERIPHERAL NERVES

The terminal branches of the brachial plexus (the musculocutaneous, median, ulnar, and radial nerves) provide the entire nerve supply to the limb below the shoulder. Of these, only the musculocutaneous and radial nerves distribute to the muscles of the upper arm.

MUSCULOCUTANEOUS NERVE

The *musculocutaneous nerve* (C4 to C7), a branch of the *lateral cord* of the brachial plexus, arises opposite the lower border of the pectoralis minor muscle. This nerve is the principal motor nerve of the anterior (flexor) compartment of the arm. It continues into the forearm as a cutaneous nerve, the lateral antebrachial cutaneous nerve. The nerve lies between the axillary artery and the coracobrachialis muscle, which it perforates and supplies. Continuing downward, it runs between the biceps brachii and brachialis muscles, supplying branches to both heads of the biceps brachii muscle and most of the brachialis muscle and often communicating with the median nerve. In this part of its course, it inclines gradually toward the lateral side of the arm; at about the level of the elbow joint, it passes between the biceps brachii and the brachioradialis muscles to pierce the deep fascia and become the *lateral antebrachial cutaneous nerve.*

The branch supplying the coracobrachialis muscle derives its fibers from C7 and usually arises from the main nerve before that nerve penetrates the muscle. Occasionally, the branch comes directly from the lateral cord of the brachial plexus. The branches to both heads of the biceps brachii muscle and to the brachialis muscle arise from the nerve after it has emerged from the coracobrachialis muscle.

The branch supplying the brachialis muscle subdivides and descends to help in the innervation of the elbow joint; other filaments supply the brachial artery and the deep brachial artery and its nutrient humeral branch. Fibers innervating the periosteum on the distal anterior aspect of the humerus are reputedly distributed with these vascular filaments.

The lateral antebrachial cutaneous nerve passes deep to the cephalic vein and soon divides into anterior and posterior branches. The *anterior branch* descends along the anterior aspect of the radial side of the forearm to the wrist and ends at the base of the thenar eminence.

Anterior view

Note: Only muscles innervated by musculocutaneous nerve shown

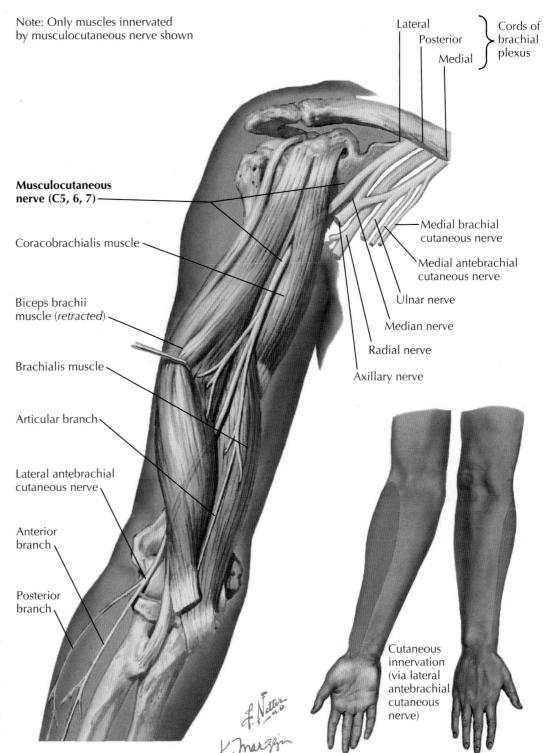

Lateral
Posterior
Medial
} Cords of brachial plexus

Musculocutaneous nerve (C5, 6, 7)

Coracobrachialis muscle

Biceps brachii muscle (*retracted*)

Brachialis muscle

Articular branch

Lateral antebrachial cutaneous nerve

Anterior branch

Posterior branch

Medial brachial cutaneous nerve

Medial antebrachial cutaneous nerve

Ulnar nerve

Median nerve

Radial nerve

Axillary nerve

Cutaneous innervation (via lateral antebrachial cutaneous nerve)

Anterior (palmar) view   **Posterior (dorsal) view**

At the wrist, it lies in front of the radial artery and gives off branches that penetrate the deep fascia to supply this part of the artery. The terminal branches of the anterior branch of the lateral antebrachial cutaneous nerve communicate with corresponding branches from the palmar cutaneous branch of the median nerve. The *posterior branch* is smaller. It curves around the radial border of the forearm and breaks up into branches that supply a variable area of skin and fascia over the back of the forearm. These branches also communicate with branches of the posterior antebrachial cutaneous nerve and with the superficial terminal branch of the radial nerve.

The areas of skin supplied by the lateral antebrachial cutaneous nerve include sensory receptors, hairs, arrectores pilorum muscles, glands, and vessels. However, these terminal cutaneous branches show considerable individual variation in the territories they supply.

Plate 2.15

Upper Limb: PART I

RADIAL NERVE

The *radial nerve* (C5 to C8, T1) is the largest branch of the brachial plexus and is the main continuation of its *posterior cord*. In the axilla, it lies behind the outer end of the axillary artery on the subscapularis, latissimus dorsi, and teres major muscles. Leaving the axilla, it enters the arm between the brachial artery and the long head of the triceps brachii muscle.

Continuing downward and accompanied by the deep brachial artery, the nerve pursues a spiral course behind the humerus, lying close to the bone in the shallow radial nerve sulcus. It passes between the long and medial and medial and lateral heads of the triceps brachii muscle and then lies deep to the lateral head. On reaching the distal third of the arm at the lateral margin of the humerus, it pierces the lateral intermuscular septum to enter the anterior compartment of the arm. Then it descends anterior to the lateral epicondyle of the humerus and the articular capsule of the elbow joint, lying deep in the furrow between the brachialis muscle medially and the brachioradialis and extensor carpi radialis longus muscles laterally. At this point, it divides into its *deep* and *superficial branches*.

In the axilla, the radial nerve gives off the small *posterior brachial cutaneous nerve* and a muscular branch to the long head of the triceps brachii muscle.

In the arm, the radial nerve supplies muscular, cutaneous, vascular, articular, and osseous branches. The first muscular branch is long and slender, arising as the nerve enters the radial nerve sulcus; it accompanies the ulnar nerve to the lower arm to supply the distal part of the medial head of the triceps brachii muscle and to furnish twigs to the elbow joint. A second, larger branch arises from the nerve as it lies in the radial nerve sulcus; it soon subdivides into smaller branches that enter the medial head of the triceps brachii muscle, with some twigs to the humeral periosteum and bone. A stouter subdivision supplies the lateral head of the triceps brachii muscle. It descends through the muscle accompanied by the medial branch of the deep brachial artery. It then penetrates and supplies the anconeus

muscle and sends branches to the humerus and the elbow joint.

Anterior to the lateral intermuscular septum, the radial nerve gives muscular branches to the lateral part of the brachialis, brachioradialis, and extensor carpi radialis longus muscles and, occasionally, to the extensor carpi radialis brevis. Vascular branches and twigs are furnished to the elbow joint.

Three cutaneous branches arise from the radial nerve above the elbow—the *posterior brachial cutaneous,*

inferior lateral brachial cutaneous, and *posterior antebrachial cutaneous nerves.*

NERVE SUPPLY TO THE ELBOW

Nerves reach the joint anteriorly from the musculocutaneous, median, and radial nerves and posteriorly from the ulnar nerve and the radial nerve branch to the anconeus muscle.

Posterior view

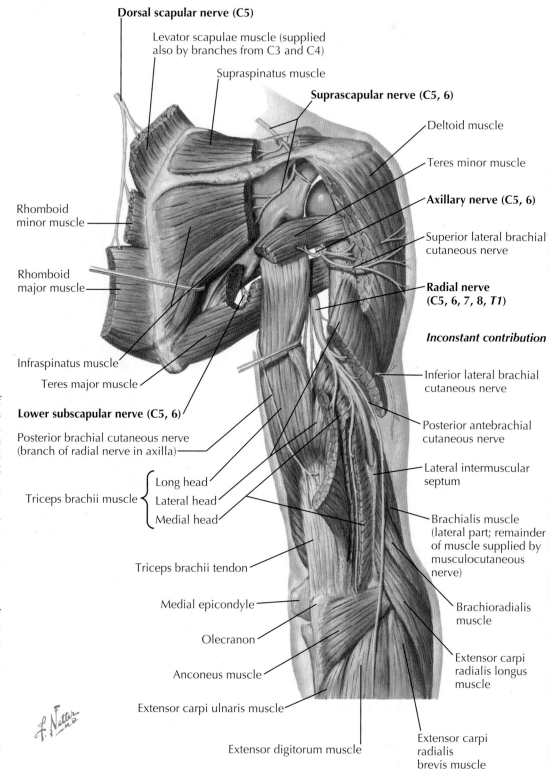

Dorsal scapular nerve (C5)

Levator scapulae muscle (supplied also by branches from C3 and C4)

Supraspinatus muscle

Suprascapular nerve (C5, 6)

Deltoid muscle

Teres minor muscle

Axillary nerve (C5, 6)

Superior lateral brachial cutaneous nerve

Radial nerve (C5, 6, 7, 8, *T1*)

Inconstant contribution

Inferior lateral brachial cutaneous nerve

Posterior antebrachial cutaneous nerve

Lateral intermuscular septum

Brachialis muscle (lateral part; remainder of muscle supplied by musculocutaneous nerve)

Brachioradialis muscle

Extensor carpi radialis longus muscle

Extensor carpi radialis brevis muscle

Rhomboid minor muscle

Rhomboid major muscle

Infraspinatus muscle

Teres major muscle

Lower subscapular nerve (C5, 6)

Posterior brachial cutaneous nerve (branch of radial nerve in axilla)

Triceps brachii muscle { Long head / Lateral head / Medial head

Triceps brachii tendon

Medial epicondyle

Olecranon

Anconeus muscle

Extensor carpi ulnaris muscle

Extensor digitorum muscle

Plate 2.16

Upper Arm and Elbow

BLOOD SUPPLY OF THE UPPER ARM

SUPERFICIAL VEINS

The subcutaneous veins of the limb are interconnected with the deep veins of the limb via perforating veins.

Certain prominent veins, unaccompanied by arteries, are found in the subcutaneous tissues of the limbs. The *cephalic* and *basilic veins,* the principal superficial veins of the upper limb, originate in venous radicals in the hand and digits.

Anastomosing longitudinal *palmar digital veins* empty at the webs of the fingers into longitudinally oriented dorsal digital veins. The *dorsal veins* of adjacent digits then unite to form relatively short *dorsal metacarpal veins,* which end in the *dorsal venous arch.* The radial continuation of the dorsal venous arch is the *cephalic vein,* which receives the dorsal veins of the thumb and then ascends at the radial border of the wrist. In the forearm, it tends to ascend at the anterior border of the brachioradialis muscle, with tributaries from the dorsum of the forearm. In the cubital space, the obliquely ascending *median cubital vein* connects the cephalic and basilic veins (see Plate 2.12). Above the cubital fossa, the cephalic vein runs in the lateral bicipital groove and then in the interval between the deltoid and pectoralis major muscles, where it is accompanied by the small deltoid branch of the thoracoacromial artery. At the deltopectoral triangle, the cephalic vein perforates the costocoracoid membrane and empties into the *axillary vein.* An *accessory cephalic vein* passes from the dorsum of the forearm spirally and laterally to join the cephalic vein at the elbow.

The *basilic vein* continues to the ulnar end of the venous arch of the dorsum of the hand. It ascends along the ulnar border of the forearm and enters the cubital fossa anterior to the medial epicondyle of the humerus. After receiving the median cubital vein, the basilic vein continues upward in the medial bicipital groove, pierces the brachial fascia a little below the middle of the arm, and enters the neurovascular compartment of the medial intermuscular septum, where it lies superficial to the brachial artery. In the distal axilla, it joins the brachial veins to form the *axillary vein.*

The *median antebrachial vein* is a frequent collecting vessel of the middle of the anterior surface of the forearm (see Plate 2.12). It terminates in the cubital fossa in the median cubital vein or in the basilic vein. It sometimes divides into a *median basilic vein* and a *median cephalic vein,* which borders the biceps brachii laterally and joins the cephalic vein. The median antebrachial vein may be large or absent.

BRACHIAL ARTERY

The brachial artery, the continuation of the axillary artery, extends from the lower border of the teres major muscle to its bifurcation opposite the neck of the radius in the lower part of the cubital fossa. The course of the vessel may be marked with the limb in right-angled abduction, when the vessel lies on a line connecting the middle of the clavicle with the midpoint between the epicondyles of the humerus. The brachial artery lies deep in the neurovascular compartment of the arm, flanked by the brachial veins on either side and by the median nerve anterior to it. The median nerve gradually crosses the artery to lie medial to it in the cubital fossa. These structures are crossed by the bicipital aponeurosis at the elbow.

BRACHIAL ARTERY IN SITU

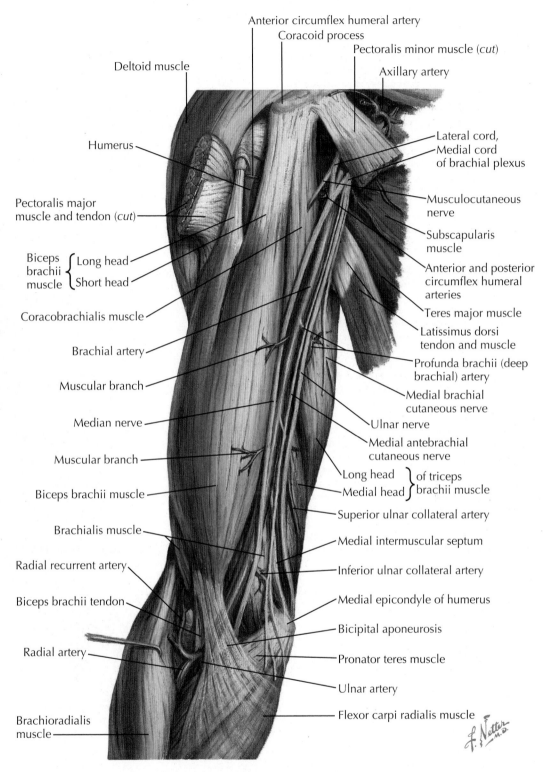

Anterior circumflex humeral artery
Coracoid process
Pectoralis minor muscle (*cut*)
Deltoid muscle
Axillary artery
Humerus
Lateral cord,
Medial cord
of brachial plexus
Pectoralis major muscle and tendon (*cut*)
Musculocutaneous nerve
Subscapularis muscle
Biceps brachii muscle { Long head / Short head }
Anterior and posterior circumflex humeral arteries
Teres major muscle
Coracobrachialis muscle
Latissimus dorsi tendon and muscle
Brachial artery
Profunda brachii (deep brachial) artery
Muscular branch
Medial brachial cutaneous nerve
Median nerve
Ulnar nerve
Medial antebrachial cutaneous nerve
Muscular branch
Long head / Medial head } of triceps brachii muscle
Biceps brachii muscle
Brachialis muscle
Superior ulnar collateral artery
Medial intermuscular septum
Radial recurrent artery
Inferior ulnar collateral artery
Biceps brachii tendon
Medial epicondyle of humerus
Bicipital aponeurosis
Radial artery
Pronator teres muscle
Ulnar artery
Flexor carpi radialis muscle
Brachioradialis muscle

f. Netter

The brachial artery is a single vessel in 80% of cases. In the other 20% of cases, a superficial brachial artery arises at the level of the upper arm and descends through the arm anterior to the median nerve. Based on its forearm distribution, this artery is a high radial artery in 10% of cases, is a high ulnar artery in 3%, and forms both radial and ulnar arteries in 7%. In the last case, the brachial artery is likely to become the common interosseous artery of the forearm.

The brachial artery provides numerous muscular branches in the arm, principally from its lateral side. An especially large branch supplies the biceps brachii muscle. The branches are named as follows:
1. The *deep brachial artery* arises from the medial and posterior aspects of the brachial artery, below the tendon of the teres major muscle. It is the largest branch of the brachial artery and accompanies the radial nerve in its diagonal course around the

Plate 2.17

Upper Limb: PART I

BLOOD SUPPLY OF THE UPPER ARM (Continued)

humerus. At the back of the humerus, the artery provides an *ascending (deltoid) branch,* which reaches up to anastomose with the descending branch of the posterior circumflex humeral artery. The deep brachial artery then divides into the middle collateral artery and the radial collateral arteries. The *middle collateral artery* plunges into the medial head of the triceps brachii muscle and descends to the anastomosis of vessels at the level of the elbow. The *radial collateral artery* continues with the radial nerve, both perforating the lateral intermuscular septum to enter the anterior compartment. The artery ends in the elbow joint anastomosis, connecting in particular with the radial recurrent artery from the radial artery. All of these branches nourish the muscles of the arm to which they are adjacent.

2. The *nutrient humeral artery* arises about the middle of the arm and enters the nutrient canal on the anteromedial surface of the humerus.

3. The *superior ulnar collateral artery* arises from the brachial artery at or a little below the middle of the arm. It pierces the medial intermuscular septum, descending behind it with the ulnar nerve. With the nerve, it passes behind the medial epicondyle of the humerus to anastomose with the inferior ulnar collateral artery and the posterior ulnar recurrent branch of the ulnar artery.

4. The *inferior ulnar collateral artery* arises from the brachial artery about 3 cm above the medial epicondyle. It divides on the brachialis muscle into anterior and posterior branches. Both of these branches reach the anastomosis around the elbow joint, anterior and posterior to it, respectively.

Brachial veins accompany the artery, one on either side of it. They are formed from the venae comitantes of the radial and ulnar arteries and have tributaries that accompany the branches of the brachial artery, draining the areas supplied by the arteries. The brachial veins contain valves and frequently anastomose with one another. At the lower border of the teres major muscle, the lateral of the two veins crosses the artery to join the more medial one; then, joined by the basilic vein, they form the axillary vein.

BLOOD SUPPLY TO THE ELBOW

The blood supply of the elbow joint comes from the anastomosis of the collateral branches of the brachial artery and the recurrent branches of the radial and ulnar arteries.

CUBITAL FOSSA

Like the axilla, the cubital fossa is a space at the bend of the elbow, where it is helpful to note the important relationships of structures that overlie the elbow joint. It is described as a triangular space, apex downward, and is bound above by a line connecting the epicondyles of the humerus. The converging side borders are muscular, the pronator teres muscle medially and the brachioradialis muscle laterally. The floor of the space is also muscular, consisting of the brachialis muscle of the arm and the supinator muscle of the forearm; deep to these muscles is the elbow joint.

The readily palpable *tendon of the biceps brachii muscle* descends centrally through the space, and its

BRACHIAL ARTERY AND ANASTOMOSES AROUND ELBOW

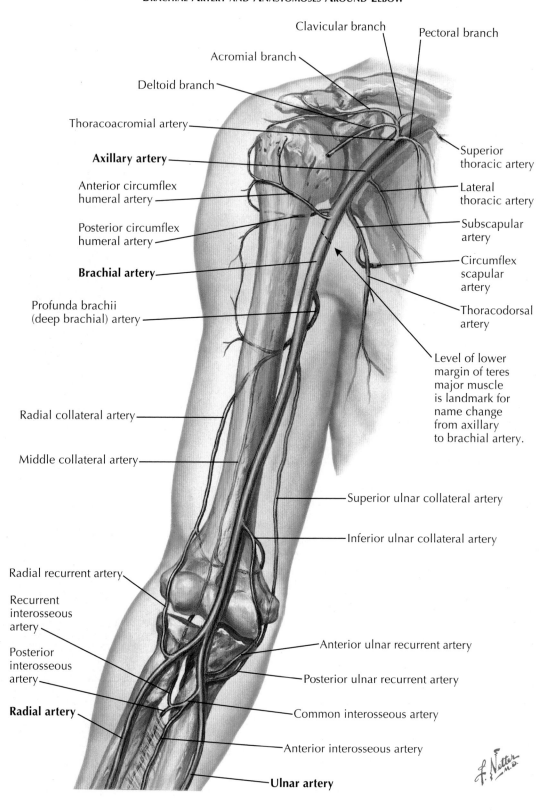

bicipital aponeurosis spans medialward across the brachial artery and median nerve to blend with the forearm fascia over the flexor muscle mass. Directly medial to the biceps brachii tendon, the *brachial artery* divides into the *radial* and *ulnar arteries* in the inferior part of the cubital fossa opposite the neck of the radius.

Although submerged between the brachioradialis and brachialis muscles, the *radial nerve* can be exposed by drawing the brachioradialis muscle lateralward and

can be followed to its bifurcation into deep and superficial branches. Superficially, the *medial cubital vein* crosses obliquely, overlying the bicipital aponeurosis, and a *medial cephalic vein* may, on occasion, lie subcutaneously toward the lateral side of the fossa. The *medial antebrachial cutaneous nerve* crosses the median cubital vein, and the *lateral antebrachial cutaneous nerve* passes deep to the median cephalic vein, if it is present.

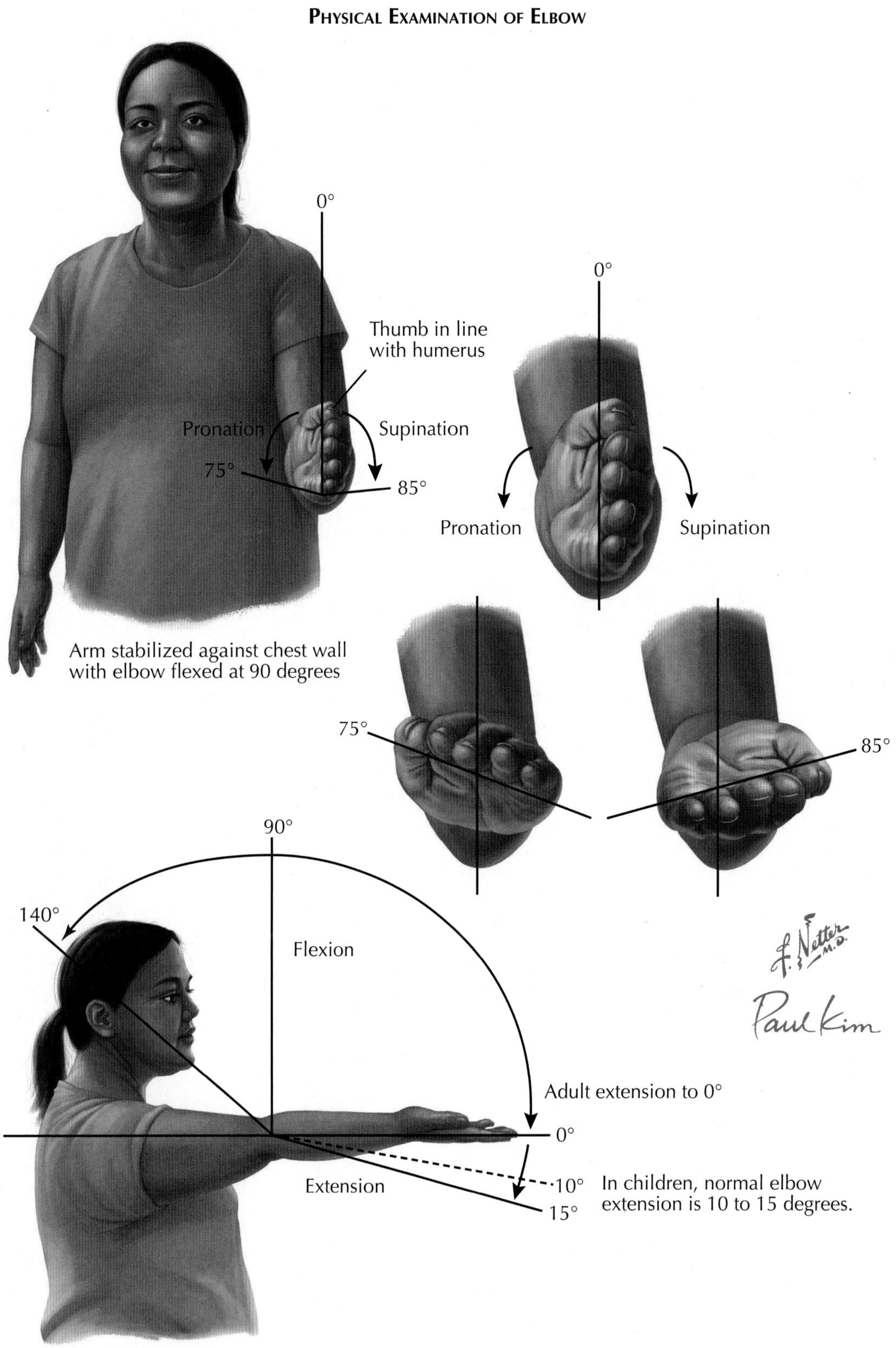

Plate 2.18

Upper Arm and Elbow

PHYSICAL EXAMINATION OF ELBOW

0°

Thumb in line with humerus

Pronation   Supination

75°   85°

Arm stabilized against chest wall with elbow flexed at 90 degrees

0°

Pronation   Supination

75°   85°

90°

Flexion

140°

Adult extension to 0°

0°

Extension

10°   In children, normal elbow extension is 10 to 15 degrees.

15°

PHYSICAL EXAMINATION OF THE UPPER ARM AND ELBOW

Physical examination of the upper arm and elbow should progress in a systematic manner from inspection to palpation to assessment of range of motion, and it should include a thorough neurovascular examination. Specific tests can also be included, when appropriate, for detecting certain pathologic processes. Findings should be compared with those from the contralateral side, and a global limb assessment should be performed to rule out overlapping or contributing disorders.

Inspection can note swelling, ecchymosis, abrasions, or lacerations from acute traumatic injuries or muscle atrophy and scars from chronic conditions or prior surgeries. The carrying angle of the elbow should be assessed to determine the presence of malalignment from prior trauma or skeletal growth disturbance. This angle is formed by the humerus and ulna with the hand and forearm fully supinated and the elbow fully extended and measures 10 to 20 degrees of valgus, with slightly more valgus on average in females than males. Valgus (cubitus valgus) or varus (cubitus varus) malalignment is diagnosed when the carrying angle is greater than or less than these normal values, respectively.

Palpation should be performed to detect sites of tenderness, deformity, and swelling or effusion that further indicate the presence of an acute or chronic injury or pathologic process. The subcutaneous nature of much of the elbow allows several important structures to be easily palpable (see Plate 2.1). Anteriorly, this includes contents of the antecubital fossa, such as the distal biceps tendon, brachial artery, and median nerve. The medial epicondyle and ulnar nerve are noted medially. Laterally, this includes the lateral epicondyle, the radial head, and the "soft spot." A joint effusion is best detected in the soft spot, a normal depression in the posterolateral aspect of the elbow that is defined by the lateral epicondyle, the tip of the olecranon, and the radial head. Finally, the tip of the olecranon and the distal triceps tendon are prominent landmarks posteriorly.

Elbow range of motion is assessed in flexion and extension, as well as with forearm pronation and supination, and includes evaluation of both active and passive motion. The normal flexion-extension arc of the elbow ranges from 0 degrees to 140 to 150 degrees, plus or minus 10 degrees. The normal pronation-supination arc ranges from 75 to 80 degrees of pronation to 80 to 85 degrees of supination. Pronation and supination should be assessed with the elbow in 90 degrees of flexion, with the thumb-up position considered neutral rotation. The functional range of elbow motion needed to complete most activities of daily living has been shown to range from 30 to 130 degrees (flexion-extension) and from 50 to 50 degrees (pronation-supination). Therefore considerable motion loss at the elbow may be tolerated. Typically, extension is the first motion lost with most pathologic conditions around the elbow.

A thorough neurovascular examination of the upper extremity should include motor and sensory testing of all relevant peripheral nerves (axillary, musculocutaneous, median, radial, ulnar), palpation of distal pulses (radial, ulnar), and assessment of capillary refill.

Plate 2.19

Upper Limb: PART I

HUMERAL SHAFT FRACTURES

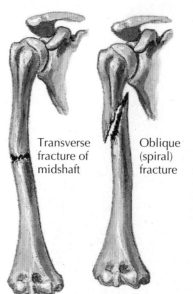
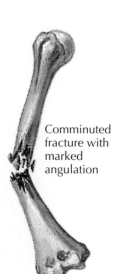

Transverse fracture of midshaft

Oblique (spiral) fracture

Comminuted fracture with marked angulation

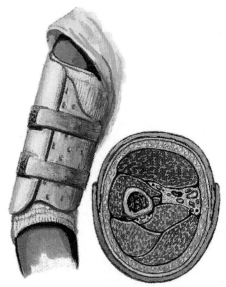

After initial swelling subsides, most fractures of shaft of humerus can be treated with functional brace of interlocking anterior and posterior components held together with Velcro straps.

HUMERAL SHAFT FRACTURES

INJURY TO THE UPPER ARM

Whenever a patient presents with a possible humeral fracture, inspect the upper arm for swelling, ecchymosis, deformity, and open wounds. Palpate the area of maximal tenderness, and assess the joint above (shoulder) and below (elbow) for injury. Always perform a thorough distal neurovascular examination. After a fracture of the humeral shaft, the arm should be supported and immobilized. When gross fracture angulation occurs, emergency care personnel should restore overall alignment of the arm by applying longitudinal traction. This is best accomplished with conscious sedation of the patient to avoid patient guarding and muscle spasm that may prevent adequate reduction of the fracture. Once the fracture is reduced, someone must maintain alignment of the fracture manually while a well-padded splint is applied to the arm to provide stability and maintain the reduction. For humeral shaft fractures, a coaptation splint typically works best. The entire injured limb can then be placed in a sling for added comfort.

FRACTURE OF SHAFT OF HUMERUS

Fractures of the humeral shaft are generally due to direct trauma and can present as different fracture patterns, such as transverse, spiral or oblique, and comminuted. Nonsurgical treatment is acceptable in most instances, but the choice of treatment is based on the type and location of the fracture, concomitant injuries, and age and condition of the patient. For closed fractures, a coaptation splint or a collar and a lightweight, hanging arm cast may be placed initially. About 10 days after injury, when the initial swelling has subsided, the patient is fitted with a fracture brace, which allows the patient to exercise the hand, wrist, elbow, and shoulder while maintaining fracture alignment.

Fractures of the humeral shaft usually heal with no significant deformity and with excellent function. Surgical fixation may be indicated for (1) segmental fractures that cannot be satisfactorily aligned, (2) associated injuries or fractures of the elbow that make early motion desirable or produce a floating elbow, (3) polytrauma that requires several weeks of bed rest (fracture alignment may be difficult to maintain if gravity cannot be used to help control it and surgical fixation can help mobilize the patient), (4) pathologic fractures, (5) open

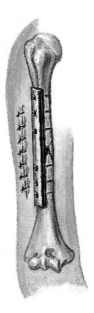

Open reduction and fixation with compression plate indicated under special conditions.

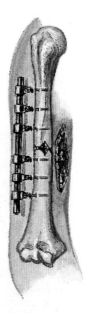

Fracture aligned and held with external fixator. Most useful for wounds requiring frequent changes of dressing.

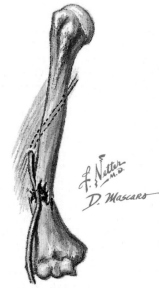

Entrapment of radial nerve in fracture of shaft of distal humerus may occur at time of fracture; must also be avoided during reduction.

fractures, (6) fractures associated with vascular injury, and (7) radial nerve palsy that develops after reduction. Radial nerve palsy can be due to nerve entrapment in the fracture site. This complication may necessitate surgical exploration and decompression of the nerve. At the same time, open reduction and internal fixation is performed to avoid further injury to the nerve by moving fracture fragments.

Internal fixation usually utilizes a compression plate. Intramedullary fixation may be performed, particularly in the case of pathologic fractures. External fixators can be used for open humeral shaft fractures. The usual indication is a large soft tissue wound that requires frequent changes of dressing. External fixation allows access to the wound while still maintaining satisfactory fracture alignment and position.

Plate 2.20

Upper Arm and Elbow

FAT PAD LESIONS

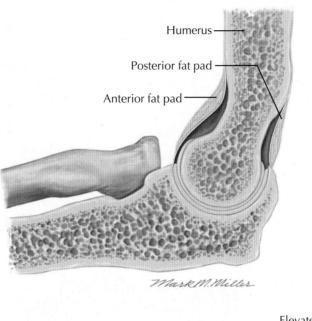

Humerus

Posterior fat pad

Anterior fat pad

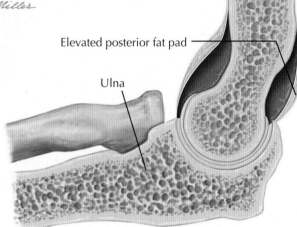

Elevated posterior fat pad

Ulna

Mark M. Miller

INJURY TO THE ELBOW

Injuries of the elbow range from nondisplaced fractures to complex fracture-dislocations. When a patient presents with an elbow injury, inspect the elbow and forearm for swelling, ecchymosis, deformity, and wounds such as abrasions or lacerations that could raise concern for an open injury. Palpate the area of maximal tenderness, and assess the joint above (shoulder) and below (wrist) for additional areas of tenderness that could suggest other injuries. Palpation can also be utilized to detect for the presence of a joint effusion associated with the injury. An effusion is, again, most easily noted by palpation over the posterolateral "soft spot" of the elbow. Elbow range of motion may be limited after an acute injury owing to pain or because of the presence of a fracture or dislocation. A thorough distal neurovascular examination is mandatory to determine whether damage has occurred to any neurovascular structures from the injury. After an elbow fracture, the elbow should be supported and immobilized with a well-padded posterior elbow splint incorporating both the upper arm and forearm. The entire injured limb can then be placed in a sling for added comfort.

Plain radiographs should initially be obtained to determine the fracture pattern and/or dislocation type after a significant elbow injury. Nondisplaced fractures may not be easy to detect on plain radiographs, but a fat pad sign may be present. In an uninjured elbow, the

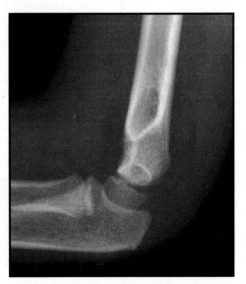

anterior fat pad of the distal humerus may be seen on a lateral radiograph, whereas the posterior fat pad is typically absent. A fracture near the elbow, such as a radial head or neck fracture or a supracondylar fracture, causes an elbow effusion that elevates both the anterior and posterior fat pads, making both evident on a lateral radiograph. Displaced fractures may be easily seen on plain radiographs, but computed tomography (CT) or magnetic resonance imaging (MRI) is often needed to better delineate the fracture pattern, particularly

Lateral radiograph of elbow in a 5-year-old female who fell from playground equipment, sustaining injury to left elbow. Radiograph shows elevation of anterior and posterior fat pads. No apparent fracture is evident on this view, but subsequent radiographs confirmed presence of a nondisplaced supracondylar humerus fracture.

when the fracture extends into the elbow joint or when multiple fracture fragments are present. MRI may also be useful to determine whether a collateral ligament injury has occurred. After an elbow dislocation, it is essential to obtain plain radiographs after the joint has been successfully reduced to confirm that the elbow is properly aligned. Multiple views should be taken, because the presence of a persistent dislocation or subluxation of the joint may be missed with only one radiographic view.

Plate 2.21   Upper Limb: PART I

DISTAL HUMERUS FRACTURES

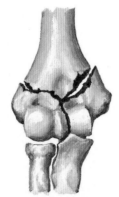

Intercondylar (T or Y) fracture of distal humerus

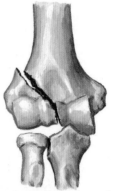

Fracture of lateral condyle of humerus. Fracture of medial condyle less common.

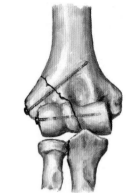

Fractured condyle fixed with one or two compression screws

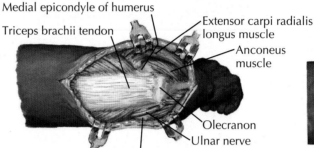

Medial epicondyle of humerus

Triceps brachii tendon

Extensor carpi radialis longus muscle

Anconeus muscle

Olecranon

Ulnar nerve

Medial epicondyle

Open (transolecranon) repair. Posterior incision skirts medial margin of olecranon, exposing triceps brachii tendon and olecranon. Ulnar nerve identified on posterior surface of medial epicondyle. Incisions made along each side of olecranon and triceps brachii tendon.

Olecranon osteotomized and reflected proximally with triceps brachii tendon

FRACTURE OF DISTAL HUMERUS

In adults, fractures of the distal humerus often require surgical fixation because they are usually caused by a high-energy injury and frequently are comminuted and/or intraarticular in location. Fracture patterns include supracondylar, transcondylar, intercondylar (T or Y), lateral or medial condyle, or epicondyle and isolated capitellar or trochlear fractures. Intraarticular fractures may be difficult to adequately assess on plain radiographs; therefore CT scans may be needed.

Surgical fixation can be with plates and screws, or screws alone, depending on the particular fracture pattern. Joint replacement has also become an option for distal humerus fractures that may be too comminuted to be stabilized with plates and screws.

COMPLEX INTRAARTICULAR FRACTURES

Comminuted intraarticular fractures of the distal humerus are among the more challenging orthopedic injuries, and their reconstruction requires considerable surgical skill. The major complications include restricted elbow motion and early degenerative joint disease.

Surgical fixation of comminuted intraarticular fractures can be problematic: the distal fragments are small, minimizing the number of available screw sites, and the fragments are primarily cancellous bone, which compromises screw purchase. In addition, the surface of the distal fracture fragments is primarily articular cartilage, which must be protected, and the complex topography

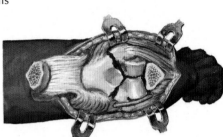

Articular surface of distal humerus reconstructed and fixed with transverse screw and buttress plates with screws. Ulnar nerve may be transposed anteriorly to prevent injury. Lateral column fixed with posterior plate and medial column fixed with plate on the medial ridge.

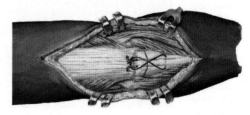

Olecranon reattached with longitudinal Kirschner wires and tension band wire wrapped around them and through hole drilled in ulna

of this region can make reconstruction of the normal anatomy difficult.

The structure of the distal humerus is conceptualized as two bony columns diverging from the shaft. The medial column includes the medial pillar of the distal humerus, the medial condyle and epicondyle, and the trochlea. The lateral column includes the lateral pillar of the distal humerus, the lateral epicondyle and condyle, and the capitellum. To approach and fix

intraarticular fractures of the distal humerus, an intraarticular osteotomy of the olecranon is usually performed and the olecranon and the aponeurosis of the triceps brachii muscle are reflected proximally, exposing the entire distal humerus. The ulnar nerve is also identified and typically transposed as part of the surgical approach. Internal fixation of the distal humerus first involves reconstructing the articular surface and holding the fragments together with transverse

Plate 2.22   Upper Arm and Elbow

TOTAL ELBOW ARTHROPLASTY FOR DISTAL HUMERUS FRACTURE

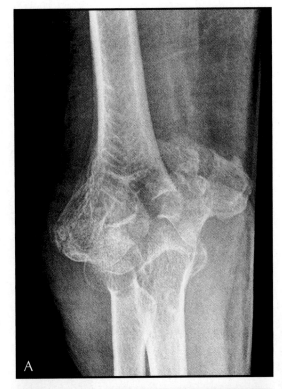

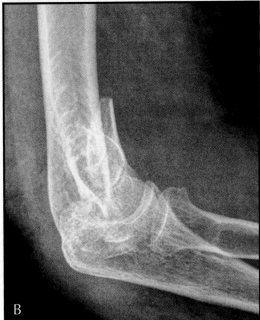

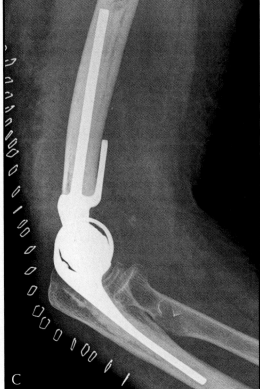

Anteroposterior (**A**) and lateral radiographs (**B**) of comminuted, distal humerus fracture. In elderly patients with poor bone quality, total elbow arthroplasty (**C**) allows early range of motion and function for these injuries.

FRACTURE OF DISTAL HUMERUS (Continued)

Kirschner wires or lag screws. The articular surface is then reattached to the shaft with plates and screws to provide stability in both the anteroposterior and mediolateral planes. Current techniques utilize bicondylar plating with precontoured plates that match the anatomy of the distal humerus. Bicondylar plating can be performed with the plates at right angles to one another (medial plate and posterolateral plate) or straight across from one another (medial plate and lateral plate). The olecranon is reattached with a precontoured plate to fit the olecranon or a tension band wire (see Plate 2.21). Newer surgical approaches have been developed and are now being utilized to avoid the need for an olecranon osteotomy while still providing enough visualization of the distal humerus from appropriate fixation. This can speed up recovery after surgery and avoids the risk of developing a nonunion at the osteotomy site.

Total elbow arthroplasty has also become an option for comminuted distal humerus fractures. In elderly patients with poor bone quality, such fractures may be unable to be stably fixed with plates and screws. Joint replacement allows early range of motion and function for these otherwise devastating elbow injuries, without requiring bony healing. In younger patients with severely comminuted distal humerus fractures that cannot be reconstructed with plates and screws, elbow hemiarthroplasty is becoming a surgical alternative in select cases. This replacement of only the humeral side of the elbow is a newer option in this patient population that is typically considered too active for a complete elbow replacement.

Early elbow range of motion is important after plating or elbow arthroplasty to avoid stiffness. Protected active and active-assisted exercises (flexion-extension, pronation-supination) are encouraged soon after surgery to maintain range of motion in the elbow joint.

FRACTURES OF LATERAL CONDYLE

Fractures of the lateral condyle can involve the capitellum alone or extend medially to involve the lateral portion of the trochlea (see Plate 2.21). Fractures of the lateral condyle are more common than those of the medial condyle and are usually displaced and require surgical fixation. As with any intraarticular fracture, open reduction and internal fixation is performed to

Plate 2.23

Upper Limb: PART I

CAPITELLUM FRACTURES

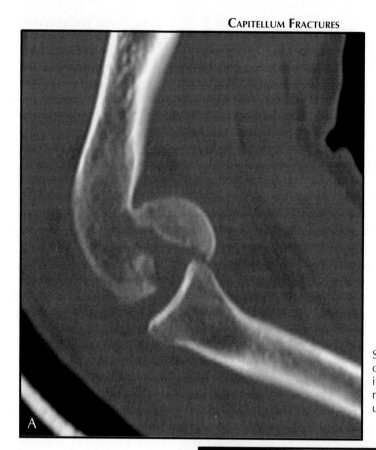

Sagittal CT (**A**) image of a type I coronal shear fracture of the capitellum that was treated with open reduction and internal fixation (**B**) using headless screws.

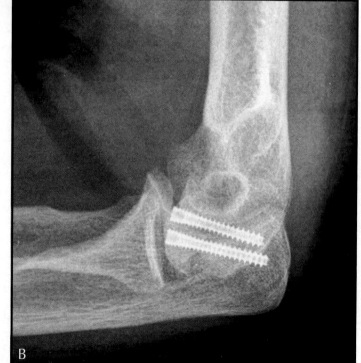

FRACTURE OF DISTAL HUMERUS (Continued)

reestablish the articular surface as accurately as possible and to allow early active motion. A plate and screws or screws alone can be used for fixation, depending on the fracture pattern. In fractures of the lateral condyle, both in adults and in children, it is important to preserve all of the soft tissue attachments, particularly posterolaterally, to maintain the blood supply to the fragment. With rigid internal fixation, the patient can begin active motion as soon as the soft tissues have healed.

FRACTURES OF CAPITELLUM

Fractures of the capitellum alone are uncommon and may be difficult to diagnose if the fracture fragment is very small. Any effusion within the elbow joint together with displacement of the fat pads on plain radiographs suggests either a capitellar fracture or other nondisplaced fracture near the elbow.

There are four types of capitellar fractures. The type I (Hahn-Steinthal) fracture is a coronal fracture that involves a large part of the osseous portion of the capitellum and is typically treated with open reduction and internal fixation with one or two screws. This method makes early joint motion possible in rehabilitation. These screws often need to be placed on the articular surface in an anterior to posterior direction and therefore are headless and countersunk. The type II (Kocher-Lorenz) fracture is a sleeve fracture that involves primarily the articular cartilage with very little underlying bone. The fragment is often too small to be fixed, and treatment includes excision of the fragment.

Type II fractures cause few subsequent problems in the elbow joint. Type III fractures are comminuted and also may be difficult to fix, and a type IV fracture is similar to a type I fracture, except that it extends more medially and includes a major portion of the trochlea.

FRACTURES OF MEDIAL EPICONDYLE

The medial epicondyle is the common origin of several flexor muscles of the hand and wrist. When the medial epicondyle is fractured, the flexor muscles pull the fragment distally. The injury is often accompanied by valgus instability of the elbow if the collateral ligament is affected and by injury to the ulnar nerve. If there is significant valgus instability of the elbow, the epicondyle must be reduced to its anatomic position and secured with a pin or a screw. During the surgical procedure, care must be taken to protect the ulnar nerve from injury, and ulnar nerve transposition may be necessary.

Plate 2.24

Upper Arm and Elbow

RADIAL HEAD AND NECK FRACTURES

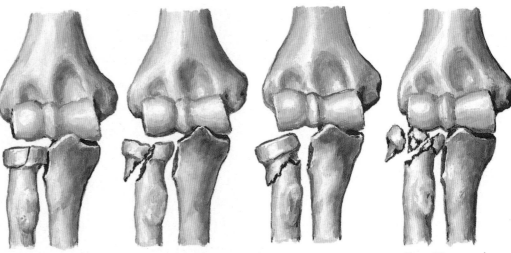

Type I: nondisplaced or minimally displaced

Type II: displaced single fragment (usually >2 mm) of the head or angulated (usually >30 degrees) of the neck

Type III: severely comminuted fractures of the radial head and neck

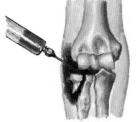

Hematoma aspirated, and 20–30 mL of lidocaine injected to permit painless testing of joint mobility

Elbow passively flexed. Blocked flexion or crepitus is indication for excision of fragments or, occasionally, entire radial head.

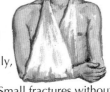

Small fractures without limitation of flexion heal well after aspiration with only sling support.

FRACTURE OF HEAD AND NECK OF RADIUS

Fractures of the radial head occur primarily in adults, whereas fractures of the radial neck are more common in children. The usual causes of these injuries are indirect trauma, such as a fall on the outstretched hand, and, less commonly, a direct blow to the elbow. Radial head and neck fractures are generally classified into four groups. In type I fractures, the fracture is nondisplaced or minimally displaced. Type II fractures refer to displaced fractures of the joint margin or neck with a single fracture line. Type III fractures are comminuted fractures of the head or neck. Type IV fractures are associated with dislocation of the elbow.

Diagnosis of a radial neck or head fracture may be difficult. Pain, effusion in the elbow, and tenderness to palpation directly over the radial head or neck are the typical manifestations. If the fracture is displaced, a "click" or crepitus over the radial head or neck is detected during forearm supination or pronation. Radiographic findings in nondisplaced fractures are minimal, and the radiograph often shows only swelling in the elbow with a fat pad sign. Any radiographic evidence of fat pad displacement accompanied by tenderness over the radial head or neck strongly suggests a fracture.

Treatment of a radial head or neck fracture depends on careful clinical and radiographic evaluation. Type I fractures can be managed nonoperatively if they appear

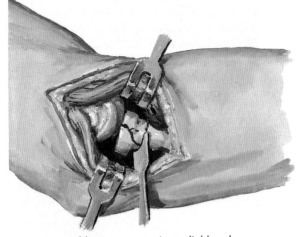

Excision of fragment or entire radial head via posterolateral incision. Radial head should be replaced with a prosthesis in patients with certain complex fractures.

Comminuted fracture of radial head with dislocation of distal radioulnar joint, proximal migration of radius, and tear of interosseous membrane (Essex-Lopresti fracture)

nondisplaced or minimally displaced on radiographs and demonstrate no evidence of a mechanical block on elbow range of motion. To determine the presence of a mechanical block, the elbow joint can be aspirated to remove the bloody effusion, followed by injection of lidocaine into the joint to relieve pain and allow a thorough examination. The examiner can then move the elbow painlessly through a full range of motion to assess the degree of flexion and extension and of pronation and supination and to detect any crepitus or blocked motion due to a displaced fragment. If the range of motion is adequate and there is no bone block or significant crepitus, then the elbow is placed in a posterior splint for a few days. After this period, the patient can remove the splint and begin active range-of-motion exercises for the injured elbow. Frequent follow-up radiographs are necessary to detect any late displacement of the fracture fragment.

Plate 2.25

Upper Limb: PART

IMAGING OF RADIAL HEAD FRACTURES

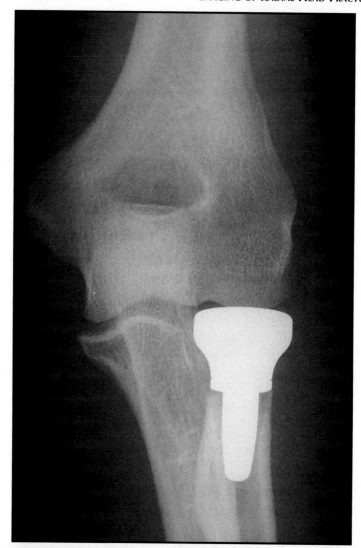

Anteroposterior radiograph of the elbow demonstrates placement of a radial head replacement following comminuted radial head fracture.

FRACTURE OF HEAD AND NECK OF RADIUS (Continued)

Controversy surrounds the treatment of displaced (type II) and comminuted (type III) fractures of the radial head or neck and fractures associated with limited range of motion due to a fracture fragment. Surgical fixation is indicated for fractures with one or two large, displaced fragments that can be effectively reduced and stabilized with a plate and/or screws or Kirschner wires. Comminuted fractures that cannot be adequately reduced and stabilized with surgery usually require excision of the radial head. When the radial head is removed, the annular ligament must be preserved to maintain the integrity of the ligament complex of the proximal radioulnar joint. Radial head implants can be placed after radial head excision, but care should be taken to avoid oversizing the prosthesis, which can limit elbow range of motion. A radial head replacement should always be used after resection of the radial head when an Essex-Lopresti injury is present (fracture of the radial head with dislocation of the distal radioulnar joint and disruption of the interosseous membrane). In an Essex-Lopresti fracture, the radius will migrate proximally if the radial head is not replaced after excision, which is very debilitating to the entire forearm complex (see Plate 2.24). Placement of a radial head implant prevents proximal migration of the radius and minimizes long-term complications.

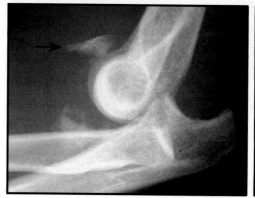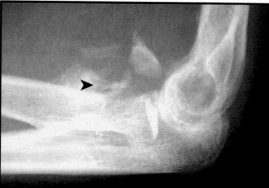

Pre- (*left*) and postreduction (*right*) lateral radiographs of the elbow demonstrate a terrible triad injury consisting of (1) an elbow dislocation with (2) a coronoid fracture (*arrow*) and (3) a radial head fracture (*arrowhead*).

Dislocations of the elbow with comminuted fractures of the radial head or neck (type IV) are serious injuries that usually involve significant soft tissue injury. Both the joint capsule and the collateral ligaments of the elbow can be damaged, and the joint injury can lead to stiffness or persistent instability, osteoarthritic changes, and myositis ossificans. If surgery is appropriate and feasible, these type IV injuries should be surgically repaired early or replaced to decrease the occurrence of complications, such as stiffness or instability and myositis ossificans. Radial head fractures can also be associated with other injuries about the elbow, such as fractures of the capitellum, coronoid process, or olecranon. The combined injury pattern of an elbow dislocation associated with both a radial head and a coronoid process fracture has been termed a *terrible triad injury.*

Plate 2.26

Upper Arm and Elbow

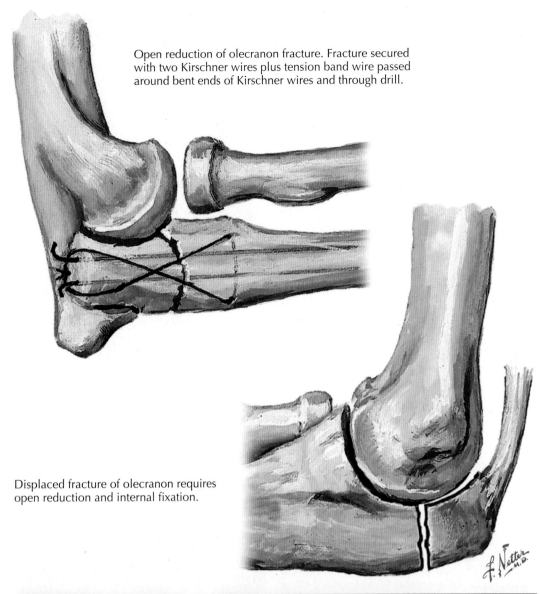

Open reduction of olecranon fracture. Fracture secured with two Kirschner wires plus tension band wire passed around bent ends of Kirschner wires and through drill.

Displaced fracture of olecranon requires open reduction and internal fixation.

FRACTURE OF OLECRANON

Olecranon fractures are caused by a direct blow to the elbow or an indirect avulsion injury, such as a fall on an outstretched hand while the triceps is contracting. Nondisplaced fractures of the olecranon can be treated with posterior splinting or a cast, but displaced fractures are best stabilized with open reduction and internal fixation. These fractures are typically intraarticular; therefore care should be taken to appropriately reduce and align the joint surface during surgical fixation, regardless of technique utilized. Fixation with a tension band wire using screws or Kirschner wires is common in more simple fracture patterns. The tension band technique acts to convert the tensile forces through the fracture that are causing displacement into compressive forces that will allow fracture reduction and healing. If the fracture is too comminuted or too distal (extends to the coronoid or proximal ulnar shaft), a tension band technique is typically not adequate for fracture stability. Interfragmentary compression utilizing plate fixation is the preferred method of treatment in this situation. Precontoured plates that match the anatomy of the olecranon are now available and routinely used. The plate is positioned along the subcutaneous border of the ulna, however, and may require removal after fracture healing owing to its very superficial location.

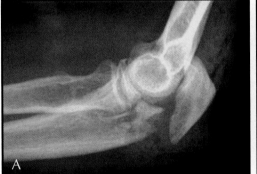
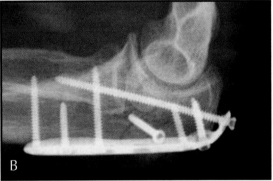

(**A**) Lateral radiograph of a displaced olecranon fracture. (**B**) A precontoured plate and screws are preferred for open reduction and internal fixation in a fracture with more distal extension.

Excision of the olecranon and triceps repair is an alternative method of treating isolated, displaced fractures if the coronoid process, collateral ligaments, and anterior soft tissues remain intact. Typically, this procedure is considered in extraarticular fractures or in fractures that are too comminuted to be stably fixed. The triceps brachii tendon covers the posterior aspect of the joint capsule before it attaches to the olecranon, and a broad expanse of the aponeurosis of the triceps brachii muscle joins the deep fascia of the forearm distal to the elbow. This expanse ensures good posterior stability of the elbow joint after olecranon excision. Up to 70% of the olecranon can be excised without resultant instability if the collateral ligaments are intact. Because the triceps brachii muscle is a primary extensor of the forearm, it must be accurately reattached to the distal fragment of the ulna after the olecranon is excised to maintain adequate elbow extension.

Plate 2.27

Upper Limb: PART I

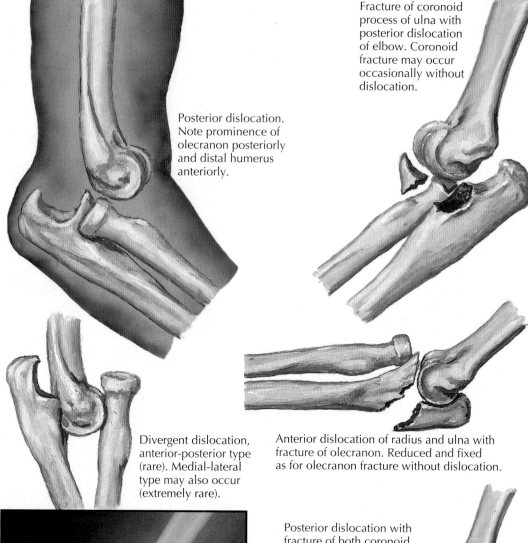

Posterior dislocation. Note prominence of olecranon posteriorly and distal humerus anteriorly.

Fracture of coronoid process of ulna with posterior dislocation of elbow. Coronoid fracture may occur occasionally without dislocation.

Divergent dislocation, anterior-posterior type (rare). Medial-lateral type may also occur (extremely rare).

Anterior dislocation of radius and ulna with fracture of olecranon. Reduced and fixed as for olecranon fracture without dislocation.

Posterior dislocation with fracture of both coronoid process and radial head. Rare but serious; poor outcome even with good treatment. May require total elbow replacement.

Lateral radiograph of posterolateral elbow dislocation

DISLOCATION OF ELBOW JOINT

Dislocations of the elbow joint are the most common dislocations after those of the shoulder and finger joints. Swelling, pain, and pseudoparalysis of the arm are acute signs and symptoms of dislocation, and elbow deformity is visible on both clinical and radiographic examinations.

Acute elbow dislocations are classified as anterior or posterior, with the direction determined by the position of the radius and ulna relative to the humerus. In addition to the anterior or posterior direction of dislocation, the forearm bones can be displaced medially or laterally. Posterior elbow dislocations are by far the most common type and usually result from a fall on an outstretched hand. The rare, but extensively studied, anterior dislocation of the elbow is usually an open injury and may lacerate the brachial artery. Rarely, the radius and ulna dislocate in different directions, an injury called a "divergent" dislocation.

Dislocations of the elbow result in a pattern of ligamentous injury that depends on the direction of dislocation. For posterior dislocations, the ligamentous injury typically starts laterally, disrupting the lateral collateral ligament complex first; it then moves medially, disrupting the anterior and posterior joint capsule, followed by the medial collateral ligament complex. Elbow dislocations are sometimes accompanied by fractures as well, including fractures of the medial or lateral epicondyle, olecranon, radial head or neck, or coronoid process of the ulna. As discussed previously, the combined injury pattern of an elbow dislocation associated with both a radial head fracture and a coronoid fracture has been termed a *terrible triad injury.* Fracture-dislocations of

the elbow, especially displaced fractures of the olecranon, coronoid process, and radial head, often require surgical fixation to ensure long-term stability and function of the joint. An avulsed medial epicondyle can become wedged inside the joint during reduction of the dislocation. Only occasionally can closed manipulation free the avulsed fragment from within the joint; arthrotomy is usually needed to remove the fragment and return it to its anatomic position.

REDUCTION OF DISLOCATION OF ELBOW JOINT

A posterior dislocation of the elbow is reduced with distal traction. While an assistant secures the proximal humerus, the examiner applies traction in the line of the forearm, holding the forearm supinated, and then gently flexes the elbow joint to allow the humerus to reduce into the olecranon fossa. If the elbow is reduced

Plate 2.28

Upper Arm and Elbow

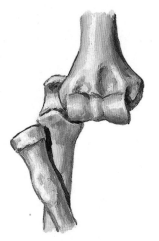

Lateral dislocation
(uncommon)

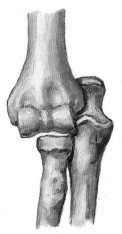

Medial dislocation
(very rare)

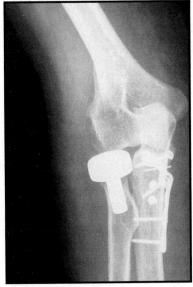

Postoperative radiograph of a terrible
triad injury of the elbow surgically
treated with radial head replacement
and open reduction and internal
fixation of the coronoid fracture

Reduction of dislocation of elbow joint

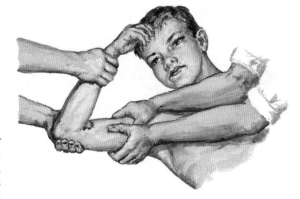

Examiner grasps patient's
wrist and applies traction
to forearm, keeping elbow extended
as far as possible; assistant supplies
countertraction. Examiner's hand at elbow
applies gentle downward pressure on proximal
forearm to release coronoid process from olecranon
fossa and also corrects medial or lateral deviation.

Elbow gently flexed as traction and countertraction maintained. Slight "click" usually heard
or felt as reduction occurs. Elbow then tested
through full range of motion. Reduction may
be accomplished without anesthesia in some
cases, but axillary block, intravenous, or even
general anesthesia is needed for some patients.
Same procedure is used for lateral, medial, or
divergent dislocation with appropriate medial,
lateral, or compressive pressure applied.

DISLOCATION OF ELBOW JOINT (Continued)

immediately after dislocation, complete muscle relaxation may not be needed; if treatment is delayed, conscious sedation, axillary block, or general anesthesia is
used to induce complete muscle relaxation. Radiographs should be obtained after reduction to confirm
that the elbow joint is concentrically aligned. The
neurovascular status of the distal limb is checked both
before and after reduction. Any changes or abnormalities suggest entrapment of a nerve or vessel during
reduction, which must be relieved promptly to prevent
a long-term deficit.

After the initial reduction, the examiner moves the
elbow through a full range of motion to assess its stability and to check for crepitus in the joint. Crepitus
strongly suggests loose fracture fragments in the joint.
If the elbow remains stable through a full range of
motion, it is immobilized in 90 degrees of flexion in a
posterior splint. The neurovascular status of the limb is
monitored frequently while the elbow is splinted to
ensure that a deficit does not develop. Most isolated
elbow dislocations are treated with splint immobilization for a short period of time (1–2 weeks) before
beginning range-of-motion exercises. The exercises
should be gentle initially but as active as symptoms
permit. The physician's assessment of the degree of
stability after reduction helps determine what range
of motion to allow and when to begin the exercise
program.

Elbow dislocations cause few long-term complications. By far the most common is residual joint stiffness,
particularly loss of extension. Although some degree of

stiffness almost always persists, early active motion can
minimize this problem. The older the patient, the earlier
active elbow movement should be started.

Myositis ossificans, another complication of elbow
dislocation, results from muscle injury at the time of
dislocation. Myositis ossificans is more likely to develop
after severe injuries, such as those that are high energy
or associated with fractures, and when treatment has
been delayed. Early passive motion is discouraged in

patients with dislocation and muscle injury because
excessive muscle stretching may precipitate the development of myositis.

Recurrent dislocations after an isolated elbow dislocation are uncommon and are thought to be due to
extensive collateral ligament damage (medial and lateral) or an occult fracture. Surgery to repair or reconstruct the collateral ligaments may be necessary in this
situation.

Plate 2.29

Upper Limb: PART I

INJURIES IN CHILDREN

Elbow fractures are more common in children than adults, and treatment can differ greatly from adults because of the healing and remodeling potential of pediatric fractures. Occult fractures are also more common in children, in part because not all of the damaged bone may be ossified. Detecting unossified fractures on plain radiographs can be difficult, and many of the epiphyses in the elbow region ossify late. Comparison radiographs of the uninjured elbow often help in identifying subtle fracture lines and displaced fracture fragments. Any child who presents with a history of fall or injury, tenderness to palpation about the elbow, and a fat pad sign on plain radiographs should be treated for an occult fracture and immobilized in a splint or cast for a minimum of 3 weeks. New callus formation at the presumed fracture site will typically be present on plain radiographs at this time to allow the diagnosis to be confirmed.

SUPRACONDYLAR FRACTURE OF HUMERUS

Supracondylar fractures of the humerus are the most common elbow fracture in children and are much more common in children and adolescents than in adults. In children, the fracture typically involves the thin bone between the coronoid fossa and the olecranon fossa of the distal humerus, proximal to the epicondyles, and the fracture line angles from an anterior distal point to a posterior proximal site. In adults, supracondylar fractures are not usually confined to the extraarticular portion of the distal humerus, as in children, but extend into the elbow joint.

The most frequent cause of supracondylar fractures of the humerus is a fall on the outstretched hand with the elbow extended. By far the most common fracture pattern is an extension-type injury with posterior displacement of the distal fragment; only 5% to 10% of supracondylar fractures are flexion-type injuries with anterior displacement of the distal fragment. Extension-type supracondylar fractures are classified as nondisplaced (type I), partially displaced with the posterior cortex still intact (type II), and completely displaced with no cortical contact between the fragments (type III).

In the evaluation of any fracture, careful assessment of the neurovascular status is important, but this assessment is even more critical in supracondylar fractures of the elbow because of the proximity of the brachial artery and median nerve to the distal spike of the proximal fragment. Neurologic injury or vascular insult and Volkmann ischemic contracture can result from this type of fracture. A direct neurovascular injury may occur from the fracture spike, or neurovascular compromise may occur from severe swelling that accompanies the injury.

Before reduction, the fractured elbow should be splinted in extension so that arterial circulation is not compromised by flexion of the distal fragment. When the injury is evaluated in the emergency department, the neurovascular status of the limb should be carefully determined and monitored. The first focus of management is on reduction of the displaced fracture fragments to alleviate any neurovascular compression if it is present. The supracondylar fracture should be reduced as soon as possible after injury, preferably with the patient under conscious sedation or general anesthesia. Closed reduction is carried out by gentle distraction in the line of the forearm until the humerus is restored to its full length. The medial or lateral angulation is

SUPRACONDYLAR HUMERUS FRACTURES

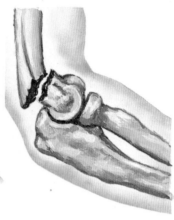

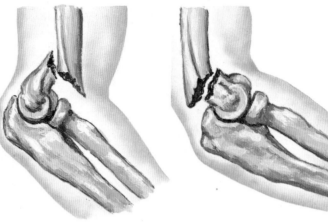

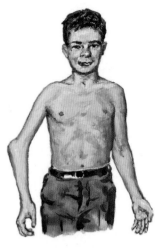

Extension type
Posterior displacement of distal fragment (most common)

Flexion type
Anterior displacement of distal fragment (uncommon)

Malunion producing cubitus varus with reversal of carrying angle is common complication

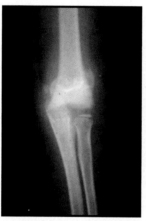
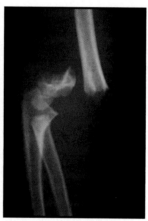

Anteroposterior (*left*) and lateral (*right*) radiographs of displaced supracondylar fracture

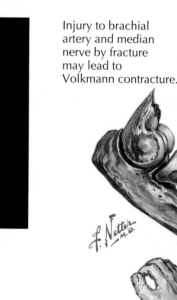

Injury to brachial artery and median nerve by fracture may lead to Volkmann contracture.

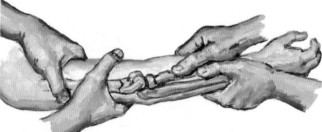

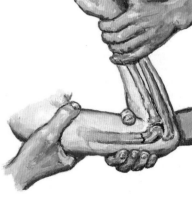

With patient under general anesthesia, reduction accomplished with traction and countertraction, plus gentle manipulative correction of medial or lateral displacement, followed by flexion of elbow beyond 90 degrees.

corrected, and in extension-type injuries the elbow is flexed greater than 90 degrees for added stability. With the elbow in extreme flexion, the posterior periosteum and the aponeurosis of the triceps brachii muscle act as a hinge to maintain the reduction of the fragments. In more stable fractures (some type II fractures), this position may be secure enough with a plaster splint or long-arm cast alone for 4 to 6 weeks to prevent redisplacement of the fracture fragments and allow healing.

In assessing the reduction achieved, displacement in the anteroposterior plane is not nearly as important as the presence of lateral or medial angulation. If the fracture heals with the distal fragment tilted medially or laterally, a significant deformity, either cubitus varus or

Plate 2.30

Upper Arm and Elbow

INJURIES IN CHILDREN (Continued)

ELBOW INJURIES IN CHILDREN

cubitus valgus, results. Varus or valgus angulation after reduction is best diagnosed on an anteroposterior radiograph or a Jones view of the elbow, which reveals a lack of contact between the two bone fragments on one cortex.

If the adequacy of the reduction or if the vascular supply of the limb is in question, the fracture should be treated either with percutaneous pin fixation performed under image intensification or with open reduction and internal fixation. Type III fractures and many type II fractures require pin fixation for stability. Image intensification allows closed reduction of the fracture and percutaneous insertion of two or three Kirschner wires. Open reduction is usually done through a lateral approach to the distal humerus. Pins can be passed in a crossed (medial and lateral pins) or divergent (all lateral pins) pattern, with care to avoid injury to the ulnar nerve when placing any medial pins. After internal fixation, the elbow can be splinted in any angle of flexion to avoid compromising the function of the brachial artery. Vascular exploration and/or repair is rarely needed but may be indicated if a pulseless, unperfused extremity does not improve after fracture reduction and operative fixation.

The major long-term complication of very severe fractures is a change in the carrying angle of the elbow, primarily cubitus varus, owing to incomplete or loss of reduction at the time of treatment. The normal carrying angle of the elbow (10–20 degrees of valgus) is decreased or reversed. Despite the abnormal appearance of the elbow, function is not typically compromised, even with a severe varus deformity. Closed or open reduction and percutaneous pinning of unstable fractures (types II and III) are used to prevent varus deformity. Angular malunions that result in a significant loss of function or cosmetic deformity are best treated with a corrective osteotomy at the site of the original fracture. The alignment of the corrective osteotomy is maintained with a plate and screws or an intramedullary nail. The osteotomy is often supplemented with cancellous bone grafts to ensure healing. Neurologic injury, although not common, does occur and can involve either the median, radial, or ulnar nerve, with median nerve injury the most common. Vascular injury is a devastating complication because it can lead to Volkmann contracture from a resulting missed compartment syndrome. Regardless of the reduction and fixation method, care should be taken once the limb is splinted or placed in a cast to closely monitor it for adequate circulation and a stable neurologic examination. Distal pulses may not always be easily palpable owing to vascular spasm from the injury, but if distal perfusion and capillary refill are normal with no evidence of compartment syndrome, the limb is likely stable. Finally, all elbow fractures can potentially result in decreased motion and stiffness.

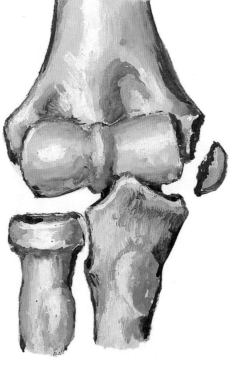

Avulsion of medial epicondyle of humerus

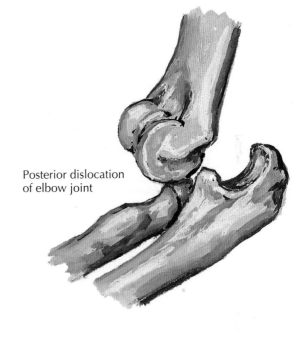

Posterior dislocation of elbow joint

Open reduction and pinning of fracture of lateral condyle

FRACTURES OF LATERAL CONDYLE

A lateral condyle fracture is the second most common elbow injury in children. Typically, it occurs as an avulsion injury of the attached extensor muscles. If not reduced well and securely fixed, this type of fracture tends to lead to significant long-term problems, including nonunion, cubitus valgus, and tardy ulnar neuropathy. Growth arrest of the lateral humerus produces a progressive valgus deformity of the joint, which, in turn, may lead to ulnar nerve palsy later in life. Nondisplaced fractures of the lateral condyle can be treated

with immobilization in a cast. However, because of a significant risk of late displacement of the fracture, the patient must be monitored with frequent radiographic examinations during the first 2 weeks after injury. Displaced fractures require open reduction and pin or screw fixation to maintain a satisfactory reduction and avoid the deformity and neurologic complications associated with this injury.

FRACTURES OF MEDIAL EPICONDYLE

This injury is the third most common elbow fracture in children. It results from a valgus stress applied to the elbow causing an avulsion injury of the medial epicondyle due to contraction of the flexor-pronator muscles. The fracture is frequently associated with a posterior or lateral dislocation of the elbow joint. Dislocation causes the strong ulnar collateral ligament to pull the epicondyle

Plate 2.31

Upper Limb: PART I

INJURIES IN CHILDREN (Continued)

fragment free from the humerus. During reduction of the dislocation, the fragment sometimes becomes trapped in the elbow joint. If not incarcerated in the joint, the fragment may be slightly displaced or rotated more than 1 cm away from the distal humerus. A significantly displaced fragment is sometimes easily palpable and freely movable on the medial aspect of the elbow joint.

Nondisplaced and minimally displaced fractures heal well with splint or cast immobilization. A displaced fragment trapped in the joint as a result of an elbow dislocation requires open reduction to restore joint congruity and stability. Significantly displaced fragments outside the joint may not heal, and some surgeons recommend open reduction and internal fixation. However, even if the fragment fails to unite, long-term complications are few.

FRACTURE OF RADIAL HEAD OR NECK

During a fall on the outstretched hand, the radial head or neck may fracture as it impacts against the capitellum, typically from a valgus stress on an extended elbow. Fractures are usually through the proximal physis and into the radial neck in a Salter II pattern. Significant angulation of the radial head fragment may occur, and if the angulation is greater than 30 degrees the fracture should be reduced with closed manipulation. Reduction is achieved using digital pressure over the angulated head while alternatively supinating and pronating the forearm. Although closed reduction is sufficient for most fractures, severely displaced or angulated fractures of the radial head require percutaneous or open reduction and internal fixation. Even completely displaced fragments should be reduced and fixed in place. In a growing child, the radial head should never be excised, because excision always leads to significant loss of elbow function.

DISLOCATION OF ELBOW JOINT

This childhood injury is less frequent in younger children but commonly seen in boys between 13 and 15 years of age and is frequently associated with athletic injuries. Apparent elbow dislocations in young children or infants should raise concern for a transphyseal fracture of the distal humerus that is the result of child abuse. Radiographs of these fractures may be confused for dislocations because of the lack of ossification of the distal humerus at this age. Most elbow dislocations in children are posterior, as in adults. Associated avulsion fractures of the elbow, particularly avulsion fractures of the medial epicondyle, can occur. With adequate anesthesia, most elbow dislocations can be reduced easily. The elbow is initially placed in a splint after reduction, and for stable, isolated injuries management is similar to that for adults.

SUBLUXATION OF RADIAL HEAD

This injury, also known as nursemaid elbow, is the most common elbow injury in children younger than 5 years and results from longitudinal traction applied to the limb. The annular ligament moves proximally and becomes interposed between the radius and ulna, causing the radial head to subluxate. Clinical findings are characteristic: the injured limb hangs dependent and the child avoids arm use, the forearm is pronated, and any attempt to flex the elbow or supinate the

SUBLUXATION OF RADIAL HEAD

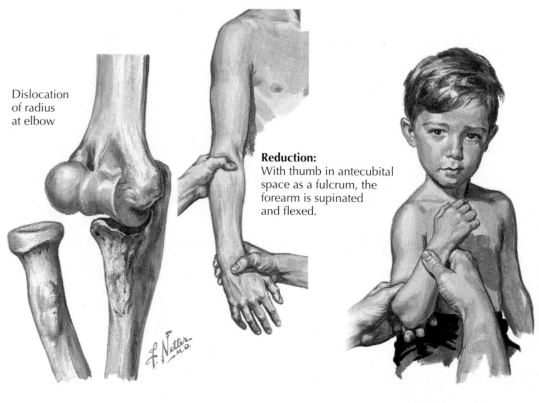

Dislocation of radius at elbow

Reduction: With thumb in antecubital space as a fulcrum, the forearm is supinated and flexed.

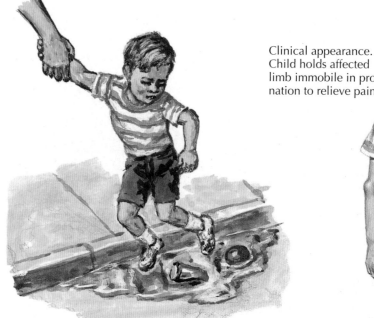

Caused by sudden sharp pull of child's forearm

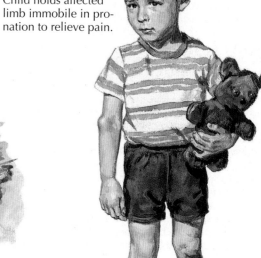

Clinical appearance. Child holds affected limb immobile in pronation to relieve pain.

forearm produces significant pain. Radiographs do not show any significant bone abnormality about the elbow. Physical examination almost always reveals localized tenderness over the radial head. In most patients, reduction can be achieved by complete supination of the forearm, pressure on the radial head, and subsequent elbow flexion. Although this causes a moment of fairly severe pain, supination causes the radial head to slide back into its normal position, and

frequently a "click" is felt as the annular ligament slides back around the radial neck. Reduction brings almost immediate and complete relief of pain, and within a few moments the child begins to use the elbow. If the closed reduction is successful, immobilization is not necessary. The physician should explain the cause of the subluxation to the child's parents and tell them to avoid longitudinal traction on the limb. The risk of recurrent subluxation is minimal.

Plate 2.32

Upper Arm and Elbow

COMPLICATIONS OF FRACTURE

A major objective in the management of fractures and dislocations is to avoid as many complications as possible. The principles of fracture treatment direct the surgeon to reduce the fracture and immobilize it with a cast, splint, or internal/external fixation devices to allow natural healing to occur. A variety of complications, either as a consequence of the injury itself or as a consequence of treatment, can produce serious and permanent problems. Acute complications such as damage to nerves and blood vessels, adult respiratory distress syndrome, and infection usually arise from the injury itself. Complications also develop during the healing process and may lead to irreparable loss of function. Chronic complications include failure of union, deformities, osteoarthritis, joint stiffness, implant failure, and reflex sympathetic dystrophy.

NEUROVASCULAR INJURY

Displacement of fracture fragments or bone ends at a dislocated joint often produces compression or laceration of adjacent vessels and nerves. Critical neurovascular structures (e.g., the brachial plexus) lie deep in the limb, close to the skeleton, which protects them from injuries. A fracture or dislocation makes nerves or vessels vulnerable to injury from sharp bone fragments or from entrapment in the fracture site.

Neurovascular complications must be identified by careful examination immediately after the injury and after any manipulation of the injured limb. Some complications are not immediately evident but do appear 24 to 48 hours after injury. Reexamination and monitoring are essential both during this period and while circumferential compression dressings and casts are in place. Prompt and sometimes aggressive treatment is required to restore function and prevent permanent loss.

Radial Nerve Palsy

The radial nerve is commonly damaged in fractures of the shaft of the humerus (see Plate 2.19). Normally protected in the spiral groove on the humeral shaft, the nerve is easily impaled by a fracture fragment or entrapped in the fracture site. Aggressive manipulation of the fracture during closed reduction may also result in nerve entrapment. Wristdrop is a common long-term consequence of this injury.

Neurovascular Injury to Elbow

A musculoskeletal injury that is frequently associated with neurovascular injury is the supracondylar fracture of the humerus in children. In the most common extension-type fracture, the humeral shaft fragment is displaced anteriorly, impinging on the critical neurovascular structures in front of the elbow. The median, radial, and ulnar nerves are all susceptible to direct injury from the displaced fracture fragment (median nerve most commonly injured), and the brachial artery may be lacerated or entrapped in the fracture site at the time of injury or during closed reduction. Distal neurovascular function must be assessed critically, and manipulative reduction must be very careful and gentle.

JOINT STIFFNESS

Effective immobilization of a fracture or dislocation in a cast or splint, if prolonged, can lead to joint stiffness, which may prove to be a bigger problem than the injury itself. Immobilization lasting more than a few weeks leads to scarring of the joint capsule and contracture of

Neurovascular injuries

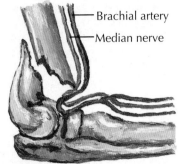
— Brachial artery
— Median nerve

Elbow injuries range from simple nondisplaced fractures to severely displaced supracondylar fractures with entrapment of median nerve or brachial artery, or both. Injured elbow always splinted in position found. Padded wire ladder splint molded to arm and secured with roller bandage.

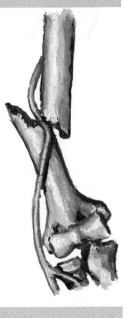
Fracture of shaft of humerus with entrapment of radial nerve in spiral groove

Joint stiffness

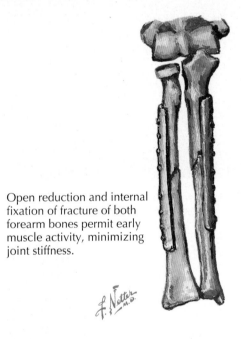

Open reduction and internal fixation of fracture of both forearm bones permit early muscle activity, minimizing joint stiffness.

Functional brace replaces cast 10–14 days after fracture of humeral shaft. Brace provides adequate support for healing yet allows full range of motion of shoulder, elbow, wrist, and fingers.

the muscles, and it also impairs the nutrition of the articular surfaces. With prolonged immobilization, adhesions develop across the articular surfaces, even in joints that had not been injured directly. In addition, prolonged immobilization results in marked atrophy of the muscles in and around the site of injury. Rehabilitation to regain motion can be a long and difficult process that may not restore full function.

Most treatment protocols, either nonoperative or operative, typically recommend beginning range of motion early in the recovery period to avoid the development of stiffness. Nonoperatively, this can be accomplished with use of functional braces that adequately immobilize the injury for healing but still allow range of motion. For example, traditional cast immobilization for a fracture of the humeral shaft requires immobilization of the shoulder and elbow joints in a shoulder spica cast. Such immobilization of both joints for 8 to 10 weeks would lead to a significant loss of function. Conversely, a functional brace allows active range of motion in the shoulder and elbow joints yet

provides adequate support of the healing fracture. A functional brace is applied 10 to 14 days after injury, once the initial swelling has subsided. The brace is adjustable and can be tightened to provide firm support about the arm and maintain acceptable alignment of the fracture. Inability to maintain stable reduction of a fracture or dislocation early in the postinjury period through nonoperative measures is an indication for open reduction and internal fixation. Surgical stabilization will then allow range-of-motion exercises without fear of loss of reduction.

When joint stiffness develops, restoring motion often requires a long-term rehabilitation program. After the patient regains joint motion with gentle passive range-of-motion exercises, active exercises are begun to strengthen the atrophied muscles. When fixed contractures fail to respond to aggressive and prolonged rehabilitation, surgical release of soft tissue may be necessary as a last resort. At the elbow joint, this includes release or excision of the contracted and thickened joint capsule.

Plate 2.33

Upper Limb: PART I

IMAGING OF OPEN AND ARTHROSCOPIC ELBOW DEBRIDEMENT

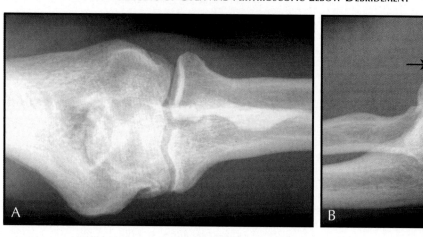

Preoperative (**A**) anteroposterior and (**B**) lateral radiographs of an arthritic elbow demonstrating osteophyte formation and a loose body (*arrow*).

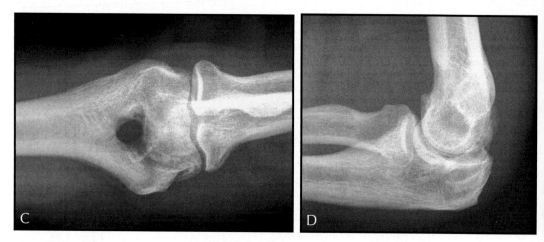

Postoperative (**C**) anteroposterior and (**D**) lateral radiographs following open elbow debridement demonstrating removal of osteophytes and the loose body.

ARTHRITIS

Primary osteoarthritis of the elbow is uncommon, unlike in the hip and knee, and the need for joint replacement in the elbow is much less common than the hip, knee, and shoulder. Elbow arthritis often develops in patients who repetitively load the joint, such as heavy laborers or athletes. It more commonly occurs in males and in the dominant extremity. Symptoms typically include pain and loss of motion. Pain typically occurs at the end ranges of motion, particularly terminal extension, from impingement due to osteophytes. Pain through the midrange of elbow motion is much less common but may develop if the articular cartilage loss is severe enough.

Other common causes of elbow arthritis include inflammatory conditions, most commonly rheumatoid arthritis, and trauma, most commonly after an intraarticular fracture. The elbow is a common site of involvement in rheumatoid arthritis, but the pharmacologic advances in treatment of this disease have made the progression of arthritis and symptoms much less severe. Although advances in implants have helped in the surgical treatment of intraarticular elbow fractures, posttraumatic arthritis can still occur.

Nonoperative management of elbow arthritis is the initial treatment and includes activity modification, range-of-motion exercises, use of braces and other support devices, intraarticular cortisone injections, and administration of nonsteroidal antiinflammatory drugs or disease-modifying antirheumatic drugs.

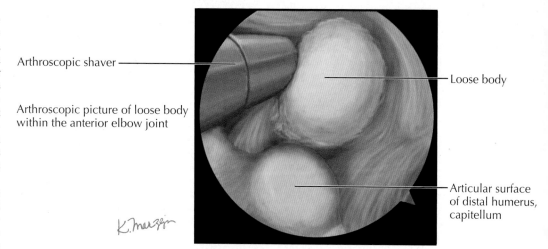

Arthroscopic shaver

Arthroscopic picture of loose body within the anterior elbow joint

Loose body

Articular surface of distal humerus, capitellum

Initial surgical treatments for elbow arthritis include open or arthroscopic debridement procedures. These surgeries are done to improve pain and range of motion and may include removal of loose bodies, osteophyte resection, capsular release or excision, and synovectomy. Recovery time can be shorter after an arthroscopic debridement, but there is a potential risk of neurovascular injury with this technique. This risk is particularly increased in patients who have undergone prior surgery in the elbow, owing to the distortion of normal anatomy. In osteoarthritis, osteophytes commonly form at the tip of the olecranon and the olecranon fossa and at the tip of the coronoid and the coronoid fossa. These bone spurs can cause impingement-type pain at the end ranges of motion, and their removal can help relieve such symptoms. Synovitis is a common source of pain

Plate 2.34

Upper Arm and Elbow

ELBOW ARTHROPLASTY OPTIONS

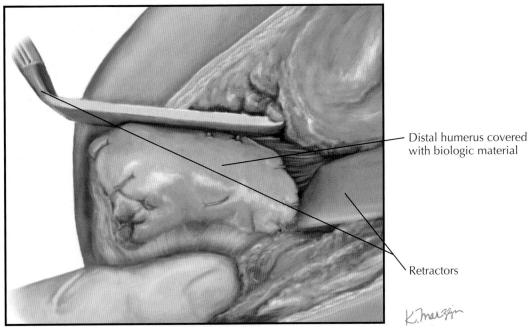

Distal humerus covered with biologic material

Retractors

Intraoperative picture of interpositional arthroplasty of the elbow

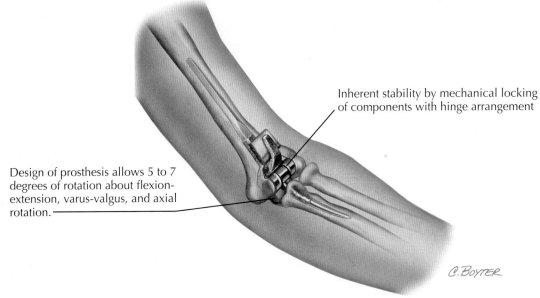

Inherent stability by mechanical locking of components with hinge arrangement

Design of prosthesis allows 5 to 7 degrees of rotation about flexion-extension, varus-valgus, and axial rotation.

ARTHRITIS (Continued)

and limited motion in a patient with rheumatoid arthritis; therefore surgical synovectomy can be beneficial and may also prevent further destruction of cartilage and bone. Finally, ulnar nerve symptoms may develop in an arthritic elbow with significant loss of range of motion, and thus ulnar nerve decompression or transposition is recommended in combination with the debridement procedure in such situations.

Although debridement procedures can provide significant symptom relief, they may not be as beneficial in patients with more advanced arthritis and their effect may wear off over time as the arthritis progresses. In these instances, surgery is aimed at reconstruction of the diseased elbow joint. Most commonly, this is in the form of a total elbow replacement, but other techniques have occasionally been employed, including interpositional arthroplasty, resection arthroplasty, and elbow arthrodesis. Interpositional arthroplasty may be an option in younger patients with severe arthritis, who may be too active for consideration of a total elbow replacement. The procedure involves covering the diseased joint surfaces with a biologic material (e.g., autogenous fascia lata, dermal allograft) to improve pain and range of motion. Resection arthroplasty is not commonly used today as a primary treatment for arthritis because of the resultant instability and dysfunction at the elbow after this procedure, although bony ankylosis can occur. It is primarily considered as a salvage procedure in cases of failed prior surgery and intractable infection.

The typical total elbow arthroplasty is an ulnohumeral replacement, with a stemmed, metallic humeral implant and a stemmed, metallic ulnar implant that articulate through a polyethylene-bearing surface. Both linked and unlinked prosthetic designs are available. Linked implants have a hinged mechanism that can be classified as constrained or semiconstrained on the basis of the absence or presence of side-to-side laxity in the implant. Linked, constrained designs had an unacceptably high failure rate and were abandoned for semiconstrained prostheses. Modern linked, semiconstrained implants allow some side-to-side laxity to decrease stress across the implant and lower the rate of component loosening.

Elbow arthrodesis is also rarely used currently, because fusion in a single position can be difficult for reasonable upper extremity function. It can be considered a salvage procedure in cases of infection and may rarely be considered an option in a young heavy laborer who may place too high a demand on an elbow replacement.

Severe, disabling arthritis is best treated with total elbow arthroplasty. Total joint replacement restores

joint motion and relieves pain by replacing the diseased articular surfaces with a plastic and metal prosthesis. The typical implant is an ulnohumeral arthroplasty, with a stemmed, metallic humeral implant and a stemmed, metallic ulnar implant that articulate through a polyethylene-bearing surface. Both linked and unlinked prosthetic designs are available. Linked implants directly connect the humeral and ulnar components

Plate 2.35

Upper Limb: PART I

IMAGING OF TOTAL ELBOW ARTHROPLASTY DESIGNS

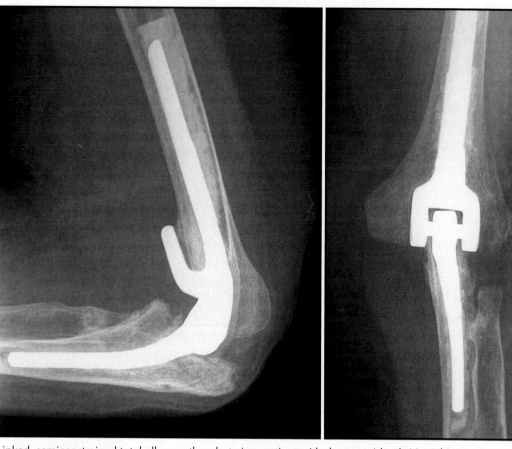

Linked, semiconstrained total elbow arthroplasty in a patient with rheumatoid arthritis. A hinge mechanism is present to link the humeral and ulnar components and provide implant stability.

ARTHRITIS (Continued)

through the bearing surface and are indicated in patients with excessive bone destruction and/or ligamentous destruction or instability. The hinge mechanism can be classified as constrained or semiconstrained on the basis of the absence or presence of side-to-side laxity in the implant. Modern linked designs have a semiconstrained articulation that allows some side-to-side laxity to decrease stress across the implant and lower the rate of component loosening. Unlinked prostheses have no direct connection between the humeral and ulnar components and therefore require the presence of adequate bone stock and intact or reconstructed collateral ligaments. If functional collateral ligaments are not present, implant failure can occur due to instability.

The most common complication of total elbow arthroplasty and the one that causes the most concern over time is implant loosening and resultant instability. Implant survival rates vary depending on the etiology of the underlying arthritis, with survival rates as high as 94% at 15 years in patients with rheumatoid arthritis but as low as 70% at 15 years in the posttraumatic population. This discrepancy is due in part to differences in age and activity level, with patients undergoing total elbow replacement for posttraumatic arthritis usually of a much younger age or higher activity level than rheumatoid arthritis patients.

Arthritic changes at the radiocapitellar joint may also need to be treated with joint replacement, either in isolation or in combination with total elbow arthroplasty.

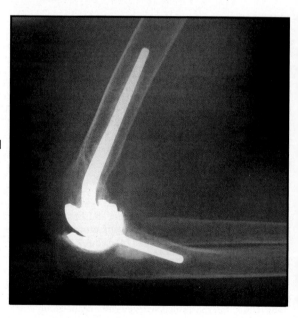

Unlinked total elbow arthroplasty, with no direct connection between the humeral and ulnar components. Adequate bone stock and ligament integrity are needed for implant stability with this design.

This is most commonly addressed with radial head resection or replacement (see Plate 2.25). Though resection of the radial head alone can provide pain relief, over time it may lead to proximal displacement of the radial shaft if the interosseous membrane and distal radioulnar joint are or become deficient. Proximal radial migration can cause pain and dysfunction, particularly with pronation-supination movements. These complications can be avoided by using a radial head replacement. Traditional implants were made of silicone, but this material has been replaced by metallic prostheses because of the high complication rate noted with silicone, particularly the generation of a significant inflammatory response from particulate debris.

Plate 2.36

Upper Arm and Elbow

CUBITAL TUNNEL SYNDROME: SITES OF COMPRESSION

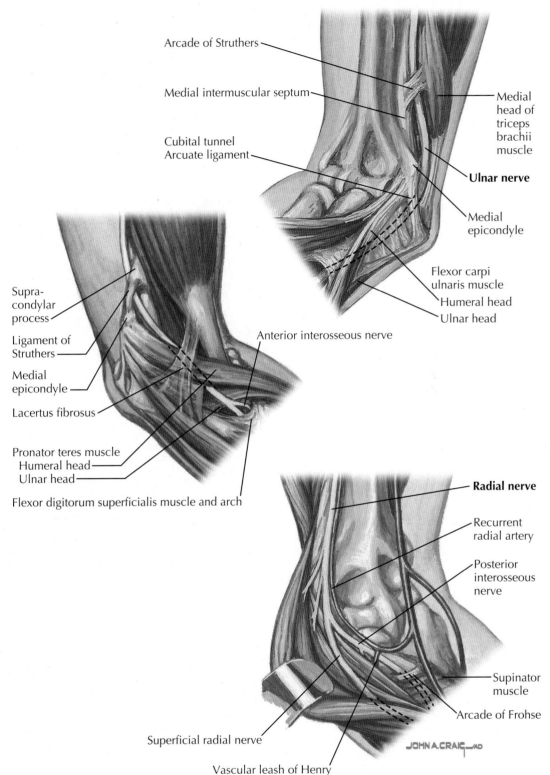

Arcade of Struthers

Medial intermuscular septum

Cubital tunnel
Arcuate ligament

Medial head of triceps brachii muscle

Ulnar nerve

Medial epicondyle

Flexor carpi ulnaris muscle
Humeral head
Ulnar head

Supra-condylar process

Ligament of Struthers

Medial epicondyle

Lacertus fibrosus

Pronator teres muscle
Humeral head
Ulnar head

Flexor digitorum superficialis muscle and arch

Anterior interosseous nerve

Radial nerve

Recurrent radial artery

Posterior interosseous nerve

Supinator muscle

Arcade of Frohse

Superficial radial nerve

Vascular leash of Henry

JOHN A. CRAIG—AD

CUBITAL TUNNEL SYNDROME

Cubital tunnel syndrome is the most common peripheral nerve compression syndrome after carpal tunnel syndrome and involves compression of the ulnar nerve at or around the elbow. The cubital tunnel is a fascial sheath that the ulnar nerve runs through just posterior to the medial epicondyle. Nerve compression can occur through the tunnel or at sites just proximal or distal to it, such as the medial intermuscular septum, the arcade of Struthers, the flexor carpi ulnaris fascia, and the deep flexor-pronator aponeurosis. A subluxating ulnar nerve may also produce symptoms similar to those of nerve compression. Other causes of ulnar nerve symptoms around the elbow can include adhesions from prior surgery; presence of an anomalous muscle (anconeus epitrochlearis); tumors; snapping of the medial triceps; bony changes from arthritis, prior fractures, or heterotopic bone; and anatomic deformities, such as cubitus valgus and cubitus varus. The arcade of Struthers is an aponeurotic band located approximately 8 cm proximal to the medial epicondyle that runs from the medial head of the triceps to the medial intermuscular septum. As the ulnar nerve crosses from the anterior to the posterior compartment in the distal part of the upper arm, it can pass underneath this band, if present. The arcade can particularly become a point of entrapment if the ulnar nerve is transposed anteriorly and the band is not released.

Symptoms of cubital tunnel syndrome include medial-sided elbow pain and paresthesias in the ulnar side of the palm and ulnar one and a half digits of the hand. A positive Tinel sign will re-create these paresthesias by tapping along the course of the ulnar nerve on the medial side of the elbow. The location of the Tinel sign may help localize the exact site of nerve compression. Direct pressure can exacerbate symptoms by increasing compression of the nerve in the cubital tunnel, whereas elbow flexion can cause traction-related deformation of the nerve that increases symptoms. Elbow flexion can also demonstrate evidence of nerve instability, because the ulnar nerve will typically dislocate or subluxate anterior to the medial epicondyle with elbow flexion and cause a snapping or clicking sensation. Snapping of the medial triceps can also create a clicking sensation at the

Plate 2.37

Upper Limb: PART I

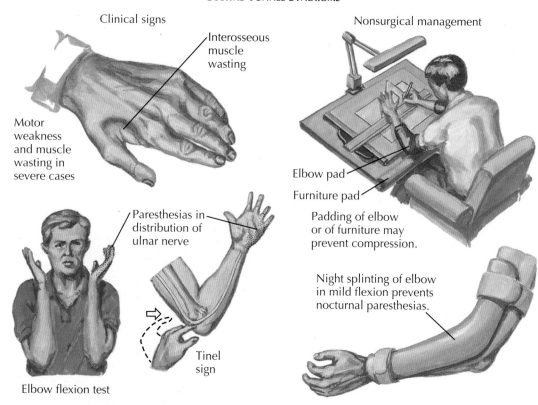

CUBITAL TUNNEL SYNDROME

Clinical signs

Interosseous muscle wasting

Motor weakness and muscle wasting in severe cases

Paresthesias in distribution of ulnar nerve

Elbow flexion test

Tinel sign

Nonsurgical management

Elbow pad

Furniture pad

Padding of elbow or of furniture may prevent compression.

Night splinting of elbow in mild flexion prevents nocturnal paresthesias.

Submuscular transposition of ulnar nerve

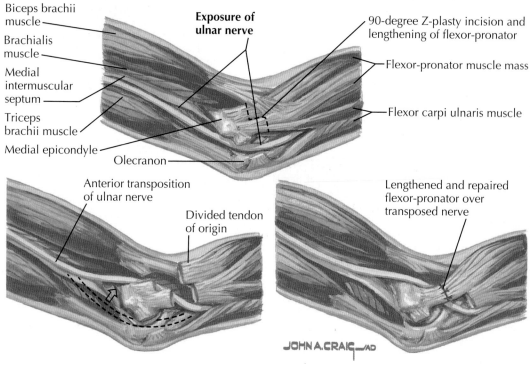

Biceps brachii muscle

Brachialis muscle

Medial intermuscular septum

Triceps brachii muscle

Medial epicondyle

Olecranon

Exposure of ulnar nerve

90-degree Z-plasty incision and lengthening of flexor-pronator

Flexor-pronator muscle mass

Flexor carpi ulnaris muscle

Anterior transposition of ulnar nerve

Divided tendon of origin

Lengthened and repaired flexor-pronator over transposed nerve

JOHN A. CRAIG—AD

CUBITAL TUNNEL SYNDROME (Continued)

elbow with range of motion and must be distinguished. With more chronic or severe cases of entrapment, motor findings can be present, including weakness and wasting of the intrinsic muscles of the hand. When symptoms of cubital tunnel syndrome are present, an electromyographic study of the extremity can be performed both to confirm that the abnormality is localized to the elbow and to determine the severity of the neuropathy. Ulnar nerve compression can occur proximally at the cervical spine or brachial plexus, as well as distally in the forearm, wrist, or hand, although much less commonly.

Nonoperative management is the initial treatment in milder cases of cubital tunnel syndrome and consists of activity modification and splinting to take pressure off the nerve, such as avoidance of repetitive or prolonged elbow flexion and use of splints that keep the elbow in a relatively extended position, particularly at night. Elbow pads can also be worn during the day to prevent compression on the nerve. Surgery is indicated when nonoperative measures fail and involves in situ decompression of the ulnar nerve or ulnar nerve transposition. In situ decompression is often used in milder cases, whereas transposition is performed in severe cases and in situations in which nerve instability is present. When performing an ulnar nerve transposition, all possible sites of nerve entrapment proximal

and distal to the cubital tunnel should be decompressed, in addition to releasing the cubital tunnel. This includes release of the arcade of Struthers if present, excision of the medial intermuscular septum, and release of the flexor carpi ulnaris and flexor digitorum superficialis fascia. Ulnar nerve transposition can be subcutaneous or submuscular and acts to decompress the nerve by placing it in a position anterior to the medial epicondyle. Subcutaneous transposition is more

commonly performed, and in this technique the nerve is stabilized anteriorly by a loose fasciodermal sling. Submuscular transposition is considered in cases of revision surgery and in patients with little to no subcutaneous fat. The flexor-pronator origin is detached with this technique to allow placement of the ulnar nerve anteriorly and adjacent to the median nerve. The flexor-pronator origin is then repaired over the transposed nerve.

Plate 2.38

Upper Arm and Elbow

EPICONDYLITIS AND OLECRANON BURSITIS

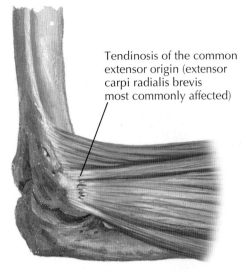

Tendinosis of the common extensor origin (extensor carpi radialis brevis most commonly affected)

Lateral epicondylitis (tennis elbow)

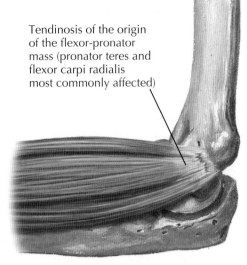

Tendinosis of the origin of the flexor-pronator mass (pronator teres and flexor carpi radialis most commonly affected)

Medial epicondylitis (golfer's elbow)

TENDON AND LIGAMENT DISORDERS AT THE ELBOW

LATERAL EPICONDYLITIS (TENNIS ELBOW)

Lateral epicondylitis, or "tennis elbow," is due to degenerative changes or tendinosis at the origin of the common extensor tendons. The most commonly affected tendon is the extensor carpi radialis brevis (ECRB), but the other common extensor tendons may also be involved. The condition does not typically occur directly at the lateral epicondyle but just distal to this point at the tendon origin. The disease process is a degenerative rather than an inflammatory condition; therefore *tendinosis* is a better descriptive term than *epicondylitis*. The condition most commonly affects patients age 30 to 60 years, and symptoms include chronic lateral elbow pain that is aggravated by wrist extension and/or forearm supination, particularly repetitive activities that involve these motions. Examination of the elbow demonstrates tenderness to palpation just distal and posterior to the lateral epicondyle, at the origin of the ECRB and other common extensor tendons. This pain is worsened by resisted wrist extension and/or resisted long finger extension (isolates the ECRB).

Nonoperative management consists of activity modification, nonsteroidal antiinflammatory drugs, cortisone injections, physical therapy, and splinting for symptom relief. Therapy is focused on both strengthening and stretching of the affected muscles. Splinting can include a wrist splint to place the extensor tendons in a resting position or a counterforce strap to unload the area of tendinosis during lifting activities. Cortisone injections can be beneficial but if too frequent can cause tissue atrophy or even rupture of the common extensor or lateral collateral ligament origin. Surgery is indicated when nonoperative measures fail and involves debridement of the area of tendinosis to remove the degenerated tissue. Arthroscopic techniques are now being used in some instances for this procedure.

MEDIAL EPICONDYLITIS (GOLFER'S ELBOW)

Medial epicondylitis, or "golfer's elbow," is due to degenerative changes or tendinosis at the origin of the flexor-pronator mass. The pronator teres and flexor carpi radialis are the most commonly involved tendons. As with lateral epicondylitis, the disease process involves the tendon origin rather than the epicondyle directly and is a degenerative rather than an inflammatory condition. Therefore tendinosis is a better description for the condition than epicondylitis. Symptoms include chronic medial elbow pain that is aggravated by wrist flexion and/or forearm pronation. Examination of the elbow demonstrates tenderness to palpation just distal and anterior to the medial epicondyle, at the origin of the flexor-pronator mass. Resisted wrist flexion and/or forearm pronation exacerbate the pain. Care must be taken to distinguish symptoms of medial epicondylitis from those that may be coming from the cubital tunnel, because both conditions may occur together. Treatment of medial epicondylitis utilizes similar strategies as treatment for lateral epicondylitis.

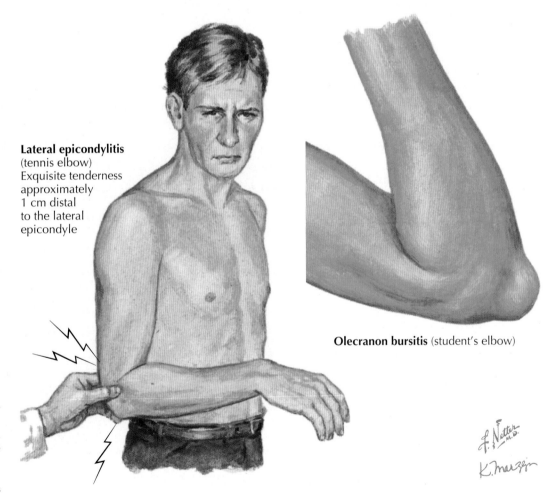

Lateral epicondylitis (tennis elbow) Exquisite tenderness approximately 1 cm distal to the lateral epicondyle

Olecranon bursitis (student's elbow)

Surgical intervention may require addressing the ulnar nerve if symptoms of cubital tunnel syndrome are also present.

OLECRANON BURSITIS

The olecranon bursa is a common site to develop bursitis because of its superficial location and the tendency to put pressure on this area from leaning on the elbow. It may develop from a direct blow, repetitive activities that aggravate the site, inflammatory conditions such as gout and rheumatoid arthritis, or infectious situations. A septic olecranon bursitis can occur from a direct inoculation or may develop secondarily as a complication of treatment for an aseptic olecranon bursitis. Pain and swelling over the olecranon process are common findings, with palpable fluctuance when a significant fluid collection is present. Worrisome signs for infection

Plate 2.39

Upper Limb: PART I

TENDON AND LIGAMENT DISORDERS AT THE ELBOW (Continued)

include warmth, erythema, and more severe pain or purulent drainage from a wound site.

Mild, aseptic cases can be managed with activity modification aimed at avoiding direct pressure on the site, with or without the use of a compressive dressing or short-term splint for further protection. Cases with a significant fluid collection should be aspirated, with the fluid sent for Gram stain, culture, and cell count if infection is a concern. Aseptic cases can be injected with cortisone after aspiration and protected with a compressive dressing or short-term extension splint to help prevent fluid reaccumulation. Septic olecranon bursitis should be treated with antibiotics in combination with serial aspirations or surgical drainage. Occasionally, surgical excision of a chronically inflamed olecranon bursa is performed, such as in inflammatory conditions like gout and rheumatoid arthritis. However, wound healing can be a concern after this procedure, with the risk of developing a nonhealing wound.

RUPTURE OF THE DISTAL BICEPS TENDON

This uncommon injury, which is associated with degenerative changes in the distal biceps tendon, is usually caused by a sudden, forceful flexion of the elbow against resistance. Rupture usually occurs at the tendon insertion on the radial tuberosity and is seen primarily in males 40 to 60 years old. Patients often report the sensation of an acute "pop" in their elbow at the time of injury, followed by the development of swelling, ecchymosis, and cosmetic deformity. If the tendon retracts proximally after rupture, an obvious defect is seen in the antecubital fossa. Occasionally, tendon retraction will not occur after injury because the bicipital aponeurosis remains intact and a clinical deformity may not be obvious. Strength testing after complete rupture typically shows a loss of elbow flexion strength of 15% to 30% and a loss of forearm supination strength of 40% to 50%. Surgical repair of the ruptured tendon is best done within the first several weeks after injury, before the tendon becomes significantly retracted, and can be performed through a single-incision or two-incision technique. Chronic injuries can be difficult to repair because the tendon may be too scarred and retracted to be brought back to bone. In such instances, a graft tissue (e.g., semitendinosus autograft or allograft, Achilles tendon allograft) may be used to span the defect, but results are much less successful than those after a primary, acute repair. Chronic injuries may do well with nonoperative management focused on physical therapy to regain as much strength and function as possible, but supination weakness is typically still noticeable.

RUPTURE OF THE DISTAL TRICEPS TENDON

Rupture of the distal triceps tendon is an even rarer injury than rupture of the distal biceps but may occur

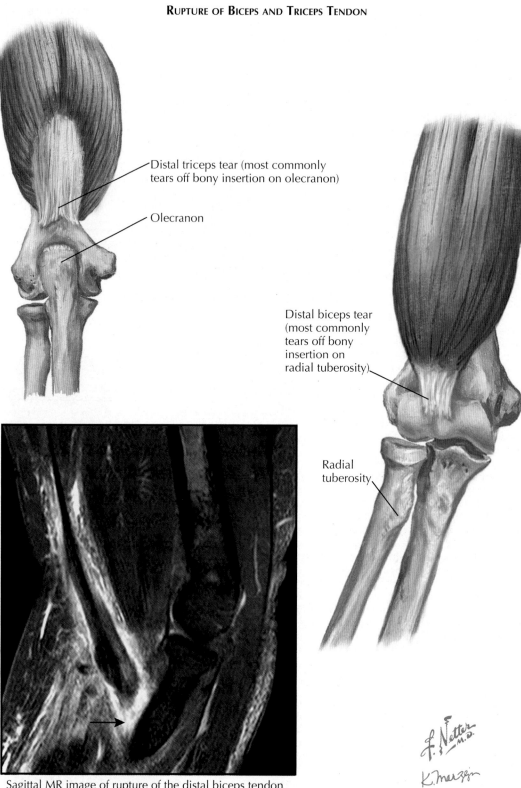

RUPTURE OF BICEPS AND TRICEPS TENDON

Distal triceps tear (most commonly tears off bony insertion on olecranon)

Olecranon

Distal biceps tear (most commonly tears off bony insertion on radial tuberosity)

Radial tuberosity

Sagittal MR image of rupture of the distal biceps tendon from the radial tuberosity (*arrow*)

more equally in both males and females. The mechanism of injury is usually caused by a sudden, forceful extension of the elbow against resistance, and rupture usually occurs at the tendon insertion on the olecranon. As with distal biceps rupture, clinical findings include swelling, ecchymosis, and cosmetic deformity. Strength testing after rupture shows a loss of elbow extension strength. This injury may be more subtle

than distal biceps rupture and may require advanced imaging, such as MRI, to confirm the diagnosis. Surgical repair of the ruptured tendon is also best done within the first several weeks after injury, before the tendon becomes significantly retracted. Chronic injuries also may require reconstructive techniques with graft tissue, such as Achilles tendon allograft, to span a defect.

Plate 2.40

Upper Arm and Elbow

TENDON AND LIGAMENT DISORDERS AT THE ELBOW (Continued)

MEDIAL ELBOW INSTABILITY

The anterior band of the medial or ulnar collateral ligament originates at the midportion of the medial epicondyle and inserts onto the coronoid or sublime tubercle of the ulna and is the primary restraint to valgus stress of the elbow (see Plate 2.6). Disruption or attenuation of this ligament will lead to medial or valgus elbow instability. Typically this is a chronic overuse injury, such as with repetitive overhead use or throwing. Rarely, isolated, acute rupture of this ligament can occur from a valgus load, such as a fall on an outstretched hand. The ligament may also be acutely injured in the setting of an elbow dislocation. In chronic throwing injuries, pain is usually gradual in onset along the medial side of the elbow and associated with the acceleration phase of pitching, when valgus stress across the elbow is greatest. Tearing typically occurs in the midsubstance of the ligament or at the distal insertion with these injuries. Associated pathologic processes may be present in throwers, including ulnar neuritis, posteromedial olecranon osteophytes, loose bodies, or osteochondritis dissecans of the capitellum. Valgus instability may be difficult to elicit in an awake patient on examination because of muscle guarding, but patients will typically complain of pain and/or apprehension with valgus stress testing.

Treatment is initially nonoperative and includes rest and activity modification, followed by a graduated rehabilitation and/or throwing program. Surgery is indicated for failure of nonoperative management and consists of ulnar collateral ligament reconstruction with autograft (i.e., palmaris longus) or allograft (i.e., semitendinosus) tendon and treatment of any associated pathologic processes, such as ulnar nerve decompression. In the rare cases of acute, isolated rupture of the ulnar collateral ligament, surgical repair of the torn ligament can be performed.

POSTEROLATERAL ROTATORY ELBOW INSTABILITY

The ulnar component of the lateral collateral ligament complex, or the lateral ulnar collateral ligament (LUCL), originates from the anteroinferior portion of the lateral epicondyle and inserts onto the supinator crest of the ulna (see Plate 2.6). This ligament is the primary restraint to varus stress of the elbow, and ligament disruption leads to posterolateral rotatory instability. Injuries to the LUCL typically occur from a varus stress to the elbow when it is in an extended and pronated position, such as in a fall on an outstretched hand. The ligament may also be acutely injured in the setting of an elbow dislocation. Rarely, iatrogenic injury can occur during elbow surgery for another reason (e.g., lateral epicondylitis debridement) or from excessive cortisone injections on the lateral side of the elbow. Traumatic

MEDIAL ELBOW AND POSTEROLATERAL ROTATORY INSTABILITY TESTS

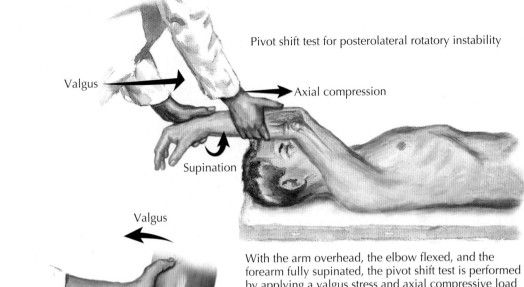

Pivot shift test for posterolateral rotatory instability

Valgus

Axial compression

Supination

With the arm overhead, the elbow flexed, and the forearm fully supinated, the pivot shift test is performed by applying a valgus stress and axial compressive load to the elbow while holding the patient's wrist and forearm. When the elbow is brought into extension with this maneuver, the radial head will subluxate or dislocate, while elbow flexion and/or pronation will reduce the radial head back into anatomic position.

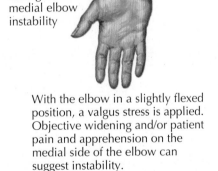

Valgus

Valgus

Valgus stress testing for medial elbow instability

With the elbow in a slightly flexed position, a valgus stress is applied. Objective widening and/or patient pain and apprehension on the medial side of the elbow can suggest instability.

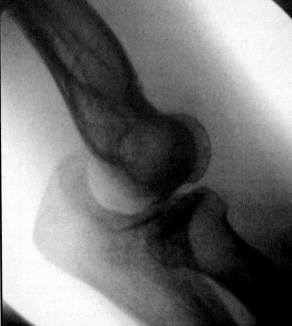

Intraoperative lateral fluoroscopic image demonstrates widening of the elbow joint due to posterolateral instability.

tearing typically occurs at the proximal origin of the ligament. Symptoms include lateral elbow pain and instability complaints, such as catching or giving way of the elbow. As with the medial side of the elbow, instability may be difficult to elicit in an awake patient on examination due to muscle guarding, but patients may complain of pain and/or apprehension with varus or posterolateral stress testing.

Treatment is initially nonoperative and includes rest, activity modification, and a rehabilitation program. A hinged elbow brace may be useful in the acute setting to provide stability while the injury is healing. Surgery is indicated for failure of nonoperative management and consists of LUCL reconstruction with a tendon graft. In cases of acute, isolated rupture of the LUCL, surgical repair of the torn ligament can be performed.

Plate 2.41

Upper Limb: PART I

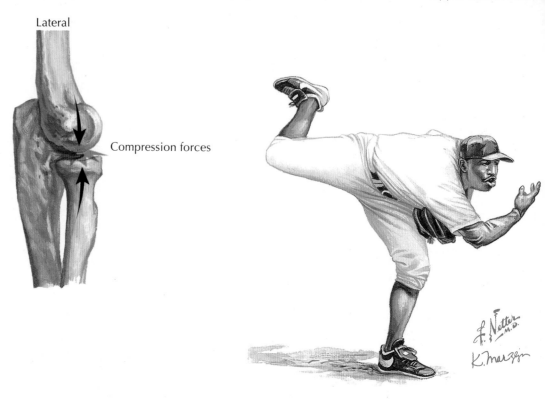

Lateral

Compression forces

Repetitive valgus loads may create compressive forces across the lateral side of the elbow at the typical site of a pathologic process in the capitellum.

OSTEOCHONDRITIS DISSECANS OF THE ELBOW

Osteochondritis dissecans typically occurs in adolescent patients from repetitive high valgus stresses to the elbow, most commonly female gymnasts and male throwers. The repetitive valgus loads may create compressive forces across the lateral side of the elbow at the typical site of a pathologic process in the capitellum. It is thought that these forces cause repetitive microtrauma and vascular insufficiency or injury to the capitellum that can lead to separation of the articular cartilage from the underlying subchondral bone. Genetic factors may also contribute in some cases. The condition occurs after the capitellum has almost completely ossified and involves both the articular cartilage and the underlying bone. If the articular cartilage becomes separated from the subchondral bone, it can become a loose body in the elbow joint.

Symptoms include activity-related lateral elbow pain that may improve with rest from the offending activity. The pain may be dull and poorly localized. Mechanical symptoms, such as clicking or locking, may be present if a loose fragment develops. On examination, tenderness to palpation is noted over the capitellum, and a joint effusion may be present. Range of motion of the elbow may produce crepitus, and patients commonly lack the terminal 10 to 30 degrees of elbow extension. Limitation of elbow flexion or of forearm pronation and supination may also occur but is less common. Plain radiographs can show lucency or fragmentation at the capitellum and a possible loose body if a fragment has broken off. If findings on plain radiographs are equivocal, advanced imaging (CT or MRI) can confirm the diagnosis. MRI

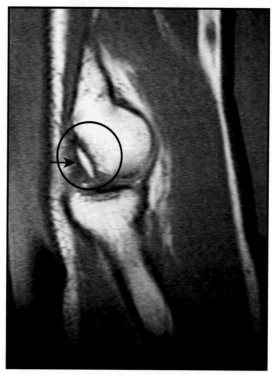

Sagittal MR image of the elbow shows a loose osteochondritis dissecans fragment of the capitellum.

is preferred and can delineate a stable versus unstable lesion by showing intervening fluid between the fragment and subchondral bone.

For intact lesions without mechanical symptoms, treatment is initially nonoperative and includes rest and activity modification, with use of nonsteroidal antiinflammatory agents as needed, followed by a graduated rehabilitation program and return to participation in the sport. Internal fixation of intact lesions may be performed either open or arthroscopically if nonoperative management fails. Displaced lesions or loose fragments typically require surgical excision of the fragment with drilling or microfracture of the capitellar defect. This can usually be done arthroscopically. Newer techniques of articular cartilage implantation are now being attempted in defects to try to restore normal articular cartilage, rather than the fibrocartilage produced by a microfracture technique.

Plate 2.42

Upper Arm and Elbow

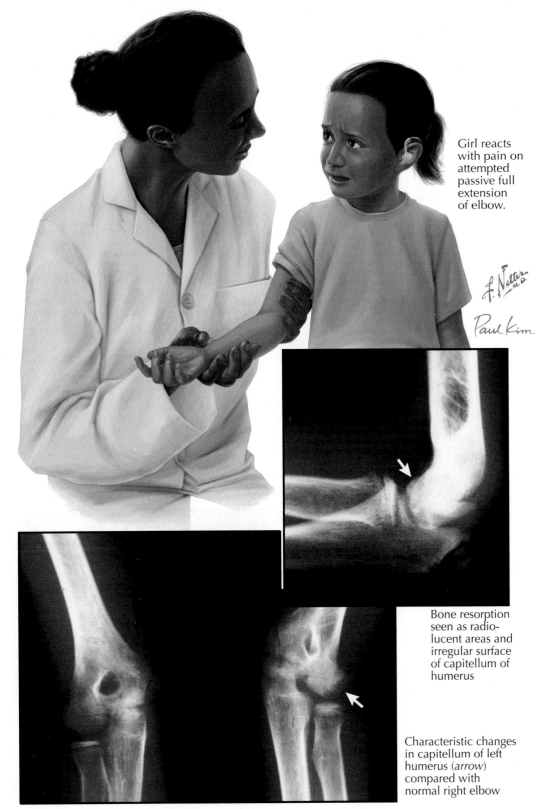

Girl reacts with pain on attempted passive full extension of elbow.

Bone resorption seen as radiolucent areas and irregular surface of capitellum of humerus

Characteristic changes in capitellum of left humerus (*arrow*) compared with normal right elbow

OSTEOCHONDROSIS OF THE ELBOW (PANNER DISEASE)

Panner disease also involves the capitellum and presents in a similar manner as a capitellar osteochondritis dissecans, but in a younger patient population and with a better long-term prognosis. Panner disease typically occurs in the dominant elbow of boys during the period of active ossification of the capitellar epiphysis between 7 and 12 years of age, with a peak at age 9 years. The pathologic process is similar to that of Legg-Calvé-Perthes disease and is believed to be caused by interference in the blood supply to the growing epiphysis, which results in resorption and eventual repair and replacement of the ossification center. The exact cause of this avascular necrosis, or bone infarct, continues to be debated, with popular theories including chronic repetitive trauma, congenital and hereditary factors, embolism (particularly fat), and endocrine disturbances. Whatever factors are responsible, the end result is avascular necrosis. Signs and symptoms are similar to those seen with osteochondritis dissecans, including dull, aching lateral elbow pain that is aggravated by use and may improve with rest. Tenderness and swelling along the lateral side of the elbow with loss of terminal elbow extension are also common. Initial radiographic changes can appear similar to osteochondritis dissecans, with fragmentation of the capitellar epiphysis, but whereas lesions of osteochondritis dissecans can often progress to loose fragments, loose bodies are rare in Panner disease. Typically, the normal radiographic appearance of the capitellum will be reconstituted over time as growth progresses.

Residual deformity of the capitellum is rare. MRI will demonstrate signal changes in the capitellar epiphysis but may be less useful than in osteochondritis dissecans owing to the lack of concern for an unstable lesion or a loose body.

Symptomatic treatment of Panner disease is sufficient, because the condition is self-limited, with the epiphysis becoming revascularized and returning to a normal configuration with time. Rest and activity modification usually relieve the pain and allow gradual return of elbow motion. Use of a long-arm cast or splint for 3 to 4 weeks may be necessary until pain, swelling, and local tenderness subside. The long-term prognosis is excellent, with complete resolution of symptoms in most patients, although a slight loss of elbow extension may persist in some.

Plate 2.43

Upper Limb: PART

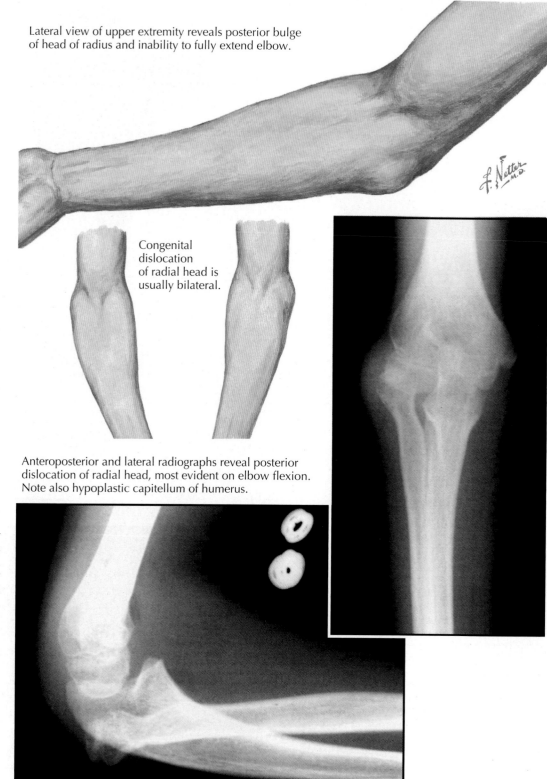

Lateral view of upper extremity reveals posterior bulge of head of radius and inability to fully extend elbow.

Congenital dislocation of radial head is usually bilateral.

Anteroposterior and lateral radiographs reveal posterior dislocation of radial head, most evident on elbow flexion. Note also hypoplastic capitellum of humerus.

CONGENITAL DISLOCATION OF RADIAL HEAD

Congenital dislocation of the radial head is typically not diagnosed until 2 to 5 years of age, when parents notice a mild limitation of elbow extension and an abnormal lateral prominence of the elbow in their child. The abnormality can be unilateral or bilateral, and the most common direction of dislocation is posterior or posterolateral, although anterior or lateral dislocations can occur. Approximately half of all cases are bilateral, and in approximately 60% of patients the deformity occurs in association with a specific syndrome or a connective tissue disorder. Therefore a search for other anomalies should be made whenever this abnormality is diagnosed. Most congenital dislocations of the radial head are asymptomatic and cause no functional disability, because the limitation of elbow motion is mild. Congenital subluxations of the radial head are less common than congenital dislocations but are more likely to be associated with pain. Anterior dislocations cause a slight decrease in flexion and supination, whereas posterior dislocations result in a slight limitation of extension and pronation.

Plain radiographs reveal the abnormality, and the radiographic features considered to be characteristic of a congenital dislocation are (1) a dislocated or subluxated radial head, (2) an underdeveloped radial head, (3) a flat or dome-shaped radial head (rather than the normal concave cup shape), (4) a more slender radius than normal, (5) a longer radius than normal, (6) an underdeveloped capitellum, and (7) a lack of anterior angulation of the distal humerus. A shortened ulna may also commonly occur with a congenital dislocation of the radial head. These associated findings may help distinguish a congenital dislocation from an acquired postnatal or traumatic dislocation, as will the presence of bilaterality and other musculoskeletal anomalies. However, a traumatic dislocation occurring in an infant and left untreated may result in deformities over time that appear similar to a congenital dislocation.

The lack of symptoms and functional limitations make treatment of congenital dislocation of the radial head largely unnecessary. Attempts at open reduction have been reported but often with recurrence. If an unacceptable appearance or pain can be attributed to the dislocation or painful arthritic changes develop, the radial head can be excised when growth is complete. This procedure relieves pain but does not usually improve range of motion because long-standing soft tissue contractures persist.

Plate 2.44

Upper Arm and Elbow

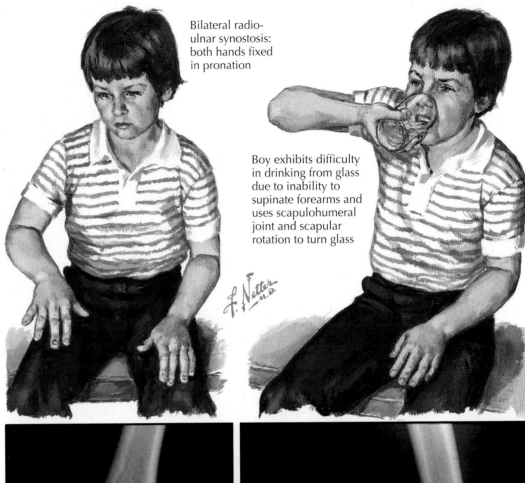

Bilateral radio-
ulnar synostosis:
both hands fixed
in pronation

Boy exhibits difficulty
in drinking from glass
due to inability to
supinate forearms and
uses scapulohumeral
joint and scapular
rotation to turn glass

Congenital Radioulnar Synostosis

Congenital radioulnar synostosis is an uncommon condition in which the proximal ends of the radius and ulna are joined, fixing the forearm in pronation. The deformity is due to a failure of the developing cartilaginous precursors of the forearm to separate during fetal development. Radioulnar synostosis is bilateral in 60% of patients and is frequently associated with other musculoskeletal abnormalities. Chromosomal abnormalities have been reported in some patients with bilateral involvement. Two types of synostosis are seen. In the first, called the headless type, the medullary canals of the radius and ulna are joined and the proximal radius is absent or malformed and fused to the ulna over a distance of several centimeters. The radius is anteriorly bowed and its diaphysis is larger and longer than that of the ulna. In the second type, the fused segment is shorter and the radius is formed normally but the radial head is dislocated anteriorly or posteriorly and fused to the diaphysis of the proximal ulna. The second type is often unilateral and sometimes associated with deformities such as syndactyly or supernumerary thumbs.

Radioulnar synostosis is present at birth but is usually not noticed until functional problems arise, most often in patients with bilateral involvement. Commonly, the only clinical finding is lack of rotation between the radius and the ulna, which fixes the forearm in a position of midpronation or hyperpronation. Range of motion in the elbow and wrist joints is usually normal or excessive, although some patients cannot completely extend the elbow. The degree of functional disability varies with the amount of fixed pronation and whether the condition is unilateral or bilateral. Unilateral deformity with less fixed pronation may be able to compensate with shoulder motion. However, in patients with bilateral involvement in which both hands are hyperpronated, many daily activities become

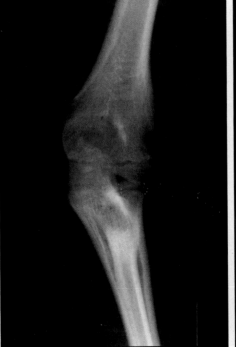
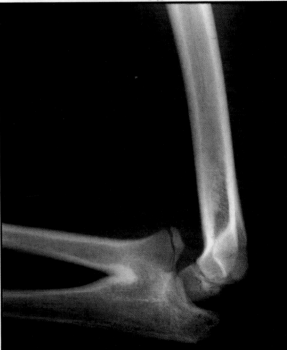

Radiographs show fusion of proximal ends of radius and ulna. Anterior dislocation of radial head apparent in view of flexed elbow (*right*).

problematic, such as turning a doorknob, buttoning clothing, drinking from a cup or eating, and performing personal hygiene.

Because the disability is so varied, treatment should be specific to the patient. Mild, unilateral abnormalities are typically left untreated. Synostosis resection to regain forearm rotation in more severe cases has not been successful, with new bone often rebridging the resected gap. In patients with hyperpronation, particularly

if bilateral, rotational osteotomy, either through the distal end of the fused area or through the radius and ulna distal to the fusion, can be performed to put the forearm in a more functional position. Typically, the dominant forearm is positioned in 0 to 20 degrees of pronation while the nondominant forearm is positioned in 20 to 30 degrees of supination. Compartment syndrome can occur as a complication of this procedure.

Plate 2.45

Upper Limb: PART I

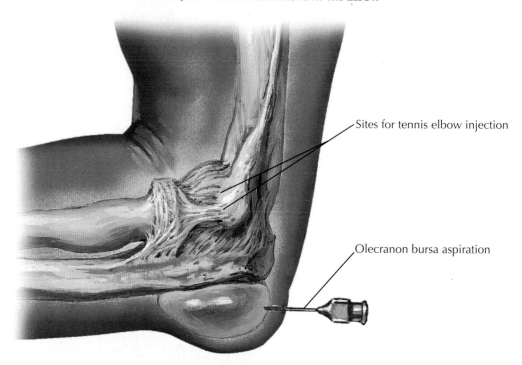

INJECTIONS AND ASPIRATIONS AT THE ELBOW

Sites for tennis elbow injection

Olecranon bursa aspiration

Elbow joint aspiration

COMMON ELBOW INJECTIONS AND BASIC REHABILITATION

Injections or aspirations about the elbow, regardless of location, should always be performed under sterile conditions. The needle site should be appropriately prepared with povidone-iodine (Betadine) or another antiseptic before injection or aspiration. Larger-gauge needles work best for aspirations (18-gauge), whereas smaller-gauge needles can be used for injections.

Injections or aspirations of the elbow joint are commonly performed through the lateral "soft spot." The soft spot is a normal depression in the posterolateral aspect of the elbow that is defined by the lateral epicondyle, the tip of the olecranon, and the radial head. If a joint effusion is present, this sulcus will develop a fullness to it and the fluid that is present in the joint can be aspirated. Typically, injection or aspiration is easiest with the elbow in a flexed position, because this is the position of maximal joint capacity. Other common sites for aspiration or injection around the elbow include the olecranon bursa for olecranon bursitis and the common extensor origin for lateral epicondylitis. The needle for an olecranon bursa injection or aspiration should be inserted into the fluctuant portion of the bursa for maximal effectiveness. For injections for lateral epicondylitis, the elbow is flexed to 90 degrees and the point of maximal tenderness along the common extensor origin is located. Ideally, the injection is fanned out from this point as the fluid goes in, because the origin of these tendons is broad.

The goal of elbow rehabilitation is to restore full, pain-free function. The elbow is prone to the development of stiffness; therefore early range of motion is a component of most rehabilitation protocols. Rehabilitation after trauma or surgery may require the use of braces or splints to protect healing tissues, while still allowing range-of-motion exercises. Four types of range of motion are typically used during elbow rehabilitation,

in the following order: active assisted, active, passive, and resisted. Exercises should include both the flexion-extension arc and the pronation-supination arc of the elbow. Active-assisted range of motion (AAROM) is typically started first after trauma or surgery, during the inflammatory phase of healing. These exercises maintain low levels of voluntary muscle activation that minimize elbow joint compression and shear forces. Active range of motion (AROM) has similar benefits to AAROM but with more voluntary muscle activation to stimulate early neuromuscular control. AROM exercises

should first be performed with gravity eliminated and then transitioned to antigravity positions. Passive range of motion (PROM) is best initiated during the remodeling phase of healing to gain permanent tissue length and motion by stretching and/or splinting. Finally, resisted range of motion (RROM) should be implemented last as healing allows, typically 8 to 12 weeks after surgery or injury. The primary goal of RROM is to restore neuromuscular control. Neuromuscular control includes strength, endurance, and coordinated muscle contractions.

Plate 2.46   Upper Arm and Elbow

SURGICAL APPROACHES TO THE UPPER ARM AND ELBOW

Anterolateral approach to humerus

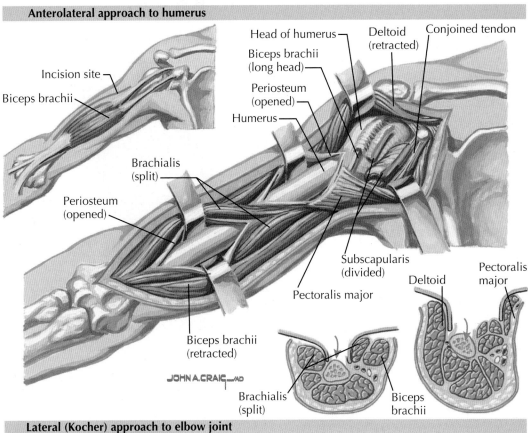

Incision site
Biceps brachii
Head of humerus
Deltoid (retracted)
Conjoined tendon
Biceps brachii (long head)
Periosteum (opened)
Humerus
Brachialis (split)
Periosteum (opened)
Subscapularis (divided)
Pectoralis major
Deltoid
Pectoralis major
Biceps brachii (retracted)
JOHN A. CRAIG—AD
Brachialis (split)
Biceps brachii

Lateral (Kocher) approach to elbow joint

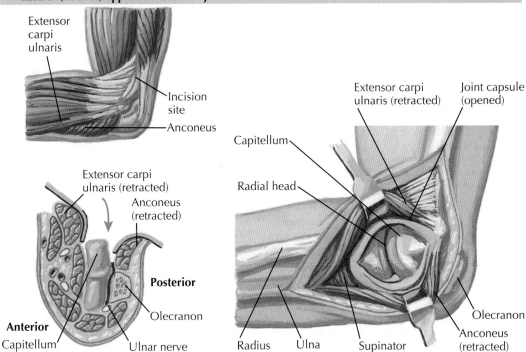

Extensor carpi ulnaris
Incision site
Anconeus
Extensor carpi ulnaris (retracted)
Anconeus (retracted)
Posterior
Olecranon
Anterior
Capitellum
Ulnar nerve
Extensor carpi ulnaris (retracted)
Joint capsule (opened)
Capitellum
Radial head
Olecranon
Anconeus (retracted)
Radius
Ulna
Supinator

SURGICAL APPROACHES TO THE UPPER ARM AND ELBOW

The most common surgical approaches to the upper arm and elbow include the anterolateral approach to the humerus, the lateral or Kocher approach to the elbow, and posterior approaches to the elbow. Arthroscopic elbow techniques are also becoming more frequently used.

The anterolateral approach to the humerus is most commonly used for plating fractures of the humeral shaft. The incision is made at the deltopectoral interval proximally and then runs along the lateral border of the biceps muscle distally. An internervous plane is utilized between the deltoid (axillary nerve) and pectoralis major (medial and lateral pectoral nerves) proximally. More distally, after retracting the biceps medially, the brachialis muscle is split longitudinally along the outer third of the muscle, utilizing an internervous plane between its medial (musculocutaneous nerve) and lateral fibers (radial nerve). Neurovascular structures at risk with this approach include the axillary nerve and anterior humeral circumflex vessels proximally, the radial nerve as it runs in the spiral groove on the posterior surface of the midshaft of the humerus and more distally as it emerges between the brachioradialis and brachialis muscles laterally, and the musculocutaneous nerve in its location on the surface of the brachialis muscle and deep to the biceps muscle. More distal fractures of the humeral shaft may be difficult to expose with the anterolateral approach, owing to the proximity

of the elbow joint. In these situations, a posterior approach to the humerus may afford better exposure. The humeral shaft can be exposed posteriorly either by splitting the triceps muscle down the midline, by taking care to identify the radial nerve, or by elevating the triceps muscle along its lateral border and reflecting all three heads of the muscle medially. The radial nerve is identified in the latter technique as it passes through the lateral intermuscular septum from posterior to anterior.

The lateral or Kocher approach to the elbow is commonly used for many procedures on the lateral side of the elbow, such as fracture fixation (radial head, capitellum), radial head replacement, and lateral collateral ligament repair or reconstruction. The approach utilizes the internervous plane between the extensor carpi ulnaris (posterior interosseous nerve) anteriorly and the anconeus (radial nerve) posteriorly. Neurovascular structures at risk include the posterior interosseous nerve and radial nerve. The posterior interosseous

Plate 2.47

Upper Limb: PART I

SURGICAL APPROACHES TO THE UPPER ARM AND ELBOW (CONTINUED)

Arthroscopy portals

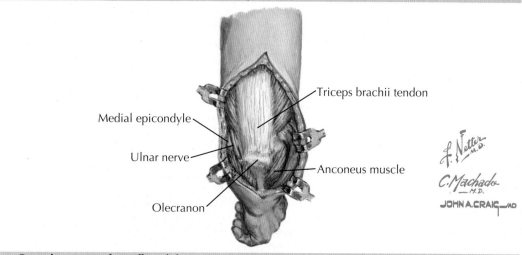

Proximal antero-lateral portal

Lateral epicondyle

Proximal anteromedial portal

Medial epicondyle

Lateral epicondyle

Triceps brachii

Posterolateral portal

Posterocentral portal

Olecranon

Direct lateral portal

Radial head

Posterior approach with olecranon osteotomy

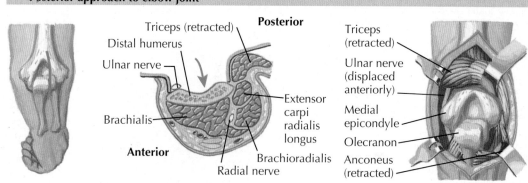

Triceps brachii tendon

Medial epicondyle

Ulnar nerve

Anconeus muscle

Olecranon

SURGICAL APPROACHES TO THE UPPER ARM AND ELBOW (Continued)

nerve can be protected by keeping the forearm pronated, and the radial nerve is avoided by not straying too far proximally or anteriorly.

Posterior approaches to the elbow can involve mobilization of the triceps tendon or leave the triceps intact. The most common method of moving the triceps is by olecranon osteotomy. This technique reflects the olecranon and triceps insertion proximally to expose the distal humerus and elbow joint. Outstanding exposure of the joint is achieved, and the approach is particularly useful in fixation of complex, intraarticular distal humerus fractures and total elbow arthroplasty. Nonunion of the olecranon osteotomy site is a risk with this technique, however. The Bryan-Morrey posterior approach is an alternative to olecranon osteotomy and involves reflection of the extensor mechanism laterally, including the triceps and anconeus. This approach can be used for similar indications as an olecranon osteotomy. Although joint exposure is not quite as good, there is no risk of osteotomy nonunion with this technique.

Elbow arthroscopy is more commonly being used as a surgical technique. Correct portal placement is essential to avoid neurovascular injuries. The proximal anterolateral and proximal anteromedial portals are most commonly utilized to visualize the anterior compartment of the elbow. The anteromedial portal is made approximately 2 cm proximal to the

Posterior approach to elbow joint

Triceps (retracted)

Distal humerus

Ulnar nerve

Brachialis

Posterior

Anterior

Extensor carpi radialis longus

Brachioradialis

Radial nerve

Triceps (retracted)

Ulnar nerve (displaced anteriorly)

Medial epicondyle

Olecranon

Anconeus (retracted)

medial epicondyle and anterior to the intermuscular septum. The ulnar nerve and medial antebrachial cutaneous nerve are at risk with this portal. The anterolateral portal is similarly made on the lateral side of the elbow, taking care to stay anterior to the humerus. The radial nerve is most at risk with this portal. The posterocentral and posterolateral portals are most commonly employed to visualize the posterior

compartment of the elbow. Both portals are made approximately 3 cm proximal to the tip of the olecranon. Finally, the direct lateral soft spot portal is made at the soft spot on the lateral side of the elbow to help with visualization and instrumentation in the lateral gutter, such as when working on a capitellar osteochondritis dissecans. The posterior antebrachial cutaneous nerve is at risk with this portal.

FOREARM AND WRIST

Plate 3.1

Upper Limb: PART I

TOPOGRAPHIC ANATOMY OF FOREARM AND WRIST

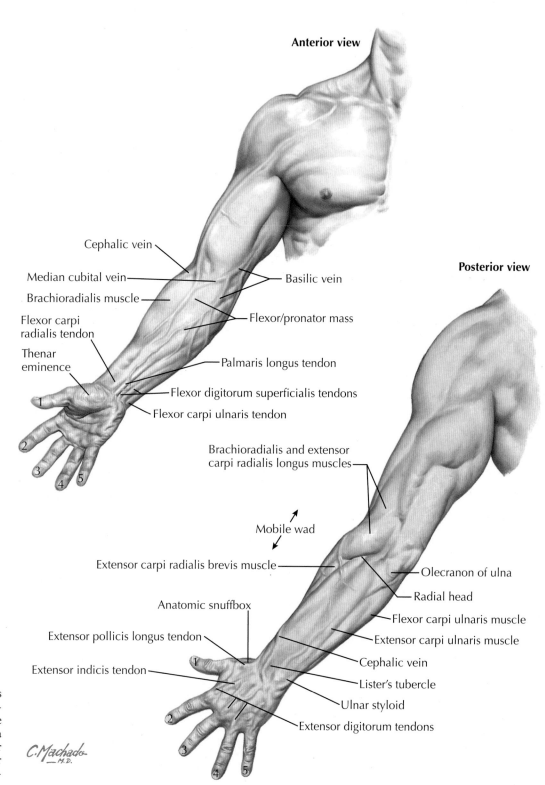

Anterior view

Posterior view

Cephalic vein

Median cubital vein

Brachioradialis muscle

Basilic vein

Flexor carpi radialis tendon

Flexor/pronator mass

Thenar eminence

Palmaris longus tendon

Flexor digitorum superficialis tendons

Flexor carpi ulnaris tendon

Brachioradialis and extensor carpi radialis longus muscles

Mobile wad

Extensor carpi radialis brevis muscle

Olecranon of ulna

Anatomic snuffbox

Radial head

Extensor pollicis longus tendon

Flexor carpi ulnaris muscle

Extensor indicis tendon

Extensor carpi ulnaris muscle

Cephalic vein

Lister's tubercle

Ulnar styloid

Extensor digitorum tendons

C. Machado — M.D.

BONES AND JOINTS OF FOREARM AND WRIST

DISTAL PARTS OF RADIUS AND ULNA

The distal end of the radius is broadened because its *carpal articular surface* is the bony contact of the forearm with the wrist and hand. This surface is concave transversely and anteroposteriorly; it is divided by a surface constriction and a slight ridging into a larger triangular portion laterally and a smaller quadrangular part medially, which are for the reception of the scaphoid and the lunate of the wrist, respectively.

The medial surface of the distal extremity of the radius is also concave and articular. As the *ulnar notch of the radius,* it receives the rounded head of the ulna. Dorsally, the distal part of the radius exhibits its *tubercle* and is otherwise somewhat ridged and grooved for the passage of the tendons of the forearm extensor muscles. Laterally, the bone ends in a downwardly projecting *styloid process.*

The distal radius (DR) and ulna have a rich vascular supply coming from the radial, ulnar, anterior interosseous, and posterior interosseous arteries. The vessels that

supply the dorsum of the distal radius can be described for the corresponding extensor tendon compartments as either intercompartmental or compartmental. Nutrient vessels branch off the main vessels and penetrate the retinaculum and underlying bone. An example is the 1,2 intercompartmental supraretinacular artery. A branch off the radial artery, it provides nutrient branches to the bone between the first and second extensor tendon

compartments. Clinically, the vessel and its corresponding branches and underlying bone can be harvested and used for vascularized bone grafting procedures in the carpus (for example, for a scaphoid nonunion advanced collapse [SNAC] with avascular proximal pole).

Ossification begins in the distal extremity of the radius at the end of the first year, and fusion takes place at age 19 to 20 years.

Plate 3.2

Forearm and Wrist

BONES OF FOREARM

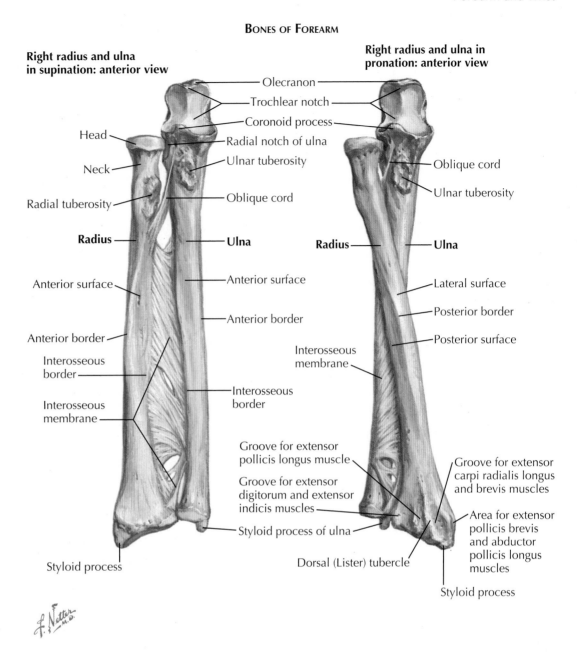

Right radius and ulna in supination: anterior view

Right radius and ulna in pronation: anterior view

Olecranon
Trochlear notch
Coronoid process
Head
Radial notch of ulna
Neck
Ulnar tuberosity
Oblique cord
Radial tuberosity
Oblique cord
Ulnar tuberosity

Radius
Ulna
Radius
Ulna

Anterior surface
Anterior surface
Lateral surface

Anterior border
Posterior border

Anterior border
Posterior surface

Interosseous border
Interosseous membrane

Interosseous membrane
Interosseous border

Groove for extensor pollicis longus muscle
Groove for extensor carpi radialis longus and brevis muscles

Groove for extensor digitorum and extensor indicis muscles
Area for extensor pollicis brevis and abductor pollicis longus muscles

Styloid process of ulna
Styloid process
Dorsal (Lister) tubercle
Styloid process

BONES AND JOINTS OF FOREARM AND WRIST (Continued)

The *ulna* has a small distal extremity. There is a small, rounded *styloid process* in line with the posterior border of the bone, and there is also a larger, rounded *head*. The distal surface of the head is smooth for contact with the articular disc of the distal radioulnar joint (DRUJ); it is continuous with the distal surface of the circumference of the head, which is received into the ulnar notch of the head of the radius.

An *ossification center* for the distal end of the ulna appears at age 5 or 6 years and fuses with the shaft at age 18 to 20 years.

CARPAL BONES

The skeleton of the wrist consists of eight small bones arranged in two rows, proximal and distal. The bones of the proximal row, from the radial to the ulnar side, are the scaphoid, lunate, triquetrum, and pisiform. Those of the distal row, in the same order, are the

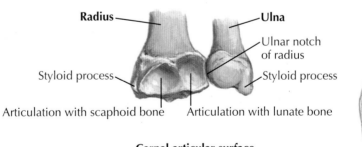

Radius
Ulna
Ulnar notch of radius
Styloid process
Styloid process
Articulation with scaphoid bone
Articulation with lunate bone

Carpal articular surface

Coronal section of radius demonstrates how thickness of cortical bone of shaft diminishes to thin layer over cancellous bone at distal end.

trapezium, trapezoid, capitate, and hamate. Fundamentally, these bones may be thought of as cubes, each of which has six surfaces. Their dorsal and palmar surfaces are nonarticular and provide for the attachment of the dorsal and palmar ligaments that hold them closely together.

The other surfaces are articular, except for the subcutaneous surfaces of the bones that form the borders

of the wrist. These surfaces also mostly lodge ligaments. The proximal articular surfaces are generally convex; the distal surfaces are usually concave. Foramina for the entrance of blood vessels are found on nonarticular areas of each bone.

The boat-shaped *scaphoid* is the largest bone of the proximal row. Its smooth radial articular surface is convex and triangular. The smooth distal surface is

Plate 3.3

Upper Limb: PART I

CARPAL BONES

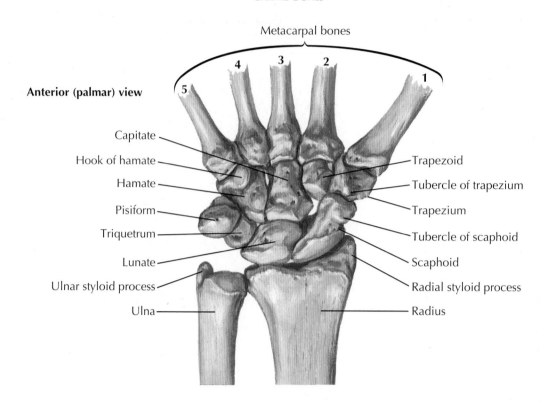

Metacarpal bones

Anterior (palmar) view

Capitate

Hook of hamate

Hamate

Pisiform

Triquetrum

Lunate

Ulnar styloid process

Ulna

Trapezoid

Tubercle of trapezium

Trapezium

Tubercle of scaphoid

Scaphoid

Radial styloid process

Radius

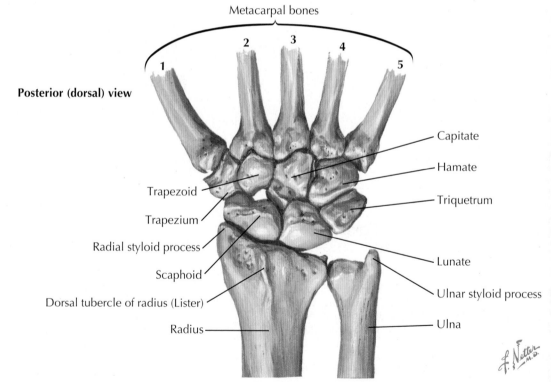

Metacarpal bones

Posterior (dorsal) view

Trapezoid

Trapezium

Radial styloid process

Scaphoid

Dorsal tubercle of radius (Lister)

Radius

Capitate

Hamate

Triquetrum

Lunate

Ulnar styloid process

Ulna

BONES AND JOINTS OF FOREARM AND WRIST (Continued)

triangular but concave and receives both the trapezium and the trapezoid. The medial surface presents two articular facets—one for the lunate and a larger inferior concavity for part of the head of the capitate.

The *lunate* is crescentic; its proximal convexity is for the more medial of the articular surfaces of the distal end of the radius. The distal surface is deeply concave for the capitate and for a small contact with the hamate. On its radial surface, this bone contacts the scaphoid; medially, it has a surface for the base of the triquetrum.

The *triquetrum* is pyramidal, with the base of the pyramid toward the lunate and the apex downward and ulnarward on the ulnar border of the wrist. The inferior surface is sinuously curved for articulation with the hamate, and the palmar surface has an oval facet for the pisiform.

The *pisiform* is small and has been likened to a pea. Its single articular facet is for the triquetrum. The

pisiform may be regarded as a sesamoid formed in the tendon of the flexor carpi ulnaris (FCU) muscle.

The *trapezium* is the radialmost bone of the distal row of carpals. Its proximomedial surface is concave for articulation with the scaphoid, and its distal surface has a saddle-shaped facet for the base of the first metacarpal. On the palmar surface of the bone is a tubercle and a deep groove, through which passes the tendon of the flexor

carpi radialis muscle. The tubercle gives attachment to the superficial lamina of the flexor retinaculum and to several thumb muscles. The medial surface of the trapezium has a large concave facet proximally for articulation with the trapezoid and has a small, flat oval surface at the distal angle of the bone for the second metacarpal.

The *trapezoid* is somewhat wedge shaped, with the broader base of the wedge dorsally. The quadrilateral

Plate 3.4

Forearm and Wrist

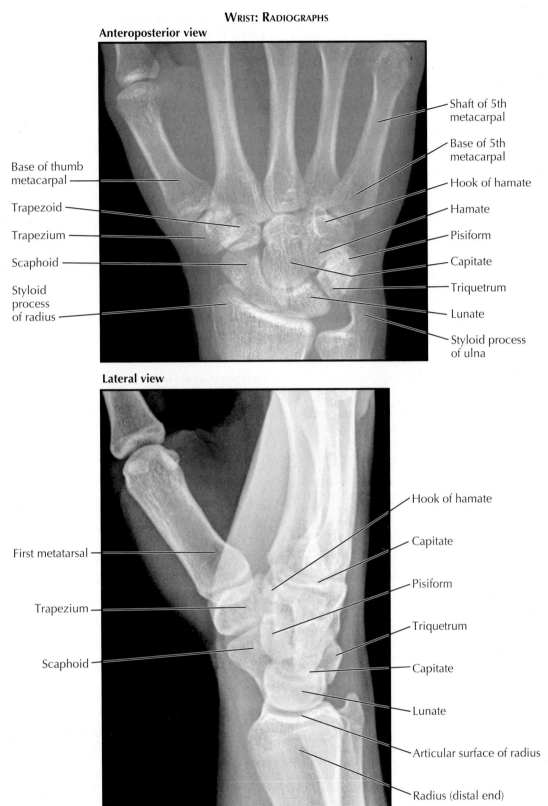

WRIST: RADIOGRAPHS

Anteroposterior view

Base of thumb metacarpal

Trapezoid

Trapezium

Scaphoid

Styloid process of radius

Shaft of 5th metacarpal

Base of 5th metacarpal

Hook of hamate

Hamate

Pisiform

Capitate

Triquetrum

Lunate

Styloid process of ulna

Lateral view

First metatarsal

Trapezium

Scaphoid

Hook of hamate

Capitate

Pisiform

Triquetrum

Capitate

Lunate

Articular surface of radius

Radius (distal end)

BONES AND JOINTS OF FOREARM AND WRIST (Continued)

proximal surface articulates with the scaphoid, whereas distally there is a large, saddle-shaped articular surface for the base of the second metacarpal. The lateral surface is convex for the trapezium, whereas the medial surface has a smooth facet for the capitate.

The *capitate* is the largest of the carpal bones and occupies the center of the wrist. Its rounded head is received into the concavity of the scaphoid and the lunate. The distal, somewhat cuboidal extremity articulates chiefly with the base of the third metacarpal, but by means of small lateral and medial facets it also makes contact with the bases of the second and third metacarpals. The lateral surface has, distally, a small, smooth facet for the distal extremity of the trapezoid, and the medial surface has an oblong articular surface for the hamate.

The *hamate* is wedge shaped and has a characteristic hook-like process, the hamulus, or hook. The apical proximal part of the wedge articulates with the lunate; the broad distal surface has two concave facets for the bases of the

fourth and fifth metacarpals. Articular surfaces laterally and medially are for the capitate and triquetrum, respectively. The hamulus gives attachment to the flexor retinaculum and the tendon of the flexor carpi ulnaris muscle and provides origin for several small finger muscles.

Ossification takes place from a single center in each bone. It begins first in the capitate and then in the hamate early in the first year; in the triquetrum, during

the third year; in the lunate, in the fourth year; in the trapezium, trapezoid, and scaphoid, in rather close sequence, in the fourth to sixth years; and in the pisiform, in the 11th or 12th year. Ossification starts earlier in the female and is completed between ages 14 and 16 years. The hamulus of the hamate may have a separate center. An os centrale, normally part of the scaphoid, may be present between the scaphoid, capitate, and trapezoid.

Plate 3.5

Upper Limb: PART I

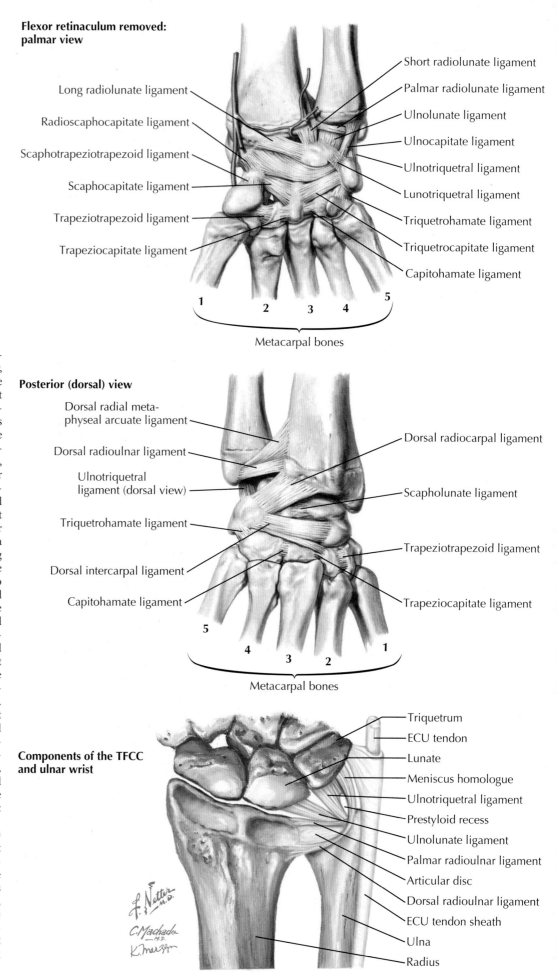

Flexor retinaculum removed: palmar view

Long radiolunate ligament
Radioscaphocapitate ligament
Scaphotrapeziotrapezoid ligament
Scaphocapitate ligament
Trapeziotrapezoid ligament
Trapeziocapitate ligament

Short radiolunate ligament
Palmar radiolunate ligament
Ulnolunate ligament
Ulnocapitate ligament
Ulnotriquetral ligament
Lunotriquetral ligament
Triquetrohamate ligament
Triquetrocapitate ligament
Capitohamate ligament

1 2 3 4 5

Metacarpal bones

Posterior (dorsal) view

Dorsal radial metaphyseal arcuate ligament
Dorsal radioulnar ligament
Ulnotriquetral ligament (dorsal view)
Triquetrohamate ligament
Dorsal intercarpal ligament
Capitohamate ligament

Dorsal radiocarpal ligament
Scapholunate ligament
Trapeziotrapezoid ligament
Trapeziocapitate ligament

5 4 3 2 1

Metacarpal bones

Components of the TFCC and ulnar wrist

Triquetrum
ECU tendon
Lunate
Meniscus homologue
Ulnotriquetral ligament
Prestyloid recess
Ulnolunate ligament
Palmar radioulnar ligament
Articular disc
Dorsal radioulnar ligament
ECU tendon sheath
Ulna
Radius

LIGAMENTS OF WRIST

The ligaments of the wrist are divided into three separate groups: the volar radiocarpal, dorsal intercapsular, and interosseous ligaments. Confusion regarding these structures often centers on the numerous different names used to identify these structures. The volar radiocarpal ligaments are the most critical of these structures and provide the majority of ligamentous stability to the carpus. The volar ligaments consist of the radioscaphocapitate ligament, the long/short radiolunate ligaments, the radioscapholunate ligaments (more of a vascular conduit), and the ulnotriquetral and ulnolunate ligaments. The radioscaphocapitate ligament is a critical restraint to ulnar translocation of the carpus and must be preserved during proximal row carpectomy and/or during radial styloidectomy. The space of Poirier is a weak point between the radioscaphocapitate and long radiolunate ligaments, where the lunate can dislocate during a lunate dislocation. During a volar approach to lunate/perilunate dislocations this space can be sutured to provide increased stability to the injured carpus. The dorsal intercapsular ligaments consist of the dorsal radiocarpal and dorsal intercarpal ligaments. These provide additional structural support to the carpus, and numerous "ligament-sparing approaches" to the wrist have been described to preserve these structures. These dorsal ligaments can also be used to correct carpal instability by being transferred to function as a capsulodesis. There are numerous intercarpal ligaments, the most critical being the scapholunate (SL) and lunotriquetral (LT) ligaments. Disruption of these intercarpal ligaments can lead to dorsiflexed or volar-flexed intercalated segment instability (DISI or VISI) deformities, respectively. Repair of these ligaments can be performed in the acute setting, whereas numerous reconstructive procedures have been described for use in the chronic setting when symptomatic.

The triangular fibrocartilage complex (TFCC) describes a confluence of soft tissue structures that stabilize the DRUJ and transmit forces across the ulnocarpal joint. The individual components include dorsal and palmar radioulnar ligaments, meniscus homologue, ulnotriquetral and ulnolunate ligaments, articular disc, and the extensor carpi ulnaris (ECU) subsheath. The dorsal and palmar radioulnar ligaments are most critical for DRUJ stability. TFCC pathology can often be diagnosed and treated with arthroscopic techniques.

Plate 3.6

Forearm and Wrist

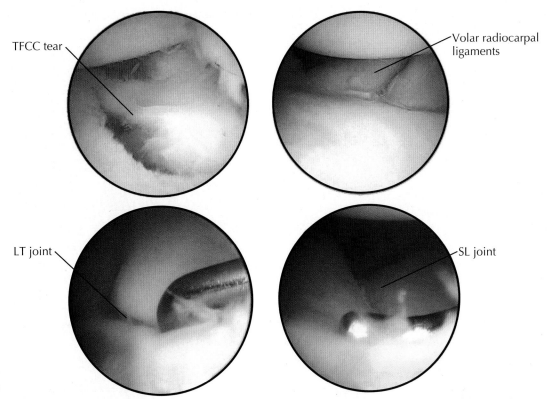

TFCC tear

Volar radiocarpal ligaments

LT joint

SL joint

Triangular fibrocartilage tear (TFCC)

Arthroscopy of Wrist

Wrist arthroscopy has rapidly evolved from an experimental diagnostic instrument to a powerful tool for both accurate diagnosis and treatment of numerous ailments. Advances in camera technology, small instrument design, safe portal identification, and, most importantly, surgeon experience and comfort have all played a role in the development of this treatment modality.

Currently, wrist arthroscopy is considered the gold standard for evaluating and often treating chronic wrist pain. TFCC injuries are a common cause of chronic ulnar-sided wrist pain. Wrist arthroscopy allows accurate identification of these injuries, determination of central versus peripheral injury, and treatment. Central TFCC tears cause painful clicking and catching in the wrist and can be debrided arthroscopically back to a stable rim of tissue. Peripheral detachment of the TFCC from the distal ulna causes ulnar-sided wrist pain with potential instability of the DRUJ and can be successfully treated with the arthroscopic passage of sutures and secure repair with gratifying results. Radiocarpal and midcarpal synovectomy, ganglion excision, scapholunate and lunotriquetral tear debridement versus repair, and loose body removal can also all be successfully treated arthroscopically. Arthroscopic visualization of both distal radius and scaphoid fracture fixation has also been reported as an adjunct to standard treatment, allowing direct visualization of intraarticular reduction and fixation.

Wrist arthroscopy requires a thorough understanding of wrist anatomy to allow safe passage of instrumentation and recognition of the anatomy and pathologic processes encountered. Arthroscopic portals are identified by their relationship to the numbered extensor tendon compartments along the dorsum of the wrist. The standard viewing portal is the 3 to 4 portal, with supplemental portals for instrumentation often occurring at the 4 to 5 interval or on either side of the extensor carpi ulnaris tendon (6R and 6U). Midcarpal arthroscopy is a critical component to any diagnostic wrist arthroscopy. The midcarpal viewing and working portals allow accurate evaluation and grading of both scapholunate and lunotriquetral instability. More advanced arthroscopists have used both palmar portals and DRUJ portals for enhanced viewing of complex intraarticular ailments.

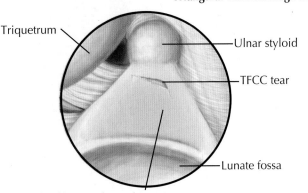

Triquetrum

Ulnar styloid

TFCC tear

Lunate fossa

Triangular fibrocartilage (disc)

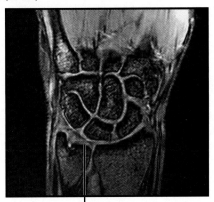

TFCC tear

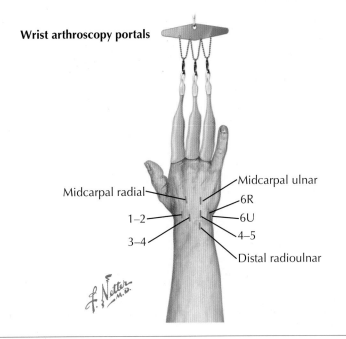

Wrist arthroscopy portals

Midcarpal ulnar

Midcarpal radial

6R

1–2

6U

3–4

4–5

Distal radioulnar

Plate 3.7

Upper Limb: PART I

MUSCLES OF FOREARM (SUPERFICIAL LAYER): ANTERIOR VIEW

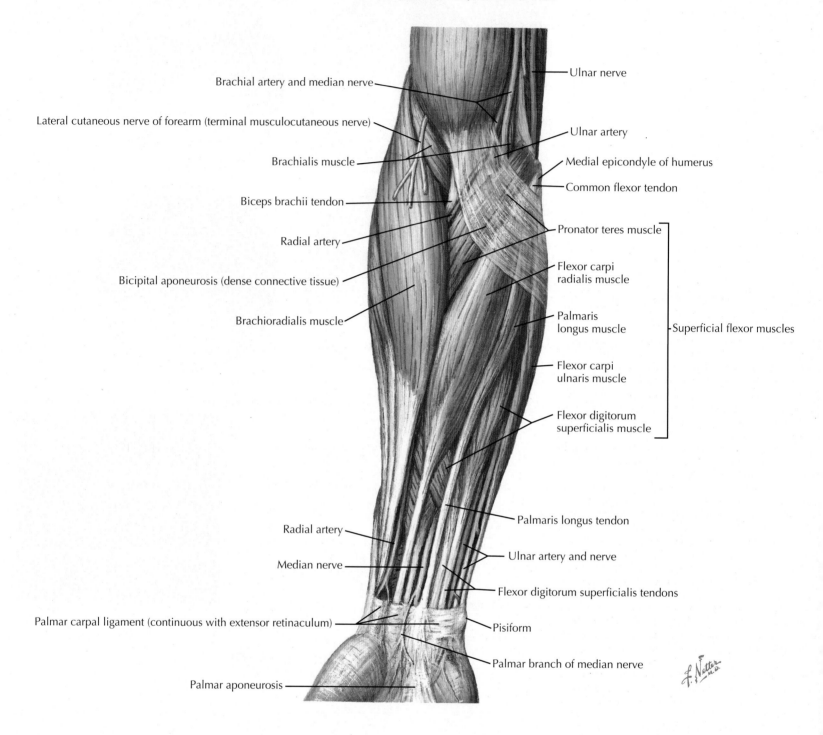

Brachial artery and median nerve

Lateral cutaneous nerve of forearm (terminal musculocutaneous nerve)

Brachialis muscle

Biceps brachii tendon

Radial artery

Bicipital aponeurosis (dense connective tissue)

Brachioradialis muscle

Ulnar nerve

Ulnar artery

Medial epicondyle of humerus

Common flexor tendon

Pronator teres muscle

Flexor carpi radialis muscle

Palmaris longus muscle

Flexor carpi ulnaris muscle

Flexor digitorum superficialis muscle

Superficial flexor muscles

Radial artery

Median nerve

Palmar carpal ligament (continuous with extensor retinaculum)

Palmar aponeurosis

Palmaris longus tendon

Ulnar artery and nerve

Flexor digitorum superficialis tendons

Pisiform

Palmar branch of median nerve

MUSCLES OF FOREARM

The forearm extends from the elbow to the wrist. It is the territory of two bones—the radius and the ulna—and of many muscles. The muscles are arranged as a flexor mass anteriorly and an extensor mass posteriorly.

There are 19 muscles in the forearm. Eleven are classified as extensor muscles; eight belong to the flexor group. These designations are simply group characteristics because certain muscles are primarily rotators of the forearm bones. Eighteen of the muscles can be grouped into *six functional groups* of *three muscles each*. The muscle excluded from these groups is the *brachioradialis,*

which is an elbow flexor with no action in the digits or at the wrist. All the groups, except for the first, are composed of muscles that move the hand and digits.

1. Rotate the radius on the ulna:
   - Pronator teres
   - Pronator quadratus
   - Supinator
2. Flex the hand at the wrist:
   - Flexor carpi radialis
   - Flexor carpi ulnaris
   - Palmaris longus
3. Flex the digits:
   - Flexor digitorum superficialis
   - Flexor digitorum profundus
   - Flexor pollicis longus

4. Extend the hand at the wrist:
   - Extensor carpi radialis longus
   - Extensor carpi radialis brevis
   - Extensor carpi ulnaris
5. Extend the digits, except the thumb:
   - Extensor digitorum
   - Extensor indicis
   - Extensor digiti minimi
6. Extend the thumb:
   - Abductor pollicis longus
   - Extensor pollicis brevis
   - Extensor pollicis longus

The muscles of the first three groups lie in the anterior compartment of the forearm; those of the last three groups are located in the posterior compartment.

Plate 3.8

Forearm and Wrist

MUSCLES OF FOREARM (INTERMEDIATE AND DEEP LAYERS): ANTERIOR VIEW

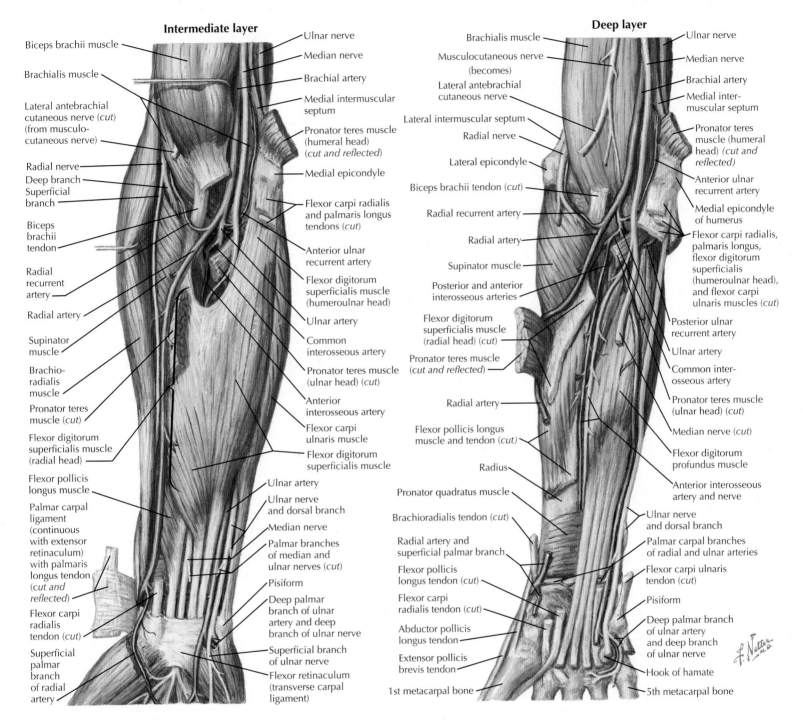

Intermediate layer

Biceps brachii muscle

Brachialis muscle

Lateral antebrachial cutaneous nerve (*cut*) (from musculo-cutaneous nerve)

Radial nerve
Deep branch
Superficial branch

Biceps brachii tendon

Radial recurrent artery

Supinator muscle

Brachio-radialis muscle

Pronator teres muscle (*cut*)

Flexor digitorum superficialis muscle (radial head)

Flexor pollicis longus muscle

Palmar carpal ligament (continuous with extensor retinaculum) with palmaris longus tendon (*cut and reflected*)

Flexor carpi radialis tendon (*cut*)

Superficial palmar branch of radial artery

Ulnar nerve
Median nerve
Brachial artery
Medial intermuscular septum
Pronator teres muscle (humeral head) (*cut and reflected*)
Medial epicondyle
Flexor carpi radialis and palmaris longus tendons (*cut*)
Anterior ulnar recurrent artery
Flexor digitorum superficialis muscle (humeroulnar head)
Ulnar artery
Common interosseous artery
Pronator teres muscle (ulnar head) (*cut*)
Anterior interosseous artery
Flexor carpi ulnaris muscle
Flexor digitorum superficialis muscle
Ulnar artery
Ulnar nerve and dorsal branch
Median nerve
Palmar branches of median and ulnar nerves (*cut*)
Pisiform
Deep palmar branch of ulnar artery and deep branch of ulnar nerve
Superficial branch of ulnar nerve
Flexor retinaculum (transverse carpal ligament)

Deep layer

Brachialis muscle
Musculocutaneous nerve (becomes)
Lateral antebrachial cutaneous nerve
Lateral intermuscular septum
Radial nerve
Lateral epicondyle
Biceps brachii tendon (*cut*)
Radial recurrent artery
Radial artery
Supinator muscle
Posterior and anterior interosseous arteries
Flexor digitorum superficialis muscle (radial head) (*cut*)
Pronator teres muscle (*cut and reflected*)
Radial artery
Flexor pollicis longus muscle and tendon (*cut*)
Radius
Pronator quadratus muscle
Brachioradialis tendon (*cut*)
Radial artery and superficial palmar branch
Flexor pollicis longus tendon (*cut*)
Flexor carpi radialis tendon (*cut*)
Abductor pollicis longus tendon
Extensor pollicis brevis tendon
1st metacarpal bone

Ulnar nerve
Median nerve
Brachial artery
Medial inter-muscular septum
Pronator teres muscle (humeral head) (*cut and reflected*)
Anterior ulnar recurrent artery
Medial epicondyle of humerus
Flexor carpi radialis, palmaris longus, flexor digitorum superficialis (humeroulnar head), and flexor carpi ulnaris muscles (*cut*)
Posterior ulnar recurrent artery
Ulnar artery
Common inter-osseous artery
Pronator teres muscle (ulnar head) (*cut*)
Median nerve (*cut*)
Flexor digitorum profundus muscle
Anterior interosseous artery and nerve
Ulnar nerve and dorsal branch
Palmar carpal branches of radial and ulnar arteries
Flexor carpi ulnaris tendon (*cut*)
Pisiform
Deep palmar branch of ulnar artery and deep branch of ulnar nerve
Hook of hamate
5th metacarpal bone

MUSCLES OF FOREARM (Continued)

FLEXOR MUSCLES

The muscles of the second and third groups and the two pronator muscles of the first group comprise the anterior antebrachial muscles. Five of these belong to a superficial layer, and three belong to a deep layer.

Superficial Layer

The muscles of this layer are listed in the order in which they lie from the radial to the ulnar side of the forearm; the flexor digitorum superficialis (FDS), however, is deep to the other four muscles:

- Pronator teres
- Flexor carpi radialis
- Palmaris longus
- Flexor carpi ulnaris
- Flexor digitorum superficialis

There is a *common tendon of origin* for these muscles, which is attached to the medial epicondyle of the humerus. The intermuscular septa and the antebrachial fascia also provide partial origins, and certain muscles have additional bony origins.

The *pronator teres muscle* has both a humeral and an ulnar head. The large humeral head arises in the medial epicondyle via the common tendon and from the adjacent fascia and intermuscular septa. The small, deep ulnar head takes origin from the medial side of the coronoid process of the ulna. It joins the deep aspect of

the humeral head, the median nerve descending between them. This obliquely descending muscle ends on the shaft of the radius at the middle of its lateral surface. The insertion is overlaid and obscured by the brachioradialis muscle.

The *flexor carpi radialis muscle* uses the common tendon of origin. Its tendon accounts for about half of the muscle's length, passes through the wrist in a compartment formed by a split in the flexor retinaculum, and ends in the base of the second metacarpal (frequently, there is an additional slip to the third metacarpal).

The *palmaris longus muscle* also uses the common tendon of origin when present (it is absent in 13% of cases). It terminates in a slender, flattened tendon, crossing the wrist superficial to the flexor retinaculum.

Plate 3.9

Upper Limb: PART I

MUSCLES OF FOREARM (SUPERFICIAL AND DEEP LAYERS): POSTERIOR VIEW

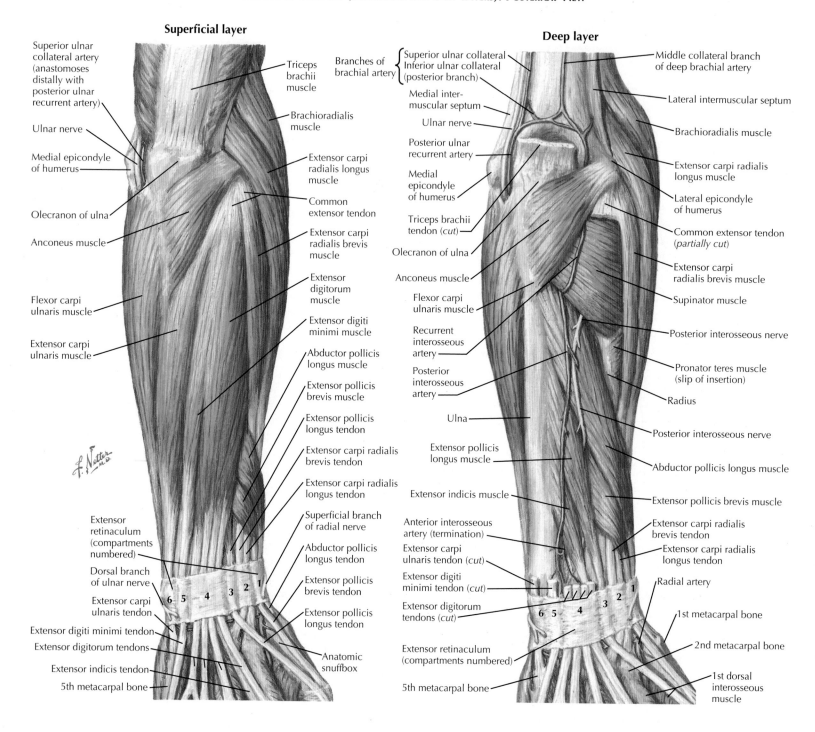

Superficial layer

Superior ulnar collateral artery (anastomoses distally with posterior ulnar recurrent artery)

Ulnar nerve

Medial epicondyle of humerus

Olecranon of ulna

Anconeus muscle

Flexor carpi ulnaris muscle

Extensor carpi ulnaris muscle

Extensor retinaculum (compartments numbered)

Dorsal branch of ulnar nerve

Extensor carpi ulnaris tendon

Extensor digiti minimi tendon

Extensor digitorum tendons

Extensor indicis tendon

5th metacarpal bone

Triceps brachii muscle

Brachioradialis muscle

Extensor carpi radialis longus muscle

Common extensor tendon

Extensor carpi radialis brevis muscle

Extensor digitorum muscle

Extensor digiti minimi muscle

Abductor pollicis longus muscle

Extensor pollicis brevis muscle

Extensor pollicis longus tendon

Extensor carpi radialis brevis tendon

Extensor carpi radialis longus tendon

Superficial branch of radial nerve

Abductor pollicis longus tendon

Extensor pollicis brevis tendon

Extensor pollicis longus tendon

Anatomic snuffbox

Deep layer

Branches of brachial artery { Superior ulnar collateral / Inferior ulnar collateral (posterior branch)

Medial intermuscular septum

Ulnar nerve

Posterior ulnar recurrent artery

Medial epicondyle of humerus

Triceps brachii tendon (cut)

Olecranon of ulna

Anconeus muscle

Flexor carpi ulnaris muscle

Recurrent interosseous artery

Posterior interosseous artery

Ulna

Extensor pollicis longus muscle

Extensor indicis muscle

Anterior interosseous artery (termination)

Extensor carpi ulnaris tendon (cut)

Extensor digiti minimi tendon (cut)

Extensor digitorum tendons (cut)

Extensor retinaculum (compartments numbered)

5th metacarpal bone

Middle collateral branch of deep brachial artery

Lateral intermuscular septum

Brachioradialis muscle

Extensor carpi radialis longus muscle

Lateral epicondyle of humerus

Common extensor tendon (partially cut)

Extensor carpi radialis brevis muscle

Supinator muscle

Posterior interosseous nerve

Pronator teres muscle (slip of insertion)

Radius

Posterior interosseous nerve

Abductor pollicis longus muscle

Extensor pollicis brevis muscle

Extensor carpi radialis brevis tendon

Extensor carpi radialis longus tendon

Radial artery

1st metacarpal bone

2nd metacarpal bone

1st dorsal interosseous muscle

MUSCLES OF FOREARM (Continued)

It constitutes, by its spreading tendinous fibers, the chief part of the *palmar aponeurosis*.

The *flexor carpi ulnaris muscle* has a humeral and an ulnar head, the humeral head coming from the common flexor tendon. The ulnar head springs from the medial border of the olecranon and the upper two-thirds of the posterior border of the ulna. The tendon of the muscle inserts on the pisiform of the wrist and, through it by two ligaments, into the hamulus of the hamate and the base of the fifth metacarpal.

The *flexor digitorum superficialis muscle* arises by a humeroulnar and a radial head of origin; these are connected by a fibrous band that crosses the median nerve and the ulnar blood vessels. The larger humeroulnar head arises from the common tendon, intermuscular septa, ulnar collateral ligament, and medial border of the coronoid process. The radial head is a thin layer arising from the upper two-thirds of the anterior border of the radius. The muscle forms two planes; the tendons of its superficial plane pass to the middle and ring fingers, and the deep lamina ends in tendons for digits 1 and 5. These tendons terminate in the palmar aspect of the shafts of the middle phalanges of digits 2 to 5 (their relationships are described in the discussion of the wrist and hand).

Deep Layer

The deep layer contains the following muscles:
- Flexor digitorum profundus
- Flexor pollicis longus
- Pronator quadratus

The *flexor digitorum profundus muscle* arises from the posterior border of the ulna (with the flexor carpi ulnaris), the proximal two-thirds of the medial surface of the ulna, and adjacent areas of the interosseous membrane. The muscle produces, near the wrist, four discrete tendons that pass side by side under the flexor retinaculum and dorsal to the tendons of the flexor digitorum superficialis muscle. The tendons terminate on the bases of the distal phalanges of digits 2 to 5. In the palm, the tendons give origin to the small lumbrical muscles.

Plate 3.10

Forearm and Wrist

CROSS-SECTIONAL ANATOMY OF RIGHT FOREARM

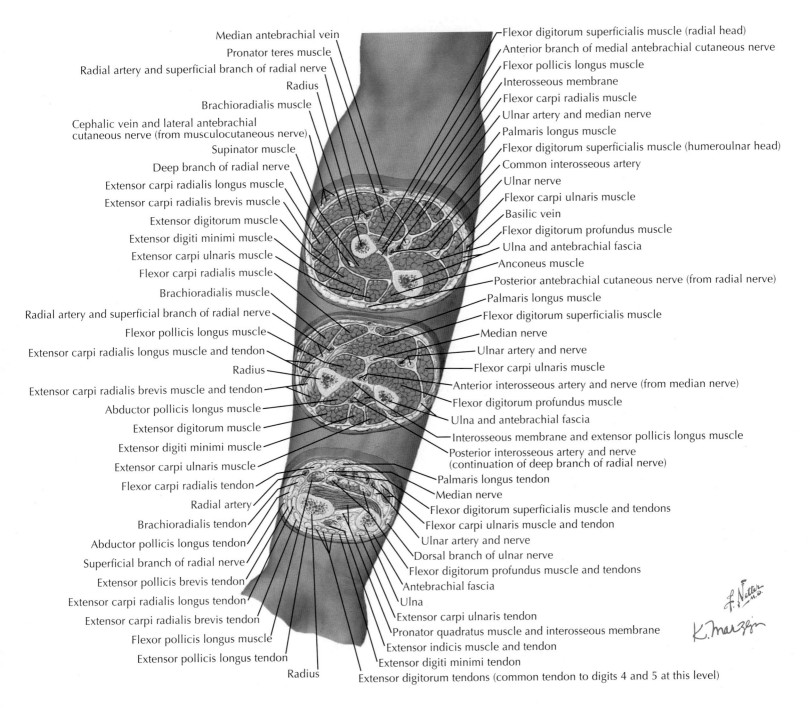

Median antebrachial vein
Pronator teres muscle
Radial artery and superficial branch of radial nerve
Radius
Brachioradialis muscle
Cephalic vein and lateral antebrachial cutaneous nerve (from musculocutaneous nerve)
Supinator muscle
Deep branch of radial nerve
Extensor carpi radialis longus muscle
Extensor carpi radialis brevis muscle
Extensor digitorum muscle
Extensor digiti minimi muscle
Extensor carpi ulnaris muscle
Flexor carpi radialis muscle
Brachioradialis muscle
Radial artery and superficial branch of radial nerve
Flexor pollicis longus muscle
Extensor carpi radialis longus muscle and tendon
Radius
Extensor carpi radialis brevis muscle and tendon
Abductor pollicis longus muscle
Extensor digitorum muscle
Extensor digiti minimi muscle
Extensor carpi ulnaris muscle
Flexor carpi radialis tendon
Radial artery
Brachioradialis tendon
Abductor pollicis longus tendon
Superficial branch of radial nerve
Extensor pollicis brevis tendon
Extensor carpi radialis longus tendon
Extensor carpi radialis brevis tendon
Flexor pollicis longus muscle
Extensor pollicis longus tendon
Radius

Flexor digitorum superficialis muscle (radial head)
Anterior branch of medial antebrachial cutaneous nerve
Flexor pollicis longus muscle
Interosseous membrane
Flexor carpi radialis muscle
Ulnar artery and median nerve
Palmaris longus muscle
Flexor digitorum superficialis muscle (humeroulnar head)
Common interosseous artery
Ulnar nerve
Flexor carpi ulnaris muscle
Basilic vein
Flexor digitorum profundus muscle
Ulna and antebrachial fascia
Anconeus muscle
Posterior antebrachial cutaneous nerve (from radial nerve)
Palmaris longus muscle
Flexor digitorum superficialis muscle
Median nerve
Ulnar artery and nerve
Flexor carpi ulnaris muscle
Anterior interosseous artery and nerve (from median nerve)
Flexor digitorum profundus muscle
Ulna and antebrachial fascia
Interosseous membrane and extensor pollicis longus muscle
Posterior interosseous artery and nerve (continuation of deep branch of radial nerve)
Palmaris longus tendon
Median nerve
Flexor digitorum superficialis muscle and tendons
Flexor carpi ulnaris muscle and tendon
Ulnar artery and nerve
Dorsal branch of ulnar nerve
Flexor digitorum profundus muscle and tendons
Antebrachial fascia
Ulna
Extensor carpi ulnaris tendon
Pronator quadratus muscle and interosseous membrane
Extensor indicis muscle and tendon
Extensor digiti minimi tendon
Extensor digitorum tendons (common tendon to digits 4 and 5 at this level)

MUSCLES OF FOREARM (Continued)

The *flexor pollicis longus muscle* arises principally from the anterior surface of the radius (just below its tuberosity nearly to the upper border of the pronator quadratus) and from the adjacent interosseous membrane. Its tendon, passing between the two sesamoids of the metacarpophalangeal (MCP) joint of the thumb, inserts on the base of the distal phalanx of the thumb.

The *pronator quadratus muscle* is a quadrilateral muscle located just above the wrist and deep to the flexor digitorum profundus and flexor pollicis longus tendons. It arises from the anterior surface of the distal

one-fourth of the ulna, its fibers running transversely across the wrist and inserting into the anterior surface of the distal fourth of the shaft of the radius.

EXTENSOR MUSCLES

The muscles of the fourth, fifth, and sixth groups, the supinator muscle of the first group, and the brachioradialis muscle make up the posterior antebrachial muscles. Six of these make up the superficial layer, and five lie in the deep layer.

Superficial Layer

The six muscles of the superficial layer are listed in the order in which they lie across the back of the forearm, from the radial to the ulnar side:

- Brachioradialis
- Extensor carpi radialis longus
- Extensor carpi radialis brevis
- Extensor digitorum
- Extensor digiti minimi
- Extensor carpi ulnaris

As for the flexor muscles, there is a common tendon of origin from the lateral epicondyle for all muscles arising below the lateral epicondyle.

The *brachioradialis muscle* arises from the upper two-thirds of the supracondylar ridge of the humerus. Its tendon appears at about the middle of the forearm and descends to insert into the lateral side of the base of the styloid process of the radius.

The *extensor carpi radialis longus muscle* arises from the lower third of the supracondylar ridge of the

Plate 3.11

Upper Limb: PART I

CROSS-SECTIONAL ANATOMY OF WRIST

Coronal view

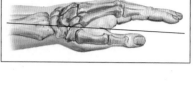

Flexor digitorum superficialis and flexor digitorum profundus tendons

1st metacarpal

Trapezium

Extensor pollicis brevis and abductor pollicis longus tendons

Radial artery

Scaphoid

Lunate

Joint capsule

Scapholunate ligament

Triangular fibrocartilage

Radius

Pronator quadratus muscle

Radial artery

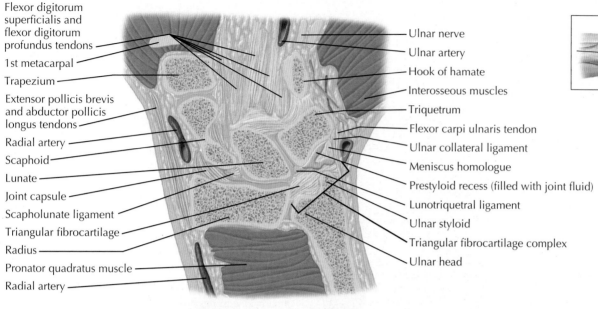

Ulnar nerve

Ulnar artery

Hook of hamate

Interosseous muscles

Triquetrum

Flexor carpi ulnaris tendon

Ulnar collateral ligament

Meniscus homologue

Prestyloid recess (filled with joint fluid)

Lunotriquetral ligament

Ulnar styloid

Triangular fibrocartilage complex

Ulnar head

Sagittal view

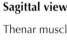

Thenar muscle

Flexor carpi radialis tendon

Transverse carpal ligament

Flexor pollicis longus tendon

Palmar aponeurosis

Joint capsule

Median nerve

Flexor digitorum superficialis tendons

Flexor digitorum profundus and flexor digitorum superficialis muscles

Pronator quadratus muscle

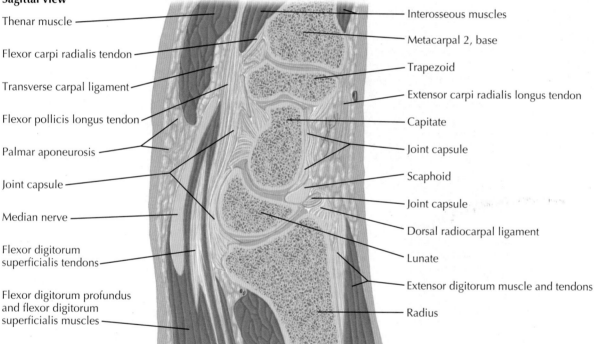

Interosseous muscles

Metacarpal 2, base

Trapezoid

Extensor carpi radialis longus tendon

Capitate

Joint capsule

Scaphoid

Joint capsule

Dorsal radiocarpal ligament

Lunate

Extensor digitorum muscle and tendons

Radius

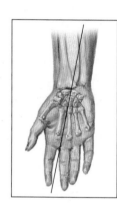

MUSCLES OF FOREARM (Continued)

humerus. It has a flat tendon that reaches into the hand to insert on the dorsum of the second metacarpal.

The *extensor carpi radialis brevis muscle* uses the common tendon of origin for the extensors. Its tendon appears in the lower third of the forearm, closely applied to the overlying tendon of the extensor carpi radialis longus, and inserts on the dorsum of the base of the third metacarpal.

The *extensor digitorum muscle* also uses the common tendon of origin for the extensors. Above the wrist, it provides four tendons that spread out on the dorsum of

the hand, joined side to side in a variable manner by intertendinous connections. Participating in the rather complex "extensor expansion" described in the section on the wrist and hand, these tendons terminate on the bases of the middle and distal phalanges of digits 2 to 5.

The *extensor digiti minimi muscle* is a slender muscle that is sometimes only incompletely separated from the extensor digitorum muscle. Its tendon joins the ulnar side of the tendon of the extensor digitorum muscle to the fifth digit for which it provides independent extensor action.

The *extensor carpi ulnaris muscle* arises by the common tendon from the lateral epicondyle but also from the middle one-half of the posterior border of the ulna. It inserts on the ulnar side of the base of the fifth metacarpal.

Deep Layer

The muscles of the deep layer are generally submerged under those of the superficial group, although certain of their tendons and parts of their fleshy bellies outcrop just above the wrist:

- Supinator
- Abductor pollicis longus
- Extensor pollicis brevis
- Extensor pollicis longus

The *supinator muscle* has a complex origin from the lateral epicondyle of the humerus, radial collateral ligament, annular ligament of the radius, and supinator crest and fossa of the ulna. Its fibers form a flat sheet, directed downward and lateralward, which wraps almost completely around the radius and inserts on the lateral surface of the upper third of this bone. As the

Plate 3.12

Forearm and Wrist

ORIGINS AND INSERTIONS OF FOREARM

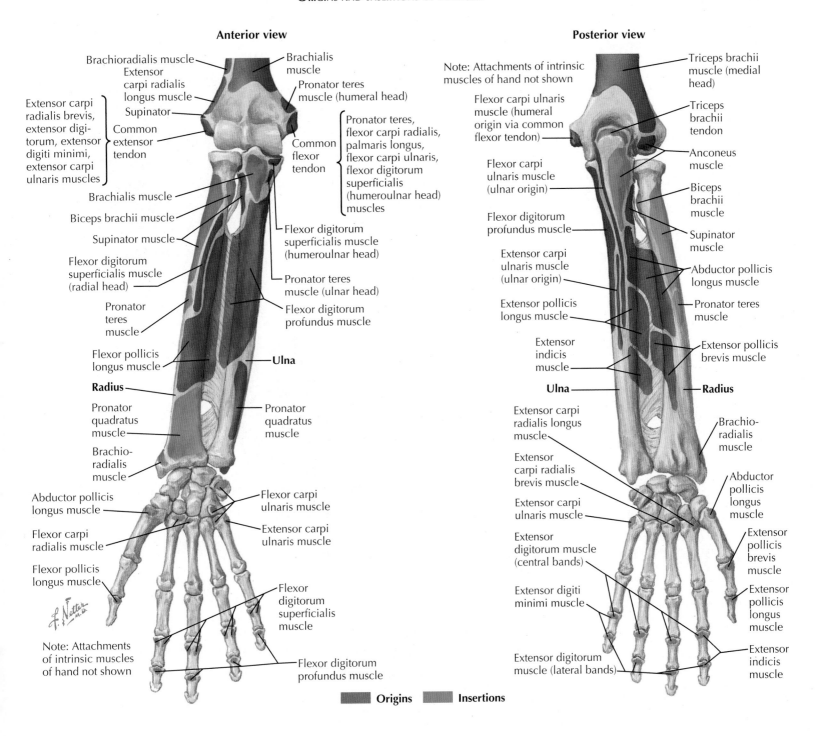

Anterior view

Brachioradialis muscle
Extensor carpi radialis longus muscle
Extensor carpi radialis brevis, extensor digitorum, extensor digiti minimi, extensor carpi ulnaris muscles
Supinator
Common extensor tendon
Brachialis muscle
Biceps brachii muscle
Supinator muscle
Flexor digitorum superficialis muscle (radial head)
Pronator teres muscle
Flexor pollicis longus muscle
Radius
Pronator quadratus muscle
Brachio-radialis muscle
Abductor pollicis longus muscle
Flexor carpi radialis muscle
Flexor pollicis longus muscle

Brachialis muscle
Pronator teres muscle (humeral head)
Common flexor tendon
Pronator teres, flexor carpi radialis, palmaris longus, flexor carpi ulnaris, flexor digitorum superficialis (humeroulnar head) muscles
Flexor digitorum superficialis muscle (humeroulnar head)
Pronator teres muscle (ulnar head)
Flexor digitorum profundus muscle
Ulna
Pronator quadratus muscle
Flexor carpi ulnaris muscle
Extensor carpi ulnaris muscle
Flexor digitorum superficialis muscle

Note: Attachments of intrinsic muscles of hand not shown

Flexor digitorum profundus muscle

Posterior view

Note: Attachments of intrinsic muscles of hand not shown
Flexor carpi ulnaris muscle (humeral origin via common flexor tendon)
Flexor carpi ulnaris muscle (ulnar origin)
Flexor digitorum profundus muscle
Extensor carpi ulnaris muscle (ulnar origin)
Extensor pollicis longus muscle
Extensor indicis muscle
Ulna
Extensor carpi radialis longus muscle
Extensor carpi radialis brevis muscle
Extensor carpi ulnaris muscle
Extensor digitorum muscle (central bands)
Extensor digiti minimi muscle
Extensor digitorum muscle (lateral bands)

Triceps brachii muscle (medial head)
Triceps brachii tendon
Anconeus muscle
Biceps brachii muscle
Supinator muscle
Abductor pollicis longus muscle
Pronator teres muscle
Extensor pollicis brevis muscle
Radius
Brachio-radialis muscle
Abductor pollicis longus muscle
Extensor pollicis brevis muscle
Extensor pollicis longus muscle
Extensor indicis muscle

◼ **Origins**   ◼ **Insertions**

MUSCLES OF FOREARM
(Continued)

muscle courses into the posterior compartment of the forearm, it is separated into superficial and deep laminae by the deep branch of the radial nerve.

The *abductor pollicis longus muscle* lies immediately distal to the supinator. It arises from the middle third of the posterior surface of the radius and the lateral part of the posterior surface of the ulna below the anconeus muscle. The fibers of the muscle converge onto its tendon, which, with the tendon of extensor pollicis brevis closely applied to its medial side, crosses the tendons of the extensor carpi radialis longus and brevis muscles

and inserts on the radial side of the base of the metacarpal of the thumb.

The *extensor pollicis brevis muscle*, with origins from the radius and the interosseous membrane distal to that of the abductor pollicis longus muscle, inserts on the base of the proximal phalanx of the thumb. It is a specialization of the distal part of the abductor pollicis longus muscle.

The *extensor pollicis longus muscle* arises from the ulna and the interosseous membrane distal to the abductor pollicis longus muscle. Its tendon passes to the ulnar side of the dorsal tubercle of the radius, then obliquely across the tendons of both radial carpal extensors, terminating on the base of the distal phalanx of the thumb.

The *extensor indicis muscle* arises just below the extensor pollicis longus from the ulna and from the interosseous membrane. In the hand, the tendon joins the ulnar side of the tendon of the digital extensor muscle for the index finger and participates with it in forming the extensor expansion over that digit.

Knowledge of the cross-sectional anatomy of the forearm is critical to understanding advanced imaging views of the forearm as well as surgical anatomy. Knowing the origins and insertions of the muscles and tendons of the forearm is helpful during operative dissection and exploration of the forearm and wrist and provides the framework to understanding the functional anatomy of the forearm and wrist.

Plate 3.13

Upper Limb: PART I

BLOOD SUPPLY OF FOREARM

The brachial artery divides into radial and ulnar arteries. Their named branches lie near the elbow and wrist, and only unnamed muscular branches arise in the middle forearm.

RADIAL ARTERY

This smaller branch continues the direct line of the brachial artery, ending at the wrist at the "pulse position." It first crosses the tendon of the pronator teres muscle and descends adjacent to the superficial branch of the radial nerve. It branches into the radial recurrent artery and muscular, palmar carpal, and superficial palmar branches.

The *radial recurrent artery* arises shortly below the origin of the radial artery. Ascending on the supinator muscle, the artery supplies this muscle and the brachioradialis and brachialis muscles and anastomoses with the radial collateral artery (see Plate 3.8).

Muscular branches supply the muscles of the radial side of the forearm. The *palmar carpal branch* arises near the distal border of the pronator quadratus muscle. It ends by anastomosing with the palmar carpal branch of the ulnar artery, the termination of the anterior interosseous artery, and recurrent branches of the deep palmar arterial arch.

The *superficial palmar branch* leaves the radial artery just before it turns from the radial border of the wrist onto the back of the hand. It descends over or through the muscles of the thumb and joins the superficial branch of the ulnar artery to form the superficial palmar arterial arch.

ULNAR ARTERY

This larger branch describes a gentle curve to the ulnar side of the forearm. It passes deep to both heads of the pronator teres and all the other superficial flexor muscles of the forearm and is crossed by the median nerve. It lies deep to the flexor carpi ulnaris muscle and enters the hand in company with the ulnar nerve.

The *anterior ulnar recurrent artery* turns upward from just below the elbow joint between the brachialis and pronator teres muscles. It supplies these muscles and anastomoses with the anterior branches of both ulnar collateral arteries.

The *posterior ulnar recurrent artery,* larger than the anterior, arises near or in common with it. It ascends between the flexor digitorum superficialis and flexor digitorum profundus muscles to supply the elbow joint. It ends in anastomoses with posterior branches of both ulnar collateral arteries and the interosseous recurrent artery and in the network of the olecranon.

The *common interosseous artery* arises from the radial side of the ulnar artery and divides into anterior and posterior interosseous arteries. The *anterior interosseous artery* descends on the anterior surface of the interosseous membrane as far as the upper border of the pronator quadratus muscle in company with veins and the anterior interosseous branch of the median nerve. It gives off nutrient arteries to the radius and ulna and a long slender median artery to the palm. At the upper border of the pronator quadratus muscle, a small *palmar carpal branch* is given off. The artery terminates in the dorsal carpal network.

The *posterior interosseous artery* passes to the back of the upper forearm, emerging between the supinator and abductor pollicis longus muscles with the deep

branch of the radial nerve. Sending twigs to the extensor muscles of the forearm, it descends to anastomose with the dorsal terminal branch of the anterior interosseous artery. An interosseous recurrent branch ascends deep to the supinator and anconeus muscles to the interval between the lateral epicondyle of the humerus and the olecranon; there, it communicates with the middle collateral, inferior ulnar collateral, and posterior ulnar recurrent arteries.

Muscular branches of the ulnar artery reach the muscles of the ulnar side of the forearm. The *palmar carpal branch* arises at the upper border of the flexor retinaculum, passes across the wrist deep to the flexor tendons, and unites with the palmar carpal branch of the radial artery. The *dorsal carpal branch* arises just above the pisiform. It winds around the border of the wrist, deep to the tendons, to help form the dorsal carpal arterial arch.

Anterior view

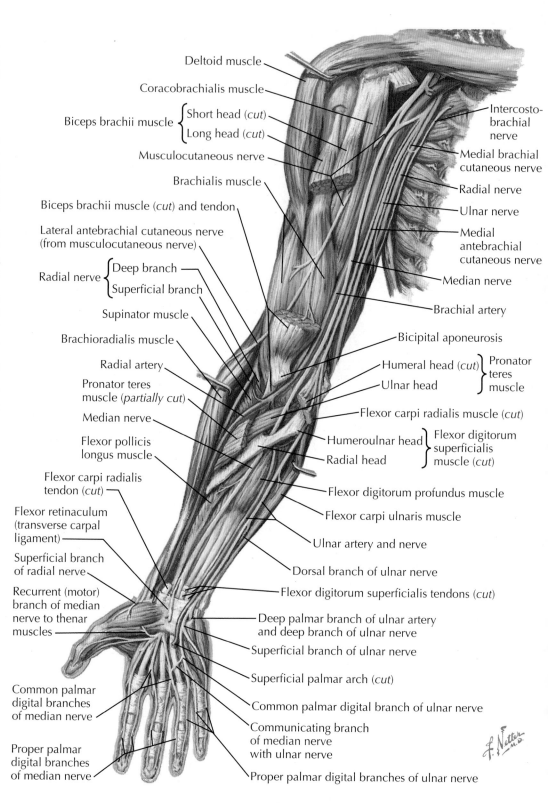

Deltoid muscle

Coracobrachialis muscle

Biceps brachii muscle { Short head (*cut*) / Long head (*cut*)

Musculocutaneous nerve

Brachialis muscle

Biceps brachii muscle (*cut*) and tendon

Lateral antebrachial cutaneous nerve (from musculocutaneous nerve)

Radial nerve { Deep branch / Superficial branch

Supinator muscle

Brachioradialis muscle

Radial artery

Pronator teres muscle (*partially cut*)

Median nerve

Flexor pollicis longus muscle

Flexor carpi radialis tendon (*cut*)

Flexor retinaculum (transverse carpal ligament)

Superficial branch of radial nerve

Recurrent (motor) branch of median nerve to thenar muscles

Common palmar digital branches of median nerve

Proper palmar digital branches of median nerve

Intercostobrachial nerve

Medial brachial cutaneous nerve

Radial nerve

Ulnar nerve

Medial antebrachial cutaneous nerve

Median nerve

Brachial artery

Bicipital aponeurosis

Humeral head (*cut*) / Ulnar head } Pronator teres muscle

Flexor carpi radialis muscle (*cut*)

Humeroulnar head / Radial head } Flexor digitorum superficialis muscle (*cut*)

Flexor digitorum profundus muscle

Flexor carpi ulnaris muscle

Ulnar artery and nerve

Dorsal branch of ulnar nerve

Flexor digitorum superficialis tendons (*cut*)

Deep palmar branch of ulnar artery and deep branch of ulnar nerve

Superficial branch of ulnar nerve

Superficial palmar arch (*cut*)

Common palmar digital branch of ulnar nerve

Communicating branch of median nerve with ulnar nerve

Proper palmar digital branches of ulnar nerve

f. Netter M.D.

Plate 3.14

Forearm and Wrist

MEDIAN NERVE

The median nerve (C[5], C6, C7, C8; T1) is formed by the union of *medial* and *lateral roots* arising from the corresponding cords of the brachial plexus.

COURSE IN ARM

The median nerve runs from the axilla into the arm, lateral to the brachial artery. At about the level of the insertion of the coracobrachialis muscle, the nerve inclines medially over the brachial artery and then descends along its medial side to the cubital fossa. Here, it lies behind the bicipital aponeurosis and the median cubital vein and in front of the insertion of the brachialis muscle and the elbow joint. (The close proximity of the vein, artery, and nerve should be remembered when performing venipuncture in this area.) The only branches given off in the arm are filaments to the brachial vessels and an inconstant twig to the pronator teres muscle.

COURSE IN FOREARM

The median nerve passes into the forearm between the humeral and ulnar heads of the pronator teres muscle, the latter separating it from the ulnar artery. It then runs deep to the aponeurotic arch between the humeroulnar and radial heads of the flexor digitorum superficialis muscle and continues downward between this muscle and the flexor digitorum profundus muscle. In the forearm, the nerve supplies branches to the pronator teres, flexor digitorum superficialis, flexor carpi radialis, and palmaris longus muscles and articular twigs to the elbow and proximal radioulnar joints.

The longest branch is the *anterior interosseous nerve*, which, accompanied by the corresponding artery, runs downward on the interosseous membrane between the flexor pollicis longus and the flexor digitorum profundus muscles; it supplies the former muscle and the lateral part of the latter and ends under the pronator quadratus, supplying this muscle and the DR, radiocarpal, and carpal joints. Vascular filaments help innervate the ulnar and anterior interosseous vessels and the nutrient vessels of the radius and ulna. A *palmar branch* arises 3 to 4 cm above the flexor retinaculum and descends over it to supply the skin of the median part of the palm and the thenar eminence. In the forearm, the median and ulnar nerves are occasionally interconnected by strands, which may explain certain anomalies in the nerve supply of the hand.

In the lower forearm, the median nerve becomes more superficial between the tendons of the palmaris longus and the flexor carpi radialis muscles. Together with the tendons of the digital flexor muscles, it enters the palm through the carpal tunnel that is bound anteriorly by the tough flexor retinaculum and posteriorly by the carpal bones. Emerging from the tunnel, the nerve splays out into its terminal muscular and palmar digital branches. The muscular branch arises close to, or is initially united with, the common palmar digital nerve to the thumb; it curves outward over or through the flexor pollicis brevis muscle to supply it before dividing to supply the abductor pollicis brevis and opponens pollicis muscles. The muscular branch may also supply all or part of the first dorsal interosseous muscle. In rare instances, it arises in the carpal tunnel and pierces the flexor retinaculum—an arrangement of potential clinical concern.

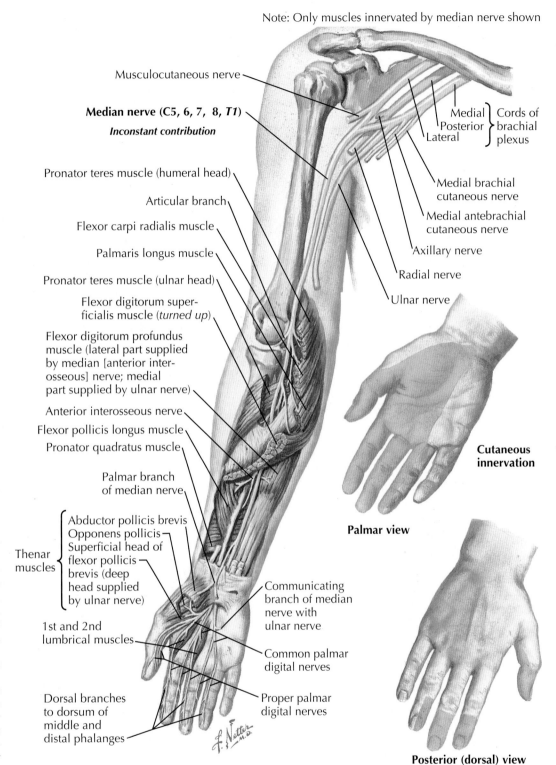

Note: Only muscles innervated by median nerve shown

Musculocutaneous nerve

Median nerve (C5, 6, 7, 8, T1)
Inconstant contribution

Medial ⎱ Cords of
Posterior ⎰ brachial
Lateral   plexus

Pronator teres muscle (humeral head)

Medial brachial cutaneous nerve

Articular branch

Medial antebrachial cutaneous nerve

Flexor carpi radialis muscle

Axillary nerve

Palmaris longus muscle

Radial nerve

Pronator teres muscle (ulnar head)

Ulnar nerve

Flexor digitorum superficialis muscle (*turned up*)

Flexor digitorum profundus muscle (lateral part supplied by median [anterior interosseous] nerve; medial part supplied by ulnar nerve)

Anterior interosseous nerve

Flexor pollicis longus muscle

Pronator quadratus muscle

Palmar branch of median nerve

Thenar muscles ⎰ Abductor pollicis brevis
Opponens pollicis
Superficial head of flexor pollicis brevis (deep head supplied by ulnar nerve)

Communicating branch of median nerve with ulnar nerve

1st and 2nd lumbrical muscles

Common palmar digital nerves

Dorsal branches to dorsum of middle and distal phalanges

Proper palmar digital nerves

Cutaneous innervation

Palmar view

Posterior (dorsal) view

The *common* and *proper palmar digital nerves* vary in their origins and distributions, but the usual arrangement is that shown in Plates 3.13 and 3.14. The proper palmar digital nerves give off dorsal twigs, which innervate the skin (including the nail beds) over the distal and dorsal aspects of the lateral three and one-half digits. Occasionally, they supply only two and one-half digits. The proper palmar digital branches to the radial side of the index finger and to the contiguous sides of the index and middle fingers also carry motor fibers to supply the first and second lumbrical muscles, respectively. Therefore the digital nerves are not concerned solely with cutaneous sensibility. They contain an admixture of efferent and afferent somatic and autonomic fibers, which transmit impulses to and from sensory endings, vessels, sweat glands, and arrectores pilorum muscles and between fascial, tendinous, osseous, and articular structures in their areas of distribution.

Plate 3.15

Upper Limb: PART

ULNAR NERVE

The ulnar nerve (C[7], C8; T1) is the main continuation of the medial cord of the brachial plexus (see Plate 3.13).

COURSE IN ARM

Initially, the ulnar nerve lies between the axillary artery and vein; as it enters the arm, it runs on the medial side of the brachial artery. At about the middle of the arm, it pierces the medial intermuscular septum and descends anterior to the medial head of the triceps brachii muscle, alongside the superior ulnar collateral artery. In the lower third of the arm, it inclines posteriorly to reach the interval between the medial humeral epicondyle and the olecranon. As the nerve enters the forearm, it lies in the groove behind the medial epicondyle, between the humeral and ulnar heads of the flexor carpi ulnaris muscle. Above the elbow, the ulnar nerve supplies no constant branches.

COURSE IN FOREARM AND HAND

The ulnar nerve runs downward on the medial side of the forearm, lying first on the ulnar collateral ligament of the elbow joint and then on the flexor digitorum profundus muscle, deep to the flexor carpi ulnaris muscle. At the elbow, the ulnar nerve and artery are separated by a considerable gap, but they are closely apposed in the lower two-thirds of the forearm, with the artery on the lateral side. At the flexor carpi ulnaris tendon, the nerve and artery emerge from under its lateral edge and are covered only by skin and fascia. They reach the hand by crossing the anterior surface of the flexor retinaculum lateral to the pisiform, and the nerve splits, under cover of the palmaris brevis muscle, into its superficial and deep terminal branches.

BRANCHES

In the forearm and hand, the ulnar nerve gives off articular, muscular, palmar, dorsal, superficial and deep terminal, and vascular branches.

Fine articular branches for the elbow joint arise from the main nerve as it runs posterior to the medial epicondyle; before splitting into its terminal branches, it supplies filaments to the wrist joint.

In the upper forearm, branches are given off to the flexor carpi ulnaris and the medial half of the flexor digitorum profundus muscles. The *palmar branch* arises 5 to 7 cm above the wrist, descends near the ulnar artery, pierces the deep fascia, and supplies the skin over the hypothenar eminence; it communicates with the medial antebrachial cutaneous nerve and the palmar branch of the median nerve. The *dorsal ulnar branch* arises 5 to 10 cm above the wrist, passes posteriorly and deep to the flexor carpi ulnaris tendon, pierces the deep fascia, and continues along the dorsomedial side of the wrist. Here it divides into branches for the areas of skin on the medial side of the back of the hand and fingers. There are usually two or three *dorsal digital nerves,* one supplying the medial side of the little finger, the second splitting into *proper dorsal digital nerves* to supply adjacent sides of the little and ring fingers, and the third (when present) supplying contiguous sides of the ring and middle fingers.

The *superficial terminal branch* supplies the palmaris brevis muscle, innervates the skin on the medial side of the palm, and gives off two palmar digital nerves. The

Note: Only muscles innervated by ulnar nerve shown

Anterior view

Cutaneous innervation

Palmar view

Posterior (dorsal) view

Flexor pollicis brevis muscle (deep head only; superficial head and other thenar muscles supplied by median nerve)

Adductor pollicis muscle

Ulnar nerve (C7, 8, T1) (no branches above elbow) *Inconstant contribution*

Medial epicondyle

Articular branch (behind condyle)

Flexor digitorum profundus muscle (medial part only; lateral part supplied by anterior interosseous branch of median nerve)

Flexor carpi ulnaris muscle (*drawn aside*)

Dorsal branch of ulnar nerve

Palmar branch

Palmar carpal ligament

Superficial branch

Deep branch

Palmaris brevis
Abductor digiti minimi } Hypothenar muscles
Flexor digiti minimi brevis }
Opponens digiti minimi }

Common palmar digital nerve

Communicating branch of median nerve with ulnar nerve

Palmar and dorsal interosseous muscles

3rd and 4th lumbrical muscles (*turned down*)

Palmar digital nerves (dorsal digital nerves are from dorsal branch)

Dorsal branches to dorsum of middle and distal phalanges

f. Netter M.D.

K. marzejon

first is the *proper palmar digital nerve* for the medial side of the little finger; the second, the *common palmar digital nerve,* communicates with the adjoining common palmar digital branch of the median nerve before dividing into the two *proper palmar digital nerves* for the adjacent sides of the little and ring fingers. Rarely, the ulnar nerve supplies two and one-half rather than one and one-half digits, and the areas supplied by the median and radial nerves are reciprocally reduced.

The *deep terminal branch* runs between and supplies the abductor and flexor muscles of the little finger,

perforates and supplies the opponens digiti minimi, and then accompanies the deep palmar arterial arch behind the flexor digitorum tendons. In the palm, it gives muscular branches to the third and fourth lumbrical and the interosseous muscles and ends by supplying the adductor pollicis muscle and, sometimes, the deep head of the flexor pollicis brevis muscle.

Variations in the nerve supplies of the palmar muscles are as common as the variations in the cutaneous distribution; they are due to the variety of interconnections between the ulnar and median nerves.

Plate 3.16

Forearm and Wrist

Anterior (palmar) view

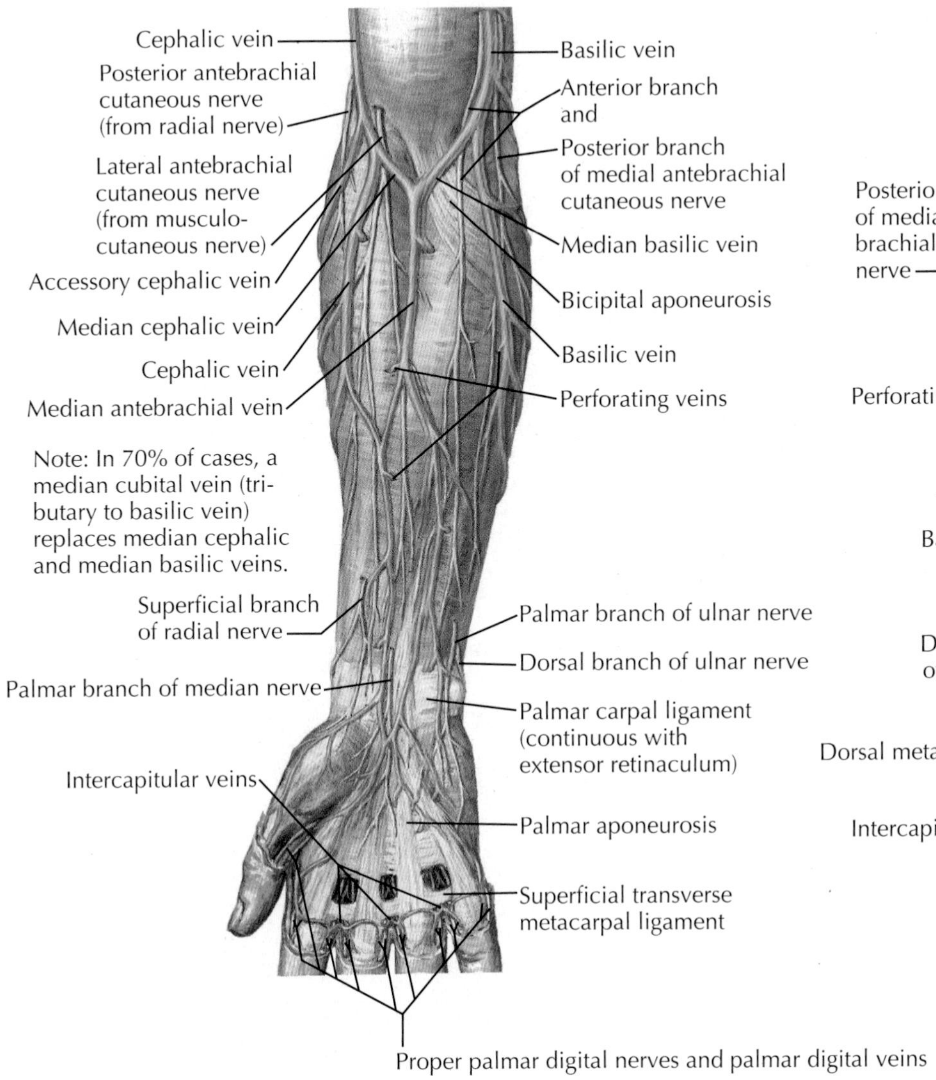

Cephalic vein
Posterior antebrachial cutaneous nerve (from radial nerve)
Lateral antebrachial cutaneous nerve (from musculo-cutaneous nerve)
Accessory cephalic vein
Median cephalic vein
Cephalic vein
Median antebrachial vein

Note: In 70% of cases, a median cubital vein (tributary to basilic vein) replaces median cephalic and median basilic veins.

Superficial branch of radial nerve
Palmar branch of median nerve
Intercapitular veins

Basilic vein
Anterior branch and
Posterior branch of medial antebrachial cutaneous nerve
Median basilic vein
Bicipital aponeurosis
Basilic vein
Perforating veins

Palmar branch of ulnar nerve
Dorsal branch of ulnar nerve
Palmar carpal ligament (continuous with extensor retinaculum)
Palmar aponeurosis
Superficial transverse metacarpal ligament

Proper palmar digital nerves and palmar digital veins

Posterior (dorsal) view

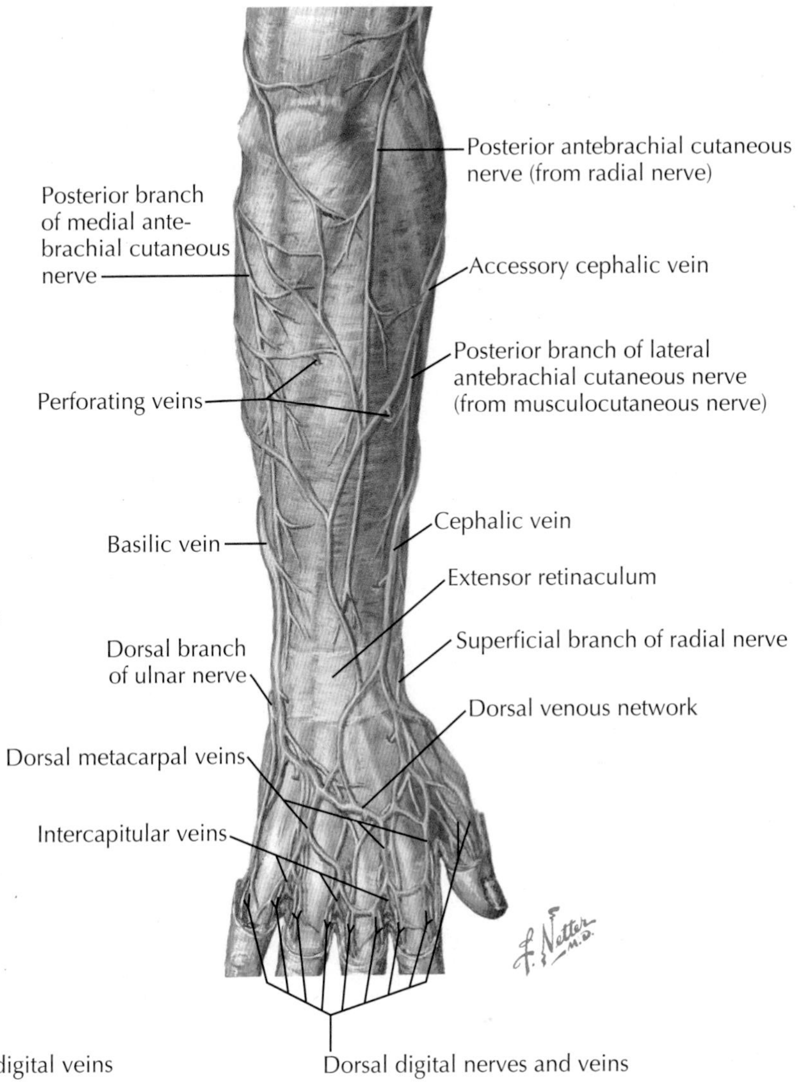

Posterior branch of medial antebrachial cutaneous nerve
Perforating veins
Basilic vein
Dorsal branch of ulnar nerve
Dorsal metacarpal veins
Intercapitular veins

Posterior antebrachial cutaneous nerve (from radial nerve)
Accessory cephalic vein
Posterior branch of lateral antebrachial cutaneous nerve (from musculocutaneous nerve)
Cephalic vein
Extensor retinaculum
Superficial branch of radial nerve
Dorsal venous network

Dorsal digital nerves and veins

CUTANEOUS NERVES

The *superficial branch of the radial nerve* arises in the cubital fossa by the division there of the radial nerve into deep and superficial branches (see Plates 3.13 and 3.16). The superficial branch, which is entirely cutaneous, courses through the forearm under cover of the brachioradialis muscle and is accompanied by the radial artery. At the distal third of the forearm, the superficial branch of the radial nerve perforates the antebrachial fascia along the lateral border of the forearm and divides into two branches.

The smaller *lateral branch* supplies the skin of the radial side and eminence of the thumb and communicates with the lateral antebrachial cutaneous nerve. The larger *medial branch* divides into four dorsal digital nerves. The first dorsal digital nerve supplies the ulnar side of the thumb; the second supplies the radial side of the index finger; the third distributes to the adjoining sides of the index and middle fingers; and the fourth supplies the adjacent sides of the middle and ring fingers.

There is usually an anastomosis on the back of the hand between the superficial branch of the radial nerve and the dorsal branch of the ulnar nerve, and there is some variability in the apparent source of the last (more median) branch of either nerve. In some such cases, the adjacent sides of the middle and ring fingers are in the territory of the ulnar nerve. Dorsal digital nerves fail to reach the extremities of the digits. They reach to the base of the nail of the thumb, to the distal interphalangeal joint of the second digit, and not quite as far as the proximal interphalangeal joints of the third and fourth digits. The distal areas of the dorsum of the digits not supplied by the radial nerve receive branches from the stout palmar digital branches of the median nerve.

The *dorsal branch of the ulnar nerve* completes the cutaneous supply of the dorsum of the hand and digits. It arises about 5 cm above the wrist, passes dorsalward from beneath the flexor carpi ulnaris tendon, and then pierces the forearm fascia. At the ulnar border of the wrist, the nerve divides into three dorsal digital branches.

The first branch courses along the ulnar side of the dorsum of the hand and supplies the ulnar side of the

little finger as far as the root of the nail. The second branch divides at the cleft between the fourth and fifth digits and supplies their adjacent sides. The third branch may divide similarly; it may supply the adjacent sides of the third and fourth digits, or it may simply anastomose with the fourth dorsal digital branch of the superficial branch of the radial nerve. The dorsal branches to the fourth digit usually extend only as far as the base of the second phalanx, with the more distal parts of the fourth and fifth digits supplied by palmar digital branches of the ulnar nerve.

The *palmar branch of the ulnar nerve* arises about the middle of the forearm, descending under the antebrachial fascia in front of the ulnar artery (see Plates 3.16 and 3.17). It perforates the fascia just above the wrist and supplies the skin of the hypothenar eminence and the medial part of the palm.

The *palmar branch of the median nerve* arises just above the wrist (see Plates 3.16 and 3.17). It perforates the palmar carpal ligament between the tendons of the palmaris longus and flexor carpi radialis muscles and distributes to the skin of the central depressed area of the palm and the medial part of the thenar eminence.

Plate 3.17

Upper Limb: PART I

Palmar view

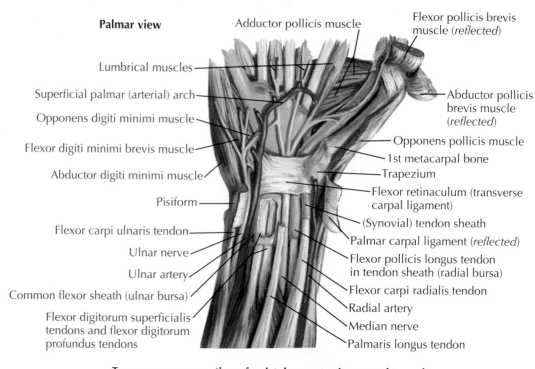

- Adductor pollicis muscle
- Flexor pollicis brevis muscle (*reflected*)
- Lumbrical muscles
- Superficial palmar (arterial) arch
- Opponens digiti minimi muscle
- Flexor digiti minimi brevis muscle
- Abductor digiti minimi muscle
- Pisiform
- Flexor carpi ulnaris tendon
- Ulnar nerve
- Ulnar artery
- Common flexor sheath (ulnar bursa)
- Flexor digitorum superficialis tendons and flexor digitorum profundus tendons
- Abductor pollicis brevis muscle (*reflected*)
- Opponens pollicis muscle
- 1st metacarpal bone
- Trapezium
- Flexor retinaculum (transverse carpal ligament)
- (Synovial) tendon sheath
- Palmar carpal ligament (*reflected*)
- Flexor pollicis longus tendon in tendon sheath (radial bursa)
- Flexor carpi radialis tendon
- Radial artery
- Median nerve
- Palmaris longus tendon

Transverse cross section of wrist demonstrating carpal tunnel

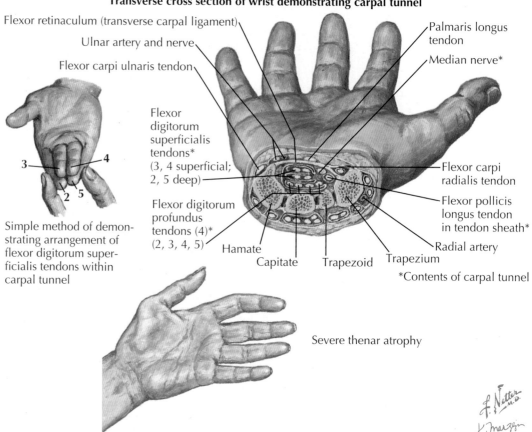

- Flexor retinaculum (transverse carpal ligament)
- Ulnar artery and nerve
- Flexor carpi ulnaris tendon
- Flexor digitorum superficialis tendons* (3, 4 superficial; 2, 5 deep)
- Flexor digitorum profundus tendons (4)* (2, 3, 4, 5)
- Hamate
- Capitate
- Trapezoid
- Trapezium
- Palmaris longus tendon
- Median nerve*
- Flexor carpi radialis tendon
- Flexor pollicis longus tendon in tendon sheath*
- Radial artery

*Contents of carpal tunnel

Simple method of demonstrating arrangement of flexor digitorum superficialis tendons within carpal tunnel

3 4
2 5

Severe thenar atrophy

Carpal Tunnel Syndrome

Carpal tunnel syndrome is the most common compression neuropathy in the upper extremity. The median nerve becomes compressed beneath the transverse carpal ligament, which is the roof of the carpal tunnel. The carpal tunnel itself contains nine flexor tendons, their associated synovium, and the median nerve.

The patient most often complains that the hand "goes to sleep." Activities such as driving the car, holding a book, or blow-drying the hair will often exacerbate these symptoms. Nighttime wakening is nearly universal as the wrist is pulled into a flexed position during sleep by the strong wrist flexors, and this is often the symptom that encourages the patient to seek medical advice.

The diagnosis of carpal tunnel syndrome is made by a careful clinical history combined with a focused physical examination. Associated conditions including diabetes mellitus, rheumatoid arthritis, gout, hypothyroidism, and pregnancy must be discussed. Physical examination first excludes more proximal nerve compression (cervical, brachial plexopathy, pronator syndrome). The Phalen test and percussion of the median nerve at the carpal tunnel can reproduce paresthesias into the radial three digits. Direct compression over the median nerve (Durkan test) has been shown to be both sensitive and specific for diagnosing carpal tunnel syndrome. Sensory testing should also be performed, as well as evaluation for thenar atrophy—signs of more advanced or prolonged median nerve compression. Electrodiagnostic testing is frequently obtained to confirm the diagnosis, grade the severity of median nerve

compression/injury, and provide prognostic information for recovery after surgical decompression.

Initial treatment consists of night splinting with the wrist in neutral, use of antiinflammatory medications when appropriate, and modification of activities. The next step in treatment employs injection of corticosteroid into the carpal canal. Eighty percent of patients report symptom improvement after injection lasting on average 3 to 9 months. Failure of conservative measures or patients presenting initially with severe

compression, thenar atrophy, and dense numbness are considered for surgical release of the carpal tunnel. Surgery can be performed either open or endoscopically with the shared goal of complete release of the transverse carpal ligament and distal antebrachial fascia. Complete relief of night symptoms occurs quickly, whereas sensory improvement takes longer to recover. Residual numbness is not uncommon in severe cases, and patients must be educated before surgical release about this potential.

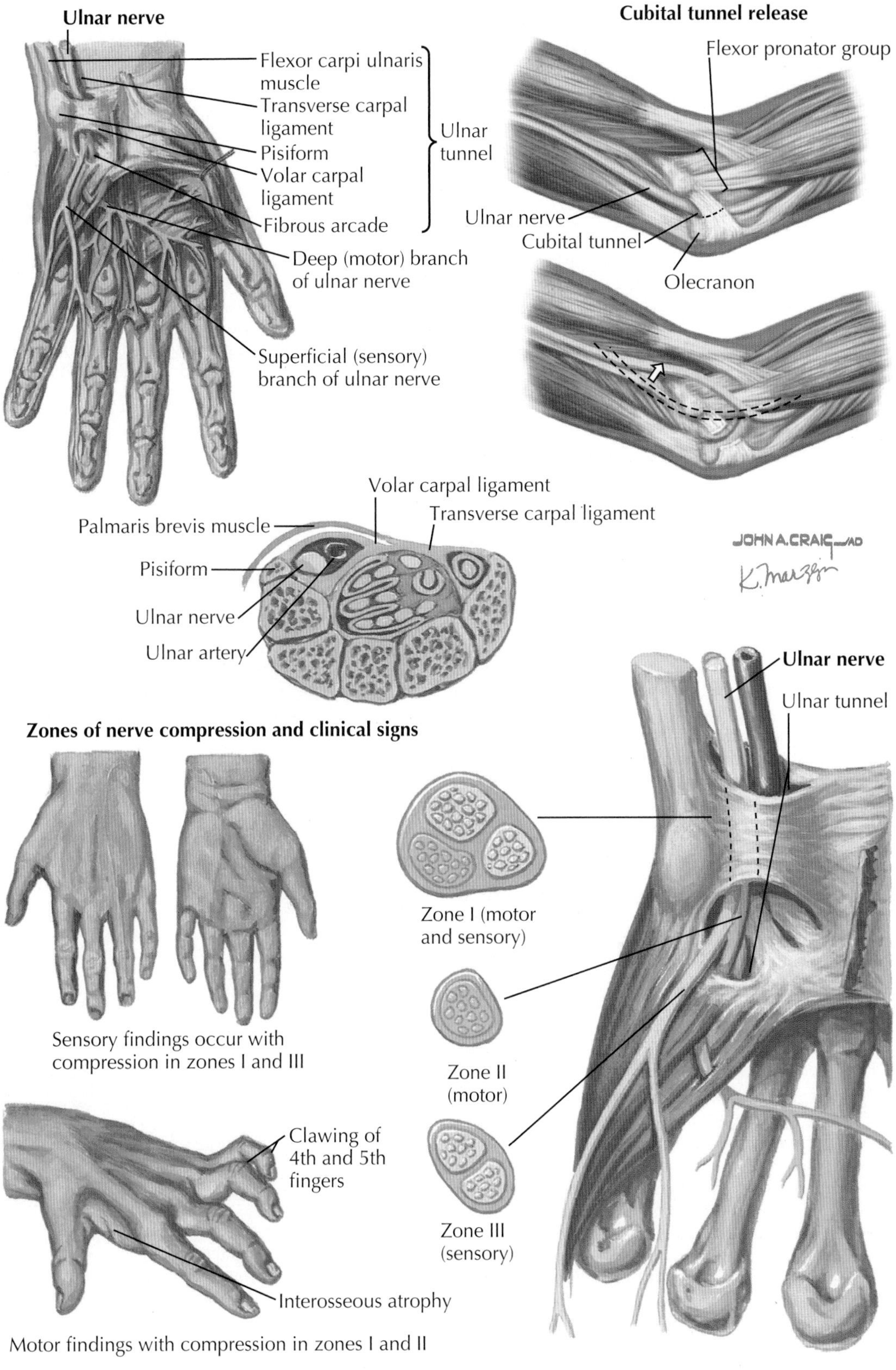

Plate 3.18

Forearm and Wrist

Ulnar nerve

Flexor carpi ulnaris muscle

Transverse carpal ligament

Pisiform

Volar carpal ligament

Fibrous arcade

} Ulnar tunnel

Deep (motor) branch of ulnar nerve

Superficial (sensory) branch of ulnar nerve

Cubital tunnel release

Flexor pronator group

Ulnar nerve

Cubital tunnel

Olecranon

Volar carpal ligament

Transverse carpal ligament

Palmaris brevis muscle

Pisiform

Ulnar nerve

Ulnar artery

JOHN A. CRAIG—AD

K. marzen

Ulnar nerve

Ulnar tunnel

Zones of nerve compression and clinical signs

Sensory findings occur with compression in zones I and III

Clawing of 4th and 5th fingers

Interosseous atrophy

Motor findings with compression in zones I and II

Zone I (motor and sensory)

Zone II (motor)

Zone III (sensory)

CUBITAL TUNNEL SYNDROME

Ulnar nerve compression at the elbow (cubital tunnel syndrome) is the second most common compression neuropathy in the upper extremity. The ulnar nerve runs posterior to the medial epicondyle and can be compressed at several points along its course. Patients initially report numbness and tingling most often in the small and ring fingers. As symptoms progress, medial elbow pain becomes more prominent, as does clumsiness in the hand. Advanced cases of ulnar nerve compression at the elbow will demonstrate atrophy of the intrinsic muscles of the hand (most obvious involving the first dorsal interosseous) and clawing of the fourth and fifth digits. Physical examination focuses on a detailed sensory examination and muscle testing of the intrinsic muscles of the hand. Instability of the ulnar nerve with elbow flexion should be evaluated. A Tinel sign over the ulnar nerve in the cubital tunnel, as well as elbow flexion/compression testing, can help localize the location of ulnar nerve compression at the level of the elbow. Electrodiagnostic testing can help make an accurate diagnosis and evaluate for more proximal and/or distal points of compression.

Initial treatment in a patient without weakness or atrophy consists of diminishing traction and compression of the ulnar nerve at the cubital tunnel. Nighttime splinting with the elbow at approximately 30 degrees, an elbow pad during the day to avoid direct trauma to the nerve, and activity modification often lead to dramatic symptom relief. Patients failing at least 3 months of consistent nonoperative treatment and/or patients presenting with more advanced symptoms should be considered for operative decompression. There are numerous surgical options from in situ decompression

to medial epicondylectomy to anterior transposition of the ulnar nerve either subcutaneously or submuscularly. Recent reports have demonstrated positive results with endoscopic ulnar nerve decompression, but further studies are needed.

Less commonly, the ulnar nerve can be compressed at the level of the wrist (at the Guyon canal). The symptoms are similar to those of cubital tunnel syndrome, but medial elbow pain and numbness along the dorsum

of the hand are absent. The ulnar nerve can be compressed at different points in reference to the hook of the hamate, and symptoms can vary from pure motor or sensory changes to combined losses. Physical examination includes a positive Tinel sign at the ulnar wrist, and careful palpation must evaluate for masses (ganglion/lipoma) and rule out hypothenar hammer syndrome. Conservative treatment is the initial management, followed by surgical decompression.

Plate 3.19

Upper Limb: PART I

EXTENSION/COMPRESSION FRACTURE OF DISTAL RADIUS (COLLES FRACTURE)

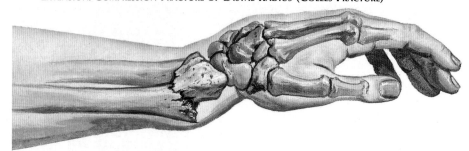

Lateral view of Colles fracture demonstrates characteristic silver fork deformity with dorsal and proximal displacement of distal fragment. Note dorsal instead of normal volar slope of articular surface of distal radius.

FRACTURE OF DISTAL RADIUS

Approximately 80% of fractures of the forearm involve the distal radius and the DRUJ. Fractures of the distal radius are common injuries in children, adults, and elderly persons, usually resulting from a fall on the outstretched hand. Significantly more force is required to fracture this part of the radius in adolescents and young adults than in older adults with severe osteoporosis. Fractures that involve the joint are usually caused by high impact.

Evaluation of any injury in the distal radius must include radiographs of the wrist, forearm, and elbow. True anteroposterior (AP), lateral, and sometimes oblique views are required to determine the extent of the injury. If intraarticular involvement is suspected, computed tomography (CT) can be performed to determine the degree of joint displacement and guide management. Fractures of the distal radius may be stable or unstable, depending on the degree of comminution and initial fracture displacement. Associated injuries to the carpal bones or ligaments of the wrist must be evaluated for and managed appropriately.

FRACTURE TYPES

Extension/Compression

The precipitating injury of the extension/compression, or Colles, fracture is a fall on the outstretched hand. The deformity is caused by dorsal displacement of the distal radius and swelling of the distal portion of the forearm and is referred to as a "silver fork" deformity. Successful treatment involves restoration of (1) the radius to its proper length, (2) the radial inclination and volar tilt of the distal radius, and (3) the congruity of the articular surface of the DR and radiocarpal joints. Loss of more than 5 mm of radial length (easily measured by using the styloid process of the ulna as a reference point) may result in disability. Restoration of the volar tilt of the distal radius is critical to long-term outcomes and diminishes the risk of altered carpal kinematics, which would lead to degenerative changes of both the radiocarpal and midcarpal joints.

If more than 50% of the metaphysis of the distal radius is comminuted, the fracture is probably unstable, and reduction is difficult to maintain in a plaster cast alone. This type of fracture is best visualized on the lateral radiograph. Definitive treatment is determined not only by the injury but also by the patient's age and occupation. Anatomic restoration is more important in younger, working patients, whereas some loss of radial

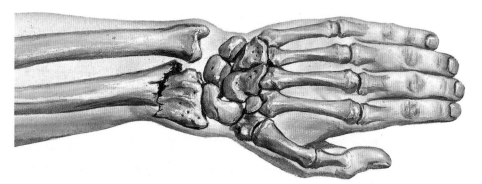

Dorsal view shows radial deviation of hand with ulnar prominence of styloid process of ulna and decrease or reverse of normal radial slope of articular surface of distal radius.

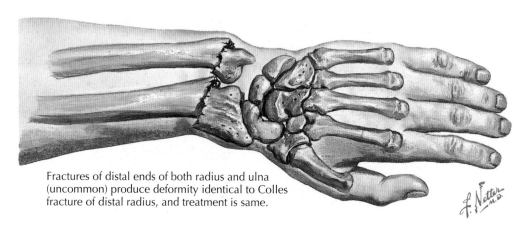

Fractures of distal ends of both radius and ulna (uncommon) produce deformity identical to Colles fracture of distal radius, and treatment is same.

length and tilt may be more acceptable in sedentary patients.

Fracture of Articular Margin of Distal Radius

Fractures of the articular margin, called Barton fractures, represent a small percentage of fractures of the distal radius. This type of fracture is best described as a fracture-dislocation of the wrist. Correct diagnosis of Barton fracture is very important because it is an inherently unstable injury and therefore difficult to manage with the traditional closed method. The injury is further defined by the direction of the dislocation. If the dorsal aspect of the articular margin, or rim, is fractured and the carpus is displaced dorsally, the injury is termed a *dorsal Barton fracture;* conversely, the more common *volar Barton fracture* refers to a fracture in which the dislocation is displaced volarly.

A fall on the outstretched hand is the most common cause of the Barton fracture. The impact wedges the lunate against either the dorsal or the volar margin of the articular surface of the radius. The lunate acts as a lever against the articular surface, causing it to fracture. The carpus is then dislocated along with the fragment of the articular margin of the radius.

Plate 3.20

Forearm and Wrist

RADIOLOGY OF DISTAL RADIUS FRACTURES

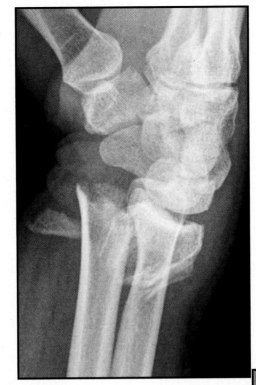

Lateral radiograph of comminuted extraarticular distal radius fracture with severe dorsal displacement and metaphyseal comminution

FRACTURE OF DISTAL RADIUS (Continued)

The stability of the closed reduction depends on the integrity of the radiocarpal ligament on the side opposite the injury. For example, the stability of the reduction of a dorsal Barton fracture is best preserved by positioning the wrist in slight extension to take advantage of the intact volar carpal ligament.

Reduction of a Barton fracture is difficult to maintain with an external fixator or with pins and plaster; therefore treatment with open reduction and internal fixation (ORIF) is usually indicated for fracture-dislocations that have large fragments. Barton fractures that involve a significant portion of the articular surface are usually unstable and must be treated with ORIF, using a small buttress plate to maintain the reduction. Buttressing the distal fragment maintains joint congruity. It is not necessary to insert screws into the distal fragment (which may be significantly comminuted) to maintain the reduction.

Fracture of Styloid Process of Radius

Most nondisplaced fractures of the styloid process of the radius can be treated with immobilization in a plaster cast. Displaced fractures must be anatomically reduced and held with either a pin, screw, or plate. Often, treatment with closed reduction and percutaneous pin fixation is sufficient. Fractures of the styloid process may be accompanied by dislocations of the lunate. Thus with any fracture of the styloid process, the carpus should be examined for other injuries. Some surgeons are using wrist arthroscopy to aid in the treatment of these injuries. Advantages of arthroscopy include direct inspection of the articular reduction and the ability to identify associated ligamentous injuries that commonly occur with this injury pattern.

Closed reduction and immobilization in a plaster cast constitute a dependable treatment for many fractures of the distal radius, but after satisfactory manipulative reduction some fractures (particularly unstable injuries in young, active adults) require operative fixation. Current fixation options include closed reduction and percutaneous pin fixation, external fixation, dorsal spanning plate, or ORIF, with a recent trend toward volar locked plating.

AP radiograph of comminuted extraarticular distal radius fracture with significant radial shortening (i.e., radius is shorter than ulna)

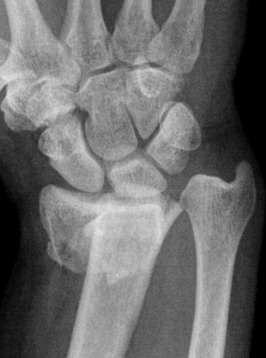

TREATMENT

The best determinants of how to treat fractures of the distal radius are the character of the fracture, whether it is stable or unstable or intraarticular or extraarticular, the lifestyle and age of the patient, and the experience of the treating surgeon.

Closed Reduction and Plaster Cast Immobilization

Colles fractures can often be reduced using manipulation or traction. After a sterile preparation of the forearm, local infiltration of lidocaine into the hematoma at the fracture site often provides adequate anesthesia for manipulating the fracture. Regional anesthesia, either an axillary or a Bier block, is also commonly used; but if the patient is very apprehensive or a more extensive

procedure is needed, then general anesthesia may be required.

Traction using fingertraps and weights is an effective method of reducing Colles fractures. The fingertraps are secured to the middle and index fingers and the thumb to suspend the arm; 10- to 15-lb weights are attached by a sling to the upper arm to provide countertraction. Gentle manual manipulation is often needed to fully reduce the fracture.

If the surgeon decides to manipulate the fracture without using fingertraps, an assistant is needed to hold the proximal forearm and provide countertraction. The fracture is then reduced with gentle longitudinal

Plate 3.21

Upper Limb: PART I

CLOSED REDUCTION AND PLASTER CAST IMMOBILIZATION OF COLLES FRACTURE

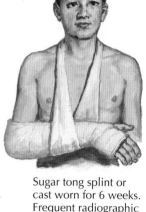

Patient supine with arm extended over table edge; elbow flexed 90 degrees and suspended in fingertraps on middle and index finger and thumb. Countertraction supplied by 10- to 15-lb weights (depending on muscularity of patient) hung from arm on padded sling. Good reduction usually occurs in 10–15 minutes. Note pneumatic cuff remains inflated during reduction to continue Bier block anesthesia.

When reduction appears satisfactory on radiographs, sugar tong splint or cast is applied over padding and molded well about wrist. Splint or cast extends from above elbow to metacarpal heads on dorsal aspect but only to midpalmar crease on volar aspect to permit finger movement. If used, cast is bivalved to allow swelling.

Sugar tong splint or cast worn for 6 weeks. Frequent radiographic monitoring necessary, especially during first 2 weeks. If slippage occurs, reduction is repeated.

F. Netter M.D.

FRACTURE OF DISTAL RADIUS (Continued)

traction. A sugar tong splint or short arm volar/radial splint is applied after reduction. To maintain the reduction, it is important to mold the plaster snugly to the forearm using three-point molding. The final position of the wrist within the splint/cast must avoid extreme positions (especially wrist flexion) because these can exacerbate nerve compression, specifically the median nerve within the carpal tunnel. Patients must be monitored on a weekly basis for the first 2 to 3 weeks with radiographs at each visit confirming maintained reduction. Six weeks of immobilization is the standard length of immobilization, followed by protected motion and progressive strengthening.

Closed Reduction and Pin Fixation

Fractures that do not remain in acceptable alignment after closed reduction require operative fixation. Patients with excellent bone quality and an intact (i.e., noncomminuted) volar cortex are candidates for closed reduction and pin fixation. The most common method is "intrafocal" pinning and uses Kirschner wires that are placed distally to proximally both through the radial styloid and dorsally into the fracture site and then engaging the volar cortex. This method is not acceptable for fractures with metaphyseal comminution or intraarticular involvement. The pins can be removed at 4 weeks, and protected motion is started. The most common complication with this treatment method is pin site infection requiring antibiotic treatment or early removal of the pins. The most concerning complication is complex regional pain syndrome arising from injury to the superficial radial nerve branches during placement of the Kirschner wire.

External Fixation

Fractures associated with severe, open soft tissue injuries or fractures that undergo either pin or plate fixation that is tenuous benefit from external fixation. The most common method of external fixation is a spanning wrist fixator. Threaded pins are placed into both the second metacarpal and the distal third of the radius and connected with clamps and bars to maintain length and neutralize forces. Newer devices have been developed that do not cross the wrist and show promise in the treatment of complex distal radius fractures. Pin track infections are common. Complex regional pain syndrome is also a risk from both sensory nerve injury and over distraction of the wrist. Dorsal spanning plate fixation avoids the complications of external fixation

Reduction by manipulation

Reduction of Colles fracture by manipulation method under local (infiltration) anesthesia:
1. Hyperextension and traction to break up impaction combined with direct thumb pressure; countertraction and fixation of forearm by assistant.

2. With continued traction, countertraction, ulnar deviation of the hand, and thumb pressure, the ends of the fragments are brought into apposition; the operator's index fingers press on the proximal fragment while the thumbs press on the distal one.

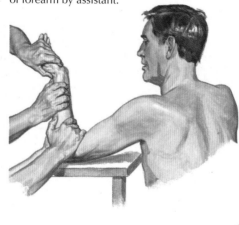

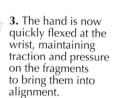

3. The hand is now quickly flexed at the wrist, maintaining traction and pressure on the fragments to bring them into alignment.

and is gaining popularity in treating distal radius fractures that more traditionally required external fixation.

Open Reduction and Internal Fixation

ORIF is arguably the current treatment of choice for most unstable, displaced distal radius fractures. Traditionally, plates and screws were placed dorsally along the distal radius, acting as a buttress plate. The intimate relationship of the extensor tendons to the bone led to high rates of extensor tendon complication requiring either hardware removal secondary to extensor tenosynovitis or tendon repair/reconstruction secondary to frank extensor tendon rupture. Locked plating technology,

in which the screw heads are threaded into the plate, allows placement of the hardware along the volar cortex of the distal radius. The overlying flexor tendons are protected from the implants by both distance and the pronator quadratus muscle. The "fixed angle construct" buttresses the articular surface with screws/pegs or tines placed immediately subchondral to the articular surface, and then the plate is fixed to the shaft of the radius. Excellent reduction can be obtained, and the rigid constructs allow early mobilization and therapy. Soft tissue irritation and injury from the hardware remain a concern and can be diminished by appropriate position along the bone and avoiding dorsal screw

Plate 3.22   Forearm and Wrist

RADIOLOGY OF OPEN REDUCTION AND INTERNAL FIXATION (ORIF)

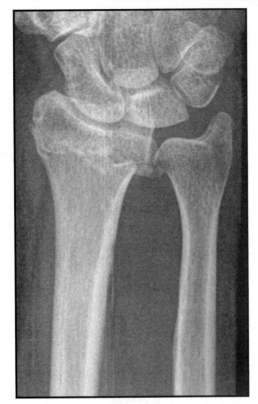

AP radiograph of a displaced intraarticular distal radius fracture

FRACTURE OF DISTAL RADIUS
(Continued)

penetration (bicortical fixation is not required with these implants). More complex injuries with comminution of the articular surface or significant volar and dorsal involvement may require ORIF with multiple plates and screws or dorsal spanning plate fixation. Fragment-specific fixation involves applying smaller implants to individual fracture fragments, leading to stable fixation and anatomic restoration of complex articular injuries.

COMPLICATIONS

The short-term complications associated with all fractures of the distal radius are significant and demand early treatment to prevent long-term residual disability. To control edema after fracture reduction and casting, the arm is elevated on pillows or in a sling above the level of the patient's heart and ice bags are applied over the cast. Severe swelling may necessitate splitting the cast, and the cast may need to be trimmed to prevent skin irritation. The physician should encourage frequent and full active range of motion of all the finger and thumb joints to prevent stiffness, which is common, and to reduce swelling. Any persistent pain under the cast should be investigated with the plaster removed entirely.

Acute injury of the median nerve after fractures of the distal radius is an uncommon but debilitating problem. After injury, fracture displacement combined with swelling occasionally distorts and compresses the median nerve, causing pain or numbness. The symptoms of median nerve compression usually subside or disappear when the fracture is reduced. If symptoms persist after reduction—particularly if the patient experiences burning pain in the median nerve distribution—prompt surgical decompression of the nerve in the carpal tunnel may be necessary. Mild residual numbness and tingling in the median nerve distribution usually subside with time or can be relieved after fracture healing with a carpal tunnel release. Sometimes, acute compartment syndrome of the forearm is associated with fractures of the distal radius. The characteristic symptom is excessive pain combined with numbness and pain on passive movement of the thumb and fingers. Compartment syndromes must be recognized promptly and should be treated with fasciotomy.

Long-term complications develop in 30% to 35% of patients. Loss of the reduction is the most common problem, which can be minimized or corrected by

AP radiograph of same wrist after ORIF with volar plate and screw fixation

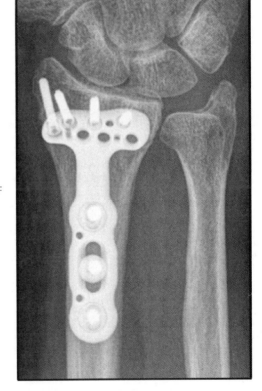

early identification of the displacement with radiographs taken at weekly intervals in the first 3 weeks after injury. Repeat closed reduction and casting may be needed; unstable fractures may require ORIF or application of an external fixator to restore and maintain alignment. After 3 weeks of healing, fractures of the distal radius have stabilized and will rarely settle with further loss of radial length. If the fracture heals with a residual deformity (usually a dorsiflexion deformity), this can be corrected with surgery. Radiocarpal and carpal instability are also associated with injuries of the distal radius. Osteoarthritis of the DRUJ may produce persistent pain. Fortunately, nonunion is

rare, but if it occurs, treatment consists of ORIF and bone grafting.

Rupture of an extensor tendon, most commonly of the thumb, is seen after fractures of the distal radius, as is stenosing tenosynovitis of the first dorsal compartment (de Quervain disease). Complex regional pain syndrome is a very debilitating complication of any musculoskeletal injury. It is frequently a result of hand and wrist fractures, but it develops most often after treatment of unstable fractures with pin fixation, external fixation, or pin and plaster fixation. Early recognition and treatment of complex regional pain syndrome are essential to restore good function.

Plate 3.23

Upper Limb: PART I

FRACTURE OF SCAPHOID: PRESENTATION AND CLASSIFICATION

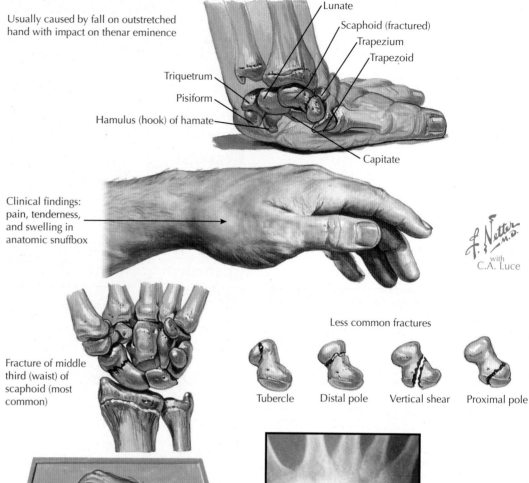

Usually caused by fall on outstretched hand with impact on thenar eminence

Lunate
Scaphoid (fractured)
Trapezium
Trapezoid
Triquetrum
Pisiform
Hamulus (hook) of hamate
Capitate

Clinical findings: pain, tenderness, and swelling in anatomic snuffbox

Fracture of middle third (waist) of scaphoid (most common)

Less common fractures

Tubercle   Distal pole   Vertical shear   Proximal pole

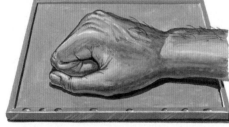
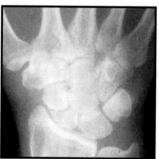

This view delineates scaphoid, but fracture may not be well visualized.

Direct posteroanterior radiograph taken with fingers clenched into fist and resting on cassette

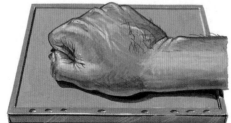
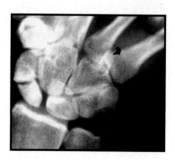

This position tends to open fracture, better visualizing it.

Radiograph also taken with clenched fist in ulnar deviation

FRACTURE OF SCAPHOID

The scaphoid acts as a link between the proximal and distal rows of the carpus and thus is quite susceptible to injury. Most fractures of the scaphoid waist result from an extension force applied to the distal pole, with the proximal pole stabilized by the strong radiocapitate and radioscaphoid ligaments. This mechanism of injury, for example, a fall on the outstretched hand, produces the most common fracture pattern—a break through the waist of the scaphoid. Other patterns include fractures of the distal tuberosity and proximal pole and vertical shear fractures of the scaphoid body.

The blood supply to the bone plays an important role in the healing process, and sometimes osteonecrosis is a complication of scaphoid fractures. The major blood supply enters the junction of the waist and distal pole on the dorsal aspect, leaving the proximal pole with a relatively poor vascular supply. Fractures through the waist of the scaphoid disrupt most of the blood supply to the proximal pole, often leading to osteonecrosis.

Fractures of the scaphoid are the most commonly missed fractures of the upper limb; yet early diagnosis is essential for successful treatment. The initial signs are tenderness and pain over the anatomic snuffbox, with some swelling and loss of the normal concavity of the dorsoradial region of the wrist. Also present is significant discomfort when the thumb is moved or the metacarpal of the thumb is compressed against the proximal carpal row.

Initial radiographs may not accurately demonstrate a fracture of the scaphoid waist. Special views are needed of the hand forming a fist and of the fist in ulnar deviation, positions that bring the scaphoid into extension. An occult fracture of the scaphoid can often be visualized by aiming the x-ray beam parallel to the suspected fracture line rather than at an acute angle to it. However, even with these special views of the wrist, some acute scaphoid fractures are not clearly seen.

If symptoms are present, even if radiographs are normal, the wrist should be immobilized in a thumb spica cast for 2 to 3 weeks. Follow-up radiographs after the plaster cast is removed often reveal a previously occult fracture. If pain persists, the cast is reapplied. Magnetic resonance imaging (MRI) is another useful tool in evaluating the wrist with a suspected occult scaphoid fracture. Immediate MRI has been shown to have high sensitivity and specificity for diagnosis of occult scaphoid fractures, as well as a favorable cost-benefit analysis compared with immobilization and repeat plain radiographs.

Most nondisplaced fractures of the scaphoid can be successfully treated by placing the limb in a thumb spica cast with the hand and wrist rigidly immobilized and the thumb in abduction. Some physicians recommend the use of an above-elbow cast, at least for the first 6 weeks of treatment, on the premise that

Plate 3.24

Forearm and Wrist

FRACTURE OF SCAPHOID: BLOOD SUPPLY AND TREATMENT

Most fractures heal well when treated with snug thumb spica cast over stockinette with wrist in 20 degrees of dorsiflexion and slight radial deviation. Cast extends to distal palmar crease on volar aspect and to knuckles on dorsal aspect. Nondisplaced fractures of waist and distal pole of scaphoid require 8–12 weeks' immobilization; displaced vertical fractures and fractures of proximal pole may need up to 18 weeks' immobilization.

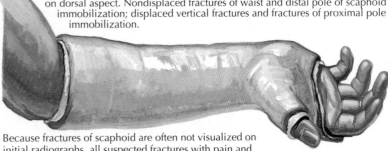

Because fractures of scaphoid are often not visualized on initial radiographs, all suspected fractures with pain and tenderness in the anatomic snuffbox immobilized as shown; radiographs are repeated in 3 weeks with cast removed. If radiographs are normal and pain or tenderness absent, cast is left off; if tenderness persists, cast is reapplied and radiography repeated in 3 weeks.

Blood supply to scaphoid enters both distal and proximal parts of bone.

Radial artery

In most persons, blood supply enters only distal part of scaphoid. Fracture through waist may lead to necrosis of proximal part.

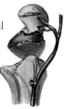

Open reduction and internal fixation

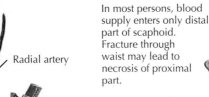

Jig holds fragments of bone in place; pilot hole drilled for trailing end of screw.

Long drill introduced to full length of screw.

Herbert jig. Device for fixing displaced fractures or nonunion of scaphoid (after Fisher).

Deep end of canal tapped for leading thread of screw.

Screw inserted through jig. Trailing end is self-tapping.

Russe bone graft for nonunion of scaphoid

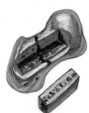

Trough created in both fragments of scaphoid, and most cancellous bone curetted

Bone autograft from ilium

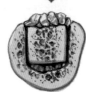

Cross section shows corticocancellous bone autograft from ilium or distal radius inserted and cancellous bone packed around it. Cast applied for 12 weeks or more as needed for good union. Success rate 85%–90%.

Longitudinal volar incision (4–5 cm). Flexor carpi radialis tendon retracted radially, other tissues ulnarly. Joint capsule opened; radiocarpal ligaments partially incised, exposing fractured scaphoid.

FRACTURE OF SCAPHOID (Continued)

above-elbow casting of scaphoid fractures may enhance union. Prompt recognition, secure immobilization, and careful follow-up remain the essentials of closed treatment. The rate of union in fractures that are immobilized initially is close to 95%. In fractures that are not immobilized initially, the nonunion rate is significantly higher. There is growing support for immediate percutaneous screw fixation of nondisplaced scaphoid fractures. Percutaneous techniques using either volar or dorsal approaches have been shown to diminish the time required for immobilization with a faster return to work and sports. However, the overall union rates between cast immobilization and surgical screw fixation are equivalent. Contemporary management of nondisplaced scaphoid fractures considers the location of the fracture (proximal, waist, distal) and individualizes treatment based on the patient's athletic, recreational, and vocational demands.

Any degree of displacement of a scaphoid fracture may be an indication of wrist instability. Displaced scaphoid fractures are often associated with ligament injuries that ultimately result in persistent wrist instability after the fracture heals. Displaced fractures should be treated with ORIF. Nonunion is much more common after displaced fractures. Therefore a scaphoid fracture with a displacement greater than 1 mm requires ORIF to ensure union and wrist function.

OPERATIVE TREATMENT

Indications for immediate operative fixation of scaphoid fractures include displaced fractures, fractures associated with carpal instability, and nonunions. Relative indications for operative fixations include delay in diagnosis (>4 weeks from injury), proximal pole fractures, and malunions.

The cannulated, headless screw, with threads of different pitches at either end, is a very effective device for stabilizing and compressing a scaphoid fracture. There

are numerous implants on the market, all with the same goal of compression across the fracture.

Acute Nondisplaced Fractures

Operative fixation of acute, nondisplaced scaphoid fractures is increasing in popularity with the introduction of less invasive surgical techniques and advances in intraoperative imaging and instrumentation. Currently,

acute scaphoid fractures can be repaired by means of open volar or dorsal approaches, percutaneous techniques, or arthroscopically assisted procedures. Common to all techniques is the use of biplanar imaging to confirm fracture reduction and central guide wire placement as well as the use of specially designed headless compression screws. Compromising accurate reduction and central screw placement, for the sake of a

Plate 3.25

Upper Limb: PART I

FRACTURE OF SCAPHOID: RADIOLOGY

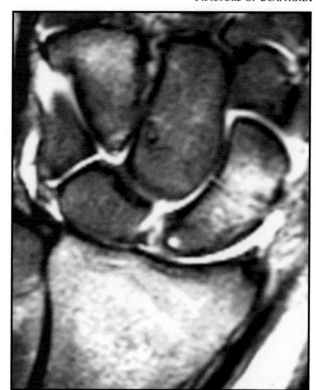

MR image of occult scaphoid fracture not seen on plain radiograph; note fracture line through the wrist of the scaphoid with surrounding bone edema.

FRACTURE OF SCAPHOID
(Continued)

percutaneous approach, must be avoided. Immediate operative fixation of acute, nondisplaced scaphoid waist fractures has entered clinical practice and is quickly becoming the standard of care. Compared with prolonged cast immobilization, the number of healed fractures is equivalent, but times to fracture healing are significantly reduced. Taras and colleagues reported return to participation in sports averaged 5.4 weeks, with successful fracture union achieved in all patients undergoing percutaneous scaphoid fixation. We counsel our athletes about the risks and benefits of all treatment regimens and advocate percutaneous fixation for all athletes requesting a rapid return to competition. Although both volar and dorsal approaches have been described, we typically use a dorsal approach to percutaneous internal fixation.

Acute Displaced Fractures

In acute, displaced scaphoid waist fractures, a volar approach to the scaphoid is used to preserve the dorsal blood supply. The fracture is reduced, with careful restoration of length and correction of the "humpback" deformity, and the cannulated, headless compression screw is applied volarly in a distal to proximal direction. The critical step is to ensure appropriate screw position (centered throughout the bone on multiple oblique views).

Acute proximal pole scaphoid fractures should be approached through a dorsal approach. Reduction is confirmed, and a cannulated, headless compression screw is placed with accurate screw placement evaluated and confirmed on multiple radiographic or fluoroscopic images.

Scaphoid Nonunion

The management of the united scaphoid fracture is challenging. Initial diagnosis must be followed by a thorough history regarding the timing of injury and further studies to (1) evaluate for carpal collapse and

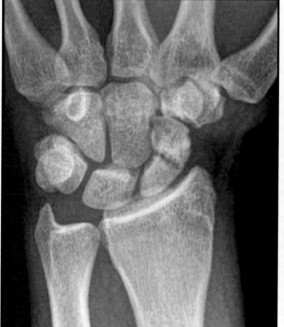

AP radiograph of scaphoid wrist nonunion

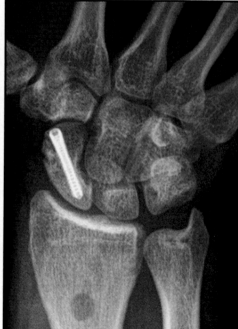

AP radiograph of same fracture after ORIF with a variable-pitch compression screw utilizing a volar approach with distal radius autograft (note harvest site in radial metaphysis)

arthritic destruction, (2) determine the vascularity of the proximal pole of the scaphoid, and (3) define the geometry of the fracture nonunion. All SNACs require debridement of the nonunion site and bone grafting. Scaphoid waist nonunions with a viable proximal pole can be managed with a volar approach to the scaphoid, debridement of the nonunion, reduction, and use of autograft bone. Proximal pole nonunions or waist

nonunions with avascular change to the proximal fragment require debridement and consideration of vascularized bone grafting either from the distal radius, thumb, or a distant site (e.g., medial femoral condyle). Any SNAC with advanced degenerative changes is best managed with some type of salvage procedure (proximal row carpectomy, limited arthrodesis, or total wrist arthrodesis).

Plate 3.26

Forearm and Wrist

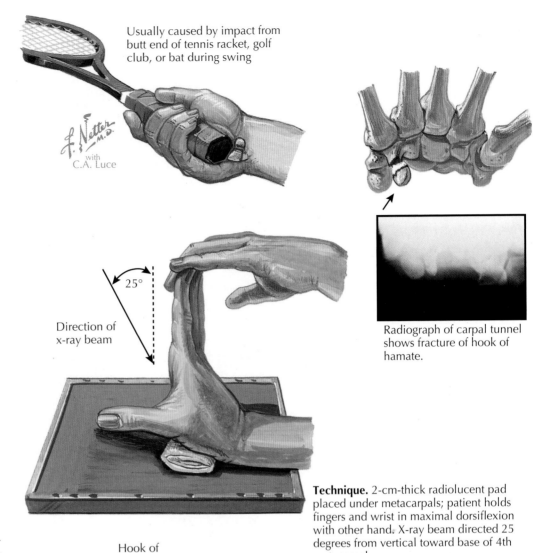

Usually caused by impact from butt end of tennis racket, golf club, or bat during swing

25°

Direction of x-ray beam

Radiograph of carpal tunnel shows fracture of hook of hamate.

Technique. 2-cm-thick radiolucent pad placed under metacarpals; patient holds fingers and wrist in maximal dorsiflexion with other hand. X-ray beam directed 25 degrees from vertical toward base of 4th metacarpal.

FRACTURE OF HAMULUS OF HAMATE

Fractures of the hamulus (hook) of the hamate are uncommon and are often missed on the initial examination. The usual cause of a hamate fracture is a fall on the outstretched hand, but this injury is also commonly seen in golfers and baseball players. For example, as a golfer hits the ground forcibly with a club, the impact may fracture the hamate.

Although the injury causes acute pain and swelling, routine anteroposterior and lateral radiographs often fail to demonstrate the fracture. The initial physical findings include a dull ache over the hypothenar eminence, tenderness over the hamate, decreased grip strength, and, occasionally, signs and symptoms of ulnar nerve impingement. The Allen test may be positive, suggesting compression of the ulnar artery. If these signs and symptoms are present but routine radiographs show no evidence of fracture, a carpal tunnel view is indicated. Often the extreme wrist extension needed to appropriately obtain a carpal tunnel view is impossible secondary to pain and swelling from the injury. Computed tomography of the carpus has become the standard of care for evaluating a suspected hook of the hamate fracture.

The rate of union after these fractures is not clearly documented, but many, if not most, probably fail to heal. Vascularity to the hamulus arises from vessels penetrating the radial base and ulnar tip, with a poor anastomosis between the two. This resultant vascular watershed predisposes even nondisplaced fractures to nonunion. As primary treatment, most authorities advocate surgical excision of the fracture fragment of the hamate. Most patients regain good function and strength after excision of the hook.

Hook of hamate fracture

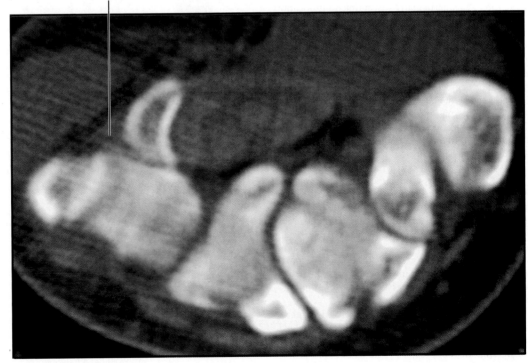

CT hook of hamate fracture

Plate 3.27

Upper Limb: PART I

DISLOCATION OF CARPUS: PRESENTATION AND TREATMENT

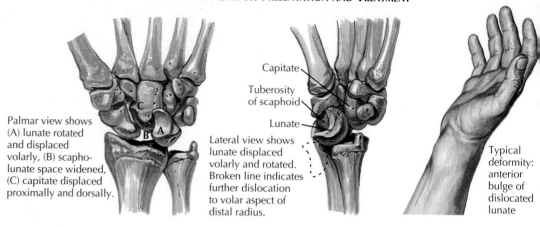

Palmar view shows (A) lunate rotated and displaced volarly, (B) scapholunate space widened, (C) capitate displaced proximally and dorsally.

Capitate

Tuberosity of scaphoid

Lunate

Lateral view shows lunate displaced volarly and rotated. Broken line indicates further dislocation to volar aspect of distal radius.

Typical deformity: anterior bulge of dislocated lunate

DISLOCATION OF CARPUS

The strong volar radiocarpal ligament between the lunate, radius, and distal row of the carpal bones provides strong support for the volar aspect of the carpus; ligament support is weaker on the dorsal side. In addition, the ligament attachments from the radius to the proximal carpal row are much stronger than the attachments from the proximal carpal row to the distal carpal row. This disparity in the support between the two carpal rows and the lack of a significant lunocapitate support make the carpus particularly susceptible to dislocation and chronic instability.

Carpal instability results from hyperextension of the wrist, as in a fall on the outstretched hand. The amount and direction of the force determine the degree of resulting instability around the lunate. The first stage, and most minor degree, of perilunate instability is the tearing of the ligament between the scaphoid and the lunate, followed by disruption of the radioscaphoid ligament. These injuries produce a scapholunate diastasis. In the second stage, with further dorsiflexion, the radiocapitate ligament ruptures, leading to dislocation of the lunate. In the third stage of injury, the radiotriquetral ligament ruptures, resulting in perilunate dislocation associated with lunotriquetral instability. In the final stage, the hand and distal row of the carpus supinate on the triquetrum, tearing the dorsal radiotriquetral ligament and causing the capitate to push the unstable lunate volarly; these events result in a volar dislocation. The signs and symptoms of a volar dislocation of the lunate include pain and swelling in the wrist. Paresthesia and dysesthesia of the median nerve are quite common associated problems.

With lunate and perilunate dislocations, the anteroposterior radiograph often shows the lunate as wedged, or pie shaped, rather than four sided. On the lateral radiograph, the lunate appears rotated out of its articulation with the head of the capitate and pointing volarly; sometimes the lunate is completely dislocated volarly.

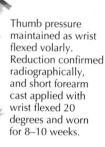

Traction applied with fingertraps and 10- to 20-lb weights hung from arm for 5–10 minutes

With hand still in traction, wrist dorsiflexed as firm thumb pressure applied over prominence of lunate. Reduction may be felt as distinct snap.

Thumb pressure maintained as wrist flexed volarly. Reduction confirmed radiographically, and short forearm cast applied with wrist flexed 20 degrees and worn for 8–10 weeks.

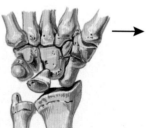

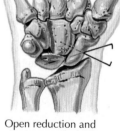

Some lunate dislocations unstable after closed reduction, as in this case. Note persistent gap between lunate and scaphoid.

Open reduction and pinning required. Pins removed in 6–8 weeks; cast worn up to 12 weeks.

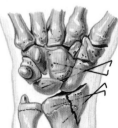

Dislocation of lunate plus fracture of styloid process of radius. Initial attempt at manipulative reduction unsuccessful.

Second closed reduction satisfactory. Styloid process of radius and lunate pinned percutaneously. Some functional disability persisted.

Plate 3.28   Forearm and Wrist

DISLOCATION OF CARPUS: RADIOLOGY

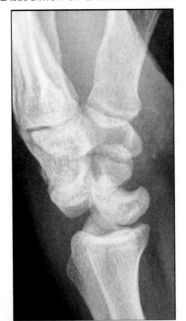

Lateral radiograph of perilunate dislocation; note how the head of the capitate no longer "sits" in the concavity of the lunate.

DISLOCATION OF CARPUS (Continued)

Initial treatment of lunate and perilunate dislocations includes a thorough neurovascular examination followed by closed reduction of the dislocation. The reduction can be performed using regional or general anesthesia. Traction is applied by placing the fingers in fingertraps and hanging a 10- to 20-lb counterweight from the upper arm. An anteroposterior radiograph should be taken of the wrist in traction to determine the degree of ligament damage and to identify any associated osteochondral fractures.

After allowing the wrist to remain distracted for approximately 10 minutes, the examiner places his or her thumb on the volar aspect of the wrist over the dislocated lunate. The injured wrist is gradually flexed volarly and pronated while thumb pressure is applied over the lunate to reduce it. If adequate closed reduction is obtained, the wrist is splinted in anticipation of definitive treatment.

Posttraumatic carpal instability is now recognized as a common complication of these injuries, and many orthopedic surgeons prefer open reduction of lunate and perilunate dislocations and stabilization of carpus injuries with wires or screws. ORIF of a lunate dislocation has several advantages. The procedure achieves and maintains anatomic reduction of the fragments and allows repair of the torn ligaments at the same time. Also, the wrist joint is debrided of any loose osteochondral fragments.

Carpus dislocations may also involve fractures of the scaphoid, triquetrum, and capitate, as well as the styloid process of the radius. In these injuries, the dislocations cause fractures rather than ligament ruptures. The best way to ensure adequate alignment and reduce the risk of late wrist instability is anatomic reduction and rigid internal fixation.

Prompt recognition and treatment of carpus instability can restore satisfactory hand and wrist function. However, decreased range of motion and early degenerative arthritis are still common complications, particularly after severe injuries.

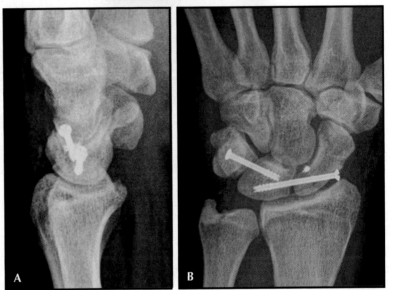

(A) Lateral and (B) anteroposterior radiographs of same patient after open reduction, compression screw fixation, and ligament repair.

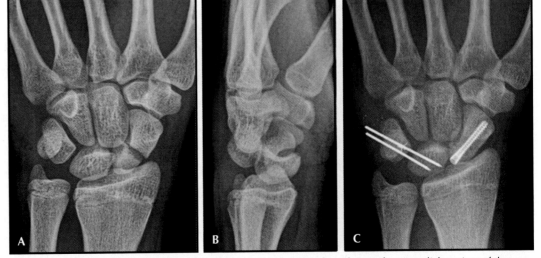

(A) Anteroposterior and (B) lateral radiographs of transscaphoid perilunate fracture-dislocation of the wrist. (C) The same patient after open reduction, compression screw fixation of the scaphoid, and pinning of the lunotriquetral joint.

Plate 3.29

Upper Limb: PART

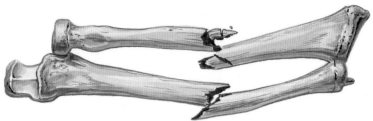

Fracture of both radius and ulna with angulation, shortening, and comminution of radius

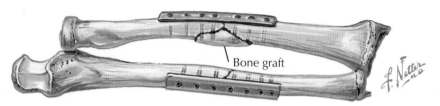

Bone graft

Open reduction and fixation with compression plates and screws through both cortices, plus bone autograft from ilium to radius. Good alignment, with restoration of radial bow and interosseous space. Postoperative immobilization in long-arm cast for 6-8 weeks.

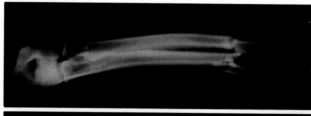

Preoperative radiograph. Fractures of shafts of both forearm bones.

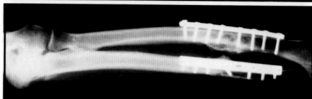

Postoperative radiograph. Compression plates applied and fragments in good alignment.

FRACTURE OF BOTH FOREARM BONES

Complications

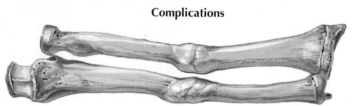

Malunion. Loss of radial bow and narrowing of interosseous space, which greatly impair pronation and supination of forearm.

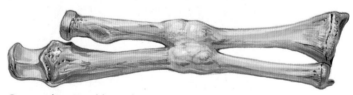

Cross union. Total loss of rotation and very difficult to correct. Separate incisions or fixation of each bone and minimal operative trauma help minimize this serious complication.

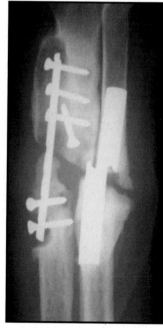

Failed ORIF

Fractures of the shafts of the radius and ulna are usually significantly displaced and are often comminuted because of the great force needed to break these strong bones. Anatomic reduction of the fractures, with full restoration of both the length and the bow of the radius, is essential to maintain maximal function of the forearm. Even when anatomic reduction is achieved, some long-term loss of supination and pronation may occur.

ORIF of fractures of both forearm bones is performed through separate incisions, maximizing the skin bridge left between the two. Both fractures must be reduced and held with clamps before either is permanently fixed; this ensures that both fractures are reduced anatomically and that the reductions are maintained. After the temporary reductions are secured, the less comminuted fracture (usually the ulna) is fixed with a compression plate and screws; the more comminuted fracture is fixed subsequently using the same technique.

Several difficulties may be encountered during the surgical procedure. Extensive comminution may make it difficult to restore the bones to their proper length. In this situation, the interosseous membrane is identified, proximally and distally, and used as a guide in restoring the bones to an adequate length. Re-creation of the anatomic bow of the radius is critical, and loss of the normal geometry will lead to permanent loss of forearm rotation. In wound closure, the fascia is left open and only the skin is closed, because tight fascial closure combined with postoperative swelling may produce a compartment syndrome.

Long-term problems associated with fractures of both forearm bones include nonunion, infection, limited motion, and synostosis between the radius and the ulna. Synostosis is rare and is usually associated with comminuted fractures at the same level in the forearm that result from crushing forces. Operative fixation through one exposure is another well-documented cause of synostosis. Nonunion can occur from inadequate fixation (e.g., using plates of insufficient strength or of improper length). One must ensure that six cortices of fixation on each side of the fracture are achieved, and one-third tubular plates (although easy to contour) are never appropriate for operative fixation of forearm fractures. Nonunion also occurs with closed reduction and plaster cast immobilization, and in the adult population, fractures of both forearm bones are an absolute indication for ORIF.

Plate 3.30   Forearm and Wrist

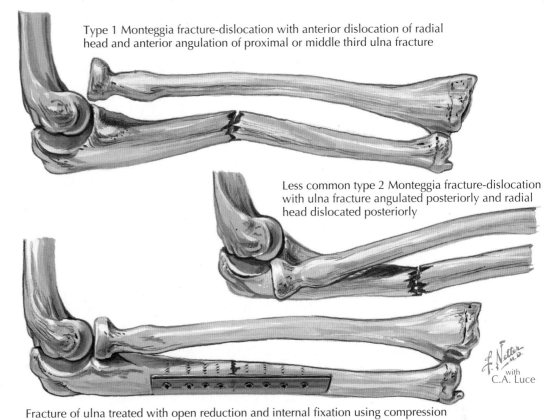

Type 1 Monteggia fracture-dislocation with anterior dislocation of radial head and anterior angulation of proximal or middle third ulna fracture

Less common type 2 Monteggia fracture-dislocation with ulna fracture angulated posteriorly and radial head dislocated posteriorly

Fracture of ulna treated with open reduction and internal fixation using compression plate and screws. After reduction of ulna, radial head spontaneously reduced.

FRACTURE OF SHAFT OF ULNA

In 1814, Monteggia described a fracture of the ulna associated with dislocation of the proximal radioulnar joint. A direct blow to, or forced pronation of, the forearm is the usual cause of this type of fracture-dislocation. Forced pronation both fractures and angulates the ulna, and then causes the radial head to dislocate.

Bado classified the patterns of dislocation that occur with Monteggia fractures. Although the radial head usually dislocates anteriorly, it can also move posteriorly, medially, or laterally. The apex of the angular deformity of the ulna usually indicates the direction of the radial head dislocation. Because of the close relationship of the proximal radius to the posterior interosseous nerve, a posterior interosseous nerve palsy is not uncommon after a Monteggia fracture.

Like the Galeazzi, or Piedmont, fracture, the Monteggia fracture in adults is difficult or impossible to treat with closed methods. Achieving a stable reduction of the radial head usually requires ORIF of the fracture of the proximal ulna.

Treatment of the Monteggia fracture is often complicated by a variety of difficulties. Occasionally during ORIF of the ulna, the radial head does not reduce. By far the most common cause for this is improper reduction of the ulna fracture, and this should always be evaluated first. Proper technique is required to ensure stable fixation and avoid nonunion and loss of reduction. When open reduction of the radial head is required, one should suspect incarcerated tissue (including the possibility of the posterior interosseous nerve), which requires removal from the radiocapitellar and proximal radioulnar joints. When an open reduction is needed, the torn annular ligament should also be repaired to help stabilize the proximal radioulnar joint. When the ulna fracture is severely comminuted, it is difficult to restore the bone to its proper length, and the reduced length creates a significant problem in reducing the radial head.

Failure to recognize and treat Monteggia fractures soon after injury can lead to restrictions in elbow and forearm motion. Late surgical treatment includes osteotomy of the ulna to restore length and geometry, as well as reconstruction of the annular ligament using the triceps brachii fascia or other local soft tissue to stabilize the proximal radius.

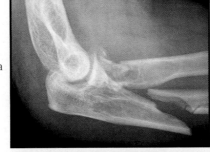

Complex Monteggia

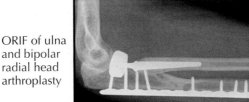

ORIF of ulna and bipolar radial head arthroplasty

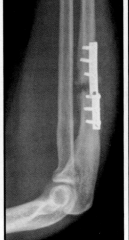

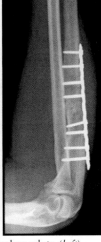

Ulnar shaft nonunion: broken plate (*left*) revision ORIF with iliac crest bone graft (ICBG) (*right*)

If radial head does not reduce after angulation of ulna is corrected, open reduction of radial head dislocation and repair of annular ligament are needed. Typically, this is done through a separate incision between the anconeus and extensor carpi ulnaris muscles.

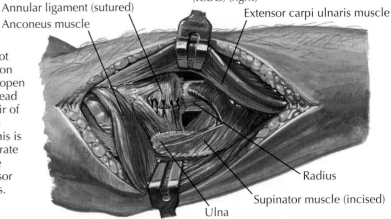

Annular ligament (sutured)
Anconeus muscle
Extensor carpi ulnaris muscle
Radius
Supinator muscle (incised)
Ulna

Plate 3.31

Upper Limb: PART I

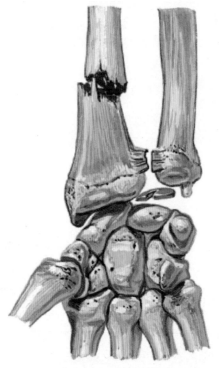

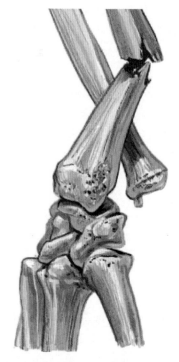

Anteroposterior view of fracture of radius
plus dislocation of DRUJ (Galeazzi fracture)

Dislocation of DRUJ better
demonstrated in lateral view

FRACTURE OF SHAFT OF RADIUS

Isolated fractures of the radial shaft are often accompanied by a disruption of the DRUJ, usually at the junction of the middle and distal thirds. The eponyms Galeazzi fracture and Piedmont fracture are frequently used to describe this type of injury. The injury is called the fracture of (surgical) necessity because of the difficulties and historically poor results associated with closed treatment methods.

Initially, Galeazzi postulated that a direct blow to the dorsolateral wrist caused this fracture-dislocation. More recent studies suggest that the usual mechanism of injury is a fall on the outstretched hand with the forearm in extreme pronation. The force across the radiocarpal joint causes fracture and shortening of the radial shaft. As further displacement occurs, the DRUJ dislocates, tearing the triangular fibrocartilage within it.

Hughston, in his classic report of 35 of 38 unsatisfactory results after closed treatment, delineated four deforming forces that lead to treatment failure: (1) the weight of the hand and the force of gravity cause subluxation of the DRUJ and dorsal angulation of the fracture; (2) the pronator quadratus muscle rotates the distal radius fragment in a volar, ulnar, and proximal direction; (3) the brachioradialis muscle rotates the distal fragment and produces shortening at the site of the radius fracture; and (4) the thumb abductors and extensors cause further shortening and displacement of the radius.

A volar surgical approach is used for ORIF of the radial shaft fracture. Retracting the flexor carpi radialis muscle ulnarly and the radial artery and brachioradialis muscle radially exposes the fracture site, which can be fixated with a compression plate. Reduction and secure fixation of the radius fracture usually reduce the DR dislocation as well.

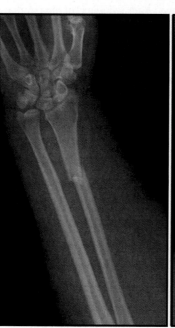

AP radiograph of the forearm demonstrating a distal third radial shaft fracture and disruption of the DRUJ Galeazzi fracture

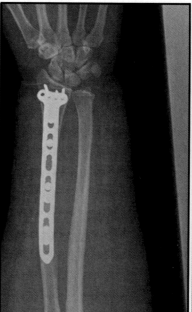

AP (left) and lateral (right) radiographs after ORIF of a Galeazzi fracture. The DRUJ is stable with the forearm in supination following ORIF of the radius.

After fixation of a radius fracture, the surgeon must look for any residual dislocation or subluxation of the DRUJ. Full passive supination of the forearm usually restores joint congruity. If the DRUJ cannot be satisfactorily aligned with closed means (e.g., supination), the joint must be surgically reduced and either pinned with Kirschner wires or with operative reattachment of the TFCC. A long-arm cast is applied, with the elbow flexed 90 degrees and the forearm in full supination. The limb is immobilized for 6 weeks to maintain the reduction. If a transfixation pin has been used to stabilize the DRUJ, it is left in place for 6 to 8 weeks.

If this fracture-dislocation is not diagnosed and appropriately treated soon after injury, later reconstructive surgery is often needed to correct the deformity of the radius and restore the function of the DRUJ. If the distal ulna cannot be adequately reduced, reconstruction or salvage excision must be undertaken.

Plate 3.32

Forearm and Wrist

GANGLION OF WRIST

A ganglion is a cystic lesion found closely associated with a joint capsule or tendon sheath. It is often seen in young adults but rarely in children; most frequently, it forms in the hand and wrist and less often in the ankle, foot, and knee. The most common site is the dorsum of the wrist just lateral to the common extensor tendons of the fingers. A ganglion usually occurs singly and may be multilocular; it consists of an outer fibrous coat and an inner synovial lining and contains a clear, colorless, gelatinous fluid.

Although the cause is uncertain, perhaps the most accepted theory is that a ganglion results from cystic degeneration of connective tissue near joints or tendon sheaths. Repeated trauma appears to be a causative factor in about 50% of cases.

CLINICAL MANIFESTATIONS

The only finding may be a slowly growing, localized swelling, but most patients report intermittent aching and mild weakness. Commonly, the patient will describe the mass waxing and waning in size and may have short-term resolution after "bumping" the mass inadvertently.

On examination, the cyst is firm, smooth, rubbery, rounded, slightly fluctuant, and, at times, tender. It is usually fixed but may be slightly movable if it involves a tendon sheath. Shining a light (pen light) through the mass confirms the fluid-filled cyst and aids in the correct diagnosis (transillumination). Clinical examination should also focus on evaluating for any carpal instability. Commonly, tears of the scapholunate interosseous ligament can lead to a dorsal ganglion cyst.

TREATMENT

Some ganglia disappear spontaneously. Treatments such as traumatic rupture, aspiration, and injections are associated with a high recurrence rate. Complete surgical excision of the ganglion and the ligamentous tissue at its base is the treatment of choice and usually prevents recurrence. Removal of the stalk and underlying swath of capsular tissue is critical to diminish recurrence. Arthroscopic techniques for removal of ganglia are gaining favor with the goals of removing the cyst with less tissue trauma and more expedient recovery.

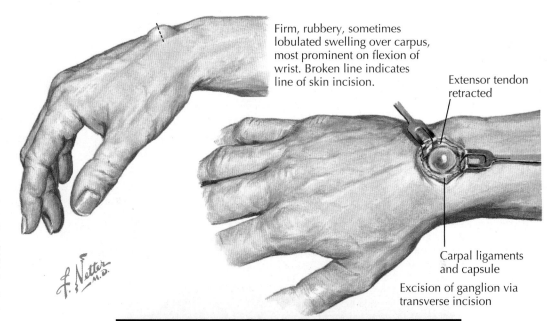

Firm, rubbery, sometimes lobulated swelling over carpus, most prominent on flexion of wrist. Broken line indicates line of skin incision.

Extensor tendon retracted

Carpal ligaments and capsule

Excision of ganglion via transverse incision

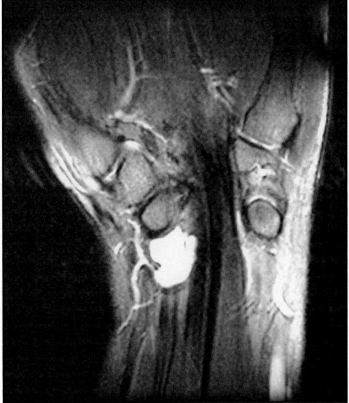

A 2-cm ganglion cyst has arisen proximal to the scaphoid on the volar aspect of the wrist. As expected from its fluid content, it returns increased signal on this fat-saturated T2-weighted sequence. (From Adam A, Dixon A, Grainger R, et al. Grainger & Allison's Diagnostic Radiology, 5th ed. Churchill Livingstone, 2007.)

Plate 3.33

Upper Limb: PART I

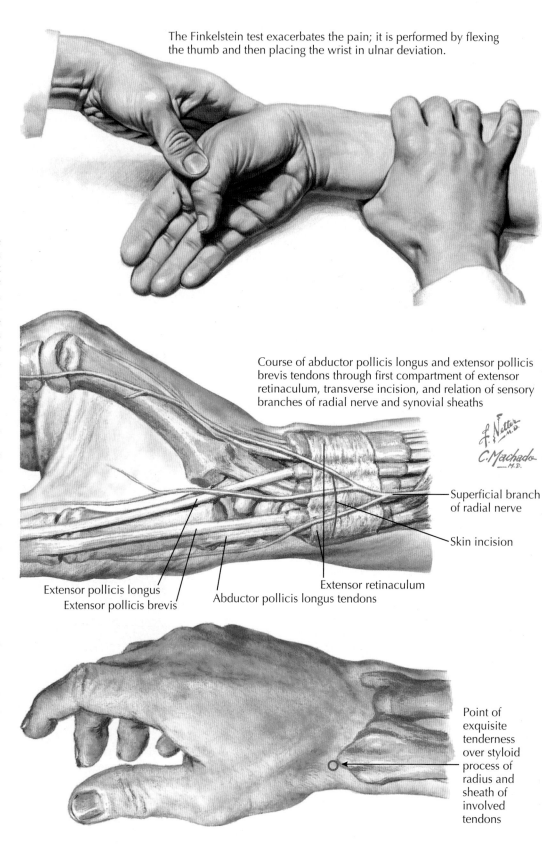

The Finkelstein test exacerbates the pain; it is performed by flexing the thumb and then placing the wrist in ulnar deviation.

Course of abductor pollicis longus and extensor pollicis brevis tendons through first compartment of extensor retinaculum, transverse incision, and relation of sensory branches of radial nerve and synovial sheaths

Superficial branch of radial nerve

Skin incision

Extensor pollicis longus
Extensor pollicis brevis
Abductor pollicis longus tendons
Extensor retinaculum

Point of exquisite tenderness over styloid process of radius and sheath of involved tendons

DE QUERVAIN DISEASE

De Quervain disease is a stenosing tenosynovitis of the abductor pollicis longus and the extensor pollicis brevis tendons at the styloid process of the radius. It is most common in women between 30 and 50 years of age. The cause remains uncertain but may be related to friction between the tendons, their fibrous sheath, and the underlying bony groove caused by movement of the thumb and wrist. The resulting inflammation causes thickening and stenosis of the synovial sheath of the first compartment of the extensor retinaculum (dorsal carpal ligament).

CLINICAL MANIFESTATIONS

Pain develops over the styloid process of the radius, radiating up the forearm and down the thumb. Occasionally, the pain occurs suddenly after a strain of the wrist. The aching pain, aggravated by use of the hand, gradually intensifies and may sometimes cause considerable weakness and disability.

Examination shows a sharp tenderness over the styloid process of the radius, and a visible swelling and palpable thickening of the fibrous sheath may be detected. Sharp pain at this site is often produced by active extension and abduction of the thumb against resistance. The Finkelstein test usually causes severe pain.

TREATMENT

Often, symptoms are relieved by injecting a corticosteroid into the sheath or placing the forearm, wrist, and thumb in a cast or removable splint for about 1 month, or both. If the pain recurs and persists after this treatment, surgery is indicated. With the use of local anesthesia, a short transverse incision is made over the sheath on the lateral aspect of the wrist; care must be taken to avoid the sensory branches of the superficial branch of the radial nerve. The thickened sheath is opened with a longitudinal incision through the first compartment, freeing the involved tendons. Great care must be exercised to locate and free all the tendons in the compartment because aberrant tendons and anatomic variations in the tendons and sheaths are common in this area. The incision is then closed. Prognosis is excellent.

Plate 3.34   Forearm and Wrist

RHEUMATOID ARTHRITIS OF WRIST

Rheumatoid arthritis is a chronic inflammatory condition involving the synovium of joints and tendons. The hand and wrist are commonly affected by this condition. The radiocarpal joint initially demonstrates painful synovitis that progresses to cartilage degeneration, ligamentous laxity, and osseous destruction. The common deformities at the wrist consist of carpal supination, volar subluxation, and ulnar translocation. The DRUJ is also frequently involved with synovitis, instability, and eventual dorsal subluxation/dislocation of the distal ulna. Extensor tenosynovitis is another common presentation, and it is often seen in conjunction with joint involvement. These deformities can also have significant effects on the joints proximal and distal to the wrist.

Clinical examination of the wrist reveals diffuse thickening, prominence of the ulnar head, extensor tenosynovitis, and possible extensor tendon lag. Extensor tenosynovitis can often be differentiated from radiocarpal synovitis by movement of the swelling with digital motion, palpation of the boundaries of the swelling, and a "dumbbell" shape to the swelling as the tenosynovium travels beneath the extensor retinaculum with swelling both proximal and distal.

Nonoperative treatment consists of medical management by the rheumatologist and selective use of splints to control symptoms. Hand therapy is critical and involves a systematic approach including education, activity modification, gentle exercise, and splinting for comfort. Failure of nonoperative treatment is often defined as failure of at least 6 months of appropriate medical management and/or progression of disease with impending or actual tendon rupture.

Surgical intervention is based on the stage and severity of the disease. Realistic goals and expectations must be discussed, with the primary goals always being to relieve pain, restore function, and halt the progress of further destruction. Patients with extensor tenosynovitis or radiocarpal/DR synovitis can be considered for synovectomy. These patients must be free of articular and bony destruction and should have failed at least 6 months of medical management. Synovectomy can greatly diminish the risk of extensor tendon rupture and can slow the process of articular and bony destruction. Patients presenting with caput ulna (dorsal subluxation of the ulnar head) or pending or actual extensor tendon rupture are managed with extensor tenosynovectomy, distal ulna excision, and tendon reconstruction (single or multiple tendon transfers). Articular destruction requires either limited versus total wrist arthrodesis or arthroplasty.

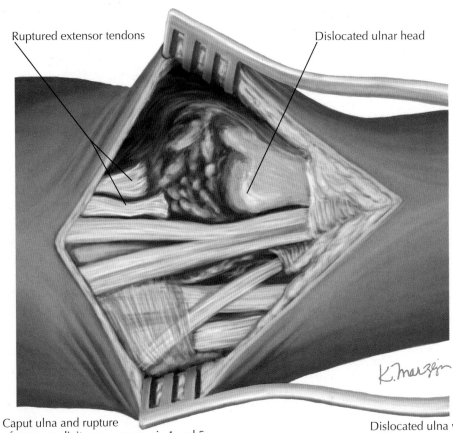

Ruptured extensor tendons   Dislocated ulnar head

K. marzyn

Caput ulna and rupture
of extensor digitorum communis 4 and 5
and extensor digitorum quinti

Dislocated ulna with
extensor tendon rupture

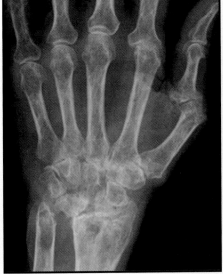

AP radiograph of the wrist in patient with severe rheumatoid arthritis. Note complete loss of radiocarpal joint space, ulnar translocation of carpus upon radial platform, and severe erosion of ulnar head.

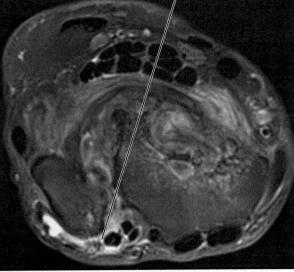

MR image of the same wrist at the level of the DRUJ. Note volar subluxation of distal radius leading to dorsal prominence of ulnar head, which led to rupture of extensor tendons to the ring and small fingers (caput ulna).

Plate 3.35

Upper Limb: PART I

ARTHRITIS OF WRIST

Primary osteoarthritis of the wrist is exceedingly rare, and most often wrist arthritis develops after trauma to the joint. Intraarticular malunion after radius fracture, scapholunate advanced collapse (SLAC), and SNAC all are common causes of articular destruction of the wrist.

SLAC and SNAC wrist share a common pathophysiology of actual or relative flexion of the scaphoid and altered loading of the radiocarpal and midcarpal articulations. There is a defined sequence of arthritic progression first involving the scaphoid and radial styloid (stage I), involvement of the entire radioscaphoid joint (stage II), capitolunate degeneration (stage III), and pancarpal arthritis (stage IV). The radiolunate joint is preserved except in the most advanced stages of disease. Nonoperative treatment consists of activity modification, nonsteroidal antiinflammatory agents, splinting, and judicious use of intraarticular corticosteroid injection. Operative treatment is reserved for those who fail conservative treatment and have pain or deformity that limits their daily activities. Surgical options can be grouped into motion-sparing versus motion-eliminating procedures. Total wrist fusion is the best option for the heavy laborer and/or patients with pancarpal degeneration. Patients with sparing of the midcarpal joint are candidates for proximal row carpectomy, which is the elimination of the scaphoid, lunate, and triquetrum. Stability is maintained by the careful preservation of the volar radioscaphocapitate ligament, and the wrist "runs" on the newly created radiocapitate articulation. Proximal row carpectomy may not be appropriate in the young or heavy laborer. When the radiolunate articulation is preserved, some form of midcarpal fusion can provide excellent pain relief and acceptable motion. Midcarpal fusion is always accompanied by scaphoid excision and then is achieved via either capitolunate arthrodesis or four-bone fusion. Total wrist arthroplasty is a motion-sparing procedure that can provide excellent pain relief and preserve motion. Current designs are appropriate for the patient with pancarpal degeneration with low demand for activities requiring wrist motion.

Radiocarpal destruction secondary to distal radius malunion can be managed with either elimination of the radiocarpal joint via radioscapholunate fusion or total wrist arthrodesis/arthroplasty. Again, the surgical decision is based on patient factors and on direct intraoperative inspection of the anticipated preserved articulations.

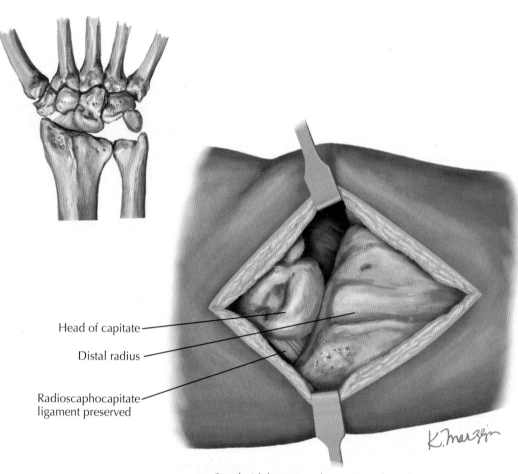

Head of capitate

Distal radius

Radioscaphocapitate ligament preserved

Scaphoid, lunate, and triquetrum have been excised.

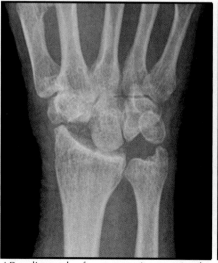

AP radiograph of postoperative proximal row carpectomy

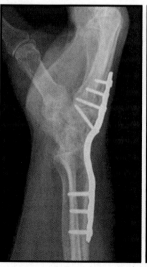

Lateral (*left*) and AP (*right*) radiographs of total wrist arthrodesis using a precontoured compression plate and screws

Plate 3.36

Forearm and Wrist

KIENBÖCK DISEASE

In Kienböck disease, also known as lunatomalacia, the collapse of the carpal lunate occurs because of avascular necrosis. The disease occurs most often in young adults between 15 and 40 years of age and is usually unilateral. The actual cause of the vascular impairment has not been determined, although several etiologic factors have been proposed: (1) single or repetitive microfractures that result in vascular embarrassment; (2) traumatic disruption of circulation or ligamentous injury with subsequent degeneration; (3) primary circulatory disease; and (4) shortening of the ulna relative to the radius, which decreases the support for the lunate. The current theory is that the disease occurs in persons with a mechanical or vascular predisposition when repetitive compression of the lunate between the capitate and distal radius disrupts the intraosseous structures. Chronic compression of the lunate (which is unavoidable in normal wrist function), effusion, and synovitis may interfere with healing and provide a mechanism for progressive collapse of the bone.

CLINICAL MANIFESTATIONS

The primary signs and symptoms of Kienböck disease are wrist pain that radiates up the forearm and stiffness, tenderness, and swelling over the lunate. Passive dorsiflexion of the middle finger produces the characteristic pain. Physical examination reveals limitation of wrist motion, usually dorsiflexion, and a striking weakness of grip. The pain and weakness increase as the lunate collapses and degenerative changes develop, making the disability both severe and chronic.

RADIOGRAPHIC FINDINGS

The avascular necrosis of the lunate may vary in degree but produces consistent and typical radiographic changes. Initial radiographic findings may be normal except for a short ulna, but sclerosis of the lunate—the radiographic hallmark of the disease—develops with time. The lunate progressively loses height and eventually fragments. Further lunate collapse leads to carpal instability and resultant degenerative joint changes, including the formation of cysts within the lunate. The degenerative changes may ultimately involve the entire wrist. The Lichtman classification uses radiographic findings to stage disease severity. This classification helps guide treatment and allows the evaluation of disease progression with time.

TREATMENT

Because the specific etiology of Kienböck disease is not fully understood, no reliable treatment has been established, although many have been proposed. Prolonged immobilization relieves symptoms, but the revascularization of the lunate does not occur readily in adults, and a decrease in range of motion in the wrist and grip strength gradually occurs. A simple excision of the lunate produces good results initially but, ultimately, the remaining carpal bones migrate, leading to joint incongruity, limited wrist motion and grip strength, and degenerative osteoarthritis.

Current surgical options aim to either unload the lunate, revascularize the lunate, or perform limited or complete wrist fusions to halt disease progress and diminish symptoms. Joint-leveling procedures (shortening the radius) have produced excellent long-term results, particularly if performed early in the disease process. Wrists that have either neutral or positive ulnar variance cannot reliably be treated with shortening of the radius. Capitate shortening has been used to unload the lunate in these situations. Vascularized bone grafting, most frequently from the dorsal radius, is often combined with these unloading procedures with the aim of improving the likelihood for lunate revascularization. Recently there have been reports of decompressing the distal radial metaphysis via a limited radial incision; this simple procedure has shown promise in earlier stages of Kienböck disease. With advancing stages of collapse and/or degenerative changes, surgical options are limited to partial versus complete wrist fusion.

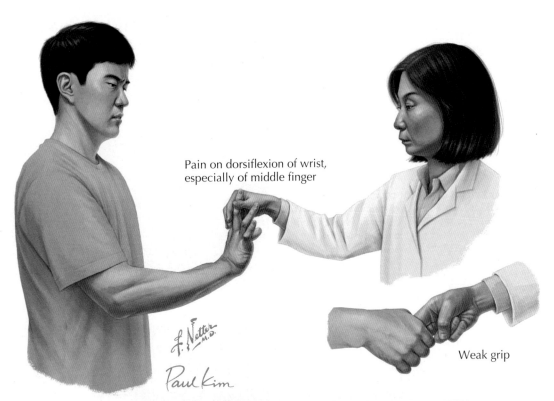

Pain on dorsiflexion of wrist, especially of middle finger

Weak grip

Lichtman classification of Kienböck disease	
Stage 1	Normal radiograph: diffuse lunate signal changes on MRI
Stage 2	Lunate sclerosis on radiograph
Stage 3	Lunate collapse
Stage 3A	+ Normal carpal alignment
Stage 3B	+ Carpal collapse with fixed scaphoid rotation
Stage 4	Lunate collapse + pancarpal arthritis

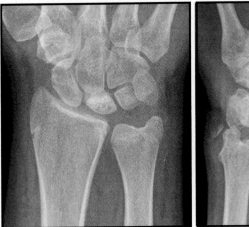

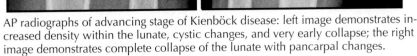

AP radiographs of advancing stage of Kienböck disease: left image demonstrates increased density within the lunate, cystic changes, and very early collapse; the right image demonstrates complete collapse of the lunate with pancarpal changes.

Plate 3.37

Upper Limb: PART I

RADIAL LONGITUDINAL DEFICIENCY

Radial longitudinal deficiency encompasses a spectrum of dysplasia and hypoplasia involving the thumb, wrist, and forearm. The severity of deformity ranges from a mild thumb hypoplasia to complete absence of the radius. Often referred to as "radial club hand," radial longitudinal deficiency more accurately describes the range of malformations encountered. The incidence is between 1 in 30,000 to 1 in 100,000 live births, with a male to female ratio of 3:2. The occurrence of bilateral involvement has been reported between 38% to 58%; and when the disorder is unilateral, the hypoplasia involves the right upper extremity twice as often as the left.

The cause of radial longitudinal deficiency remains unknown. Several factors have been proposed as potential insults to the developing limb, including intrauterine compression, vascular insufficiency, environmental insults, maternal drug exposure, and genetic mutations. Upper limb development occurs during the first 4 to 7 weeks of embryonic life and coincides with the appearance of the cardiac, renal, and hematopoietic systems. Thus single or multiple embryonic insults can result in malformations of several organ systems. Therefore all children presenting with a radial-sided dysplasia, regardless of severity, mandate thorough evaluation for associated medical conditions. Of primary concern are the cardiac, renal, gastrointestinal, and hematopoietic systems. The spectrum of these malformations ranges from mild to devastating.

ANATOMIC MANIFESTATIONS AND CLASSIFICATIONS

Thumb

The length of the average thumb extends to the distal half of the index finger's proximal phalanx in adduction, reaching the palmar surface of the small finger's proximal phalanx in opposition. Absence of thumb function, either from congenital or traumatic afflictions, has been estimated to diminish overall hand function by 40%.

Blauth classified thumb hypoplasia into five types according to thumb size, depth of the first web space, intrinsic muscle deficiency, extrinsic muscle deficiency, and bony/ligamentous joint stability. Manske and colleagues divided type III thumb hypoplasia into subtypes IIIA and IIIB, based on the presence or absence of a stable first carpometacarpal joint. This subdivision has critical implications to surgical management and separates the reconstructible thumb (IIIA) from the largely nonreconstructible thumb (IIIB).

Forearm

The forearm in radial dysplasia has a deficient skeleton, hypoplastic or absent musculature, and altered neurovascular anatomy. Forearm length and radial deviation of the hand/carpus are directly related to the severity of radial deficiency. The relative shortening of the limb remains constant throughout growth.

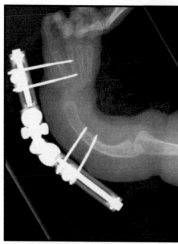

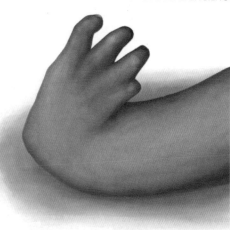

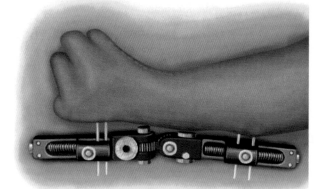

Clinical appearance of type IV radial longitudinal deficiency (note the >90-degree angulation of the wrist relative to the forearm)

Radiograph of type IV radial longitudinal deficiency (i.e., complete absence of radius)

External fixation in place after 6 weeks of soft tissue stretching

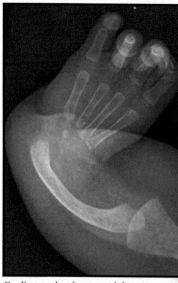

Radiograph of external fixation of the forearm to stretch the contracted soft tissue prior to radialization/centralization

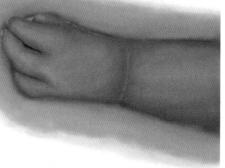

Clinical appearance after formal radicalization of the forearm

Common associated syndromes			
Syndrome	**Associated conditions**		**Inheritance**
Holt-Oram	Atrial septal defects Arrhythmias	Other upper limb abnormalities	Autosomal dominant
VACTERL	V = vertebral anomalies A = imperforate anus C = cardiac defects	TE = tracheoesophageal fistula R = renal anomalies L = limb defects	Sporadic
Fanconi anemia	Pancytopenia develops between 5 and 10 years of age		Autosomal recessive
Thrombocytopenia-absent radius (TAR)	Thrombocytopenia/anemia at birth and improves during first year of life. **Note: absent radius with normal thumb**		Autosomal recessive

Bayne and Klug classified radial dysplasia into four types based on the radiographic severity of skeletal deficiency. Type IV dysplasia is the most prevalent, defined by complete absence of the radius. The ulna is bowed with marked radial and palmar displacement of the hand. The forearm in type IV dysplasia averages 60% of the length of the contralateral normal side.

TREATMENT

The overall health of the child and the severity of the osseous and soft tissue deformities guide long-term treatment plans. Parents and families are instructed on realistic goals for improving function and cosmesis of the upper limb.

Plate 3.38   Forearm and Wrist

TYPE II HYPOPLASTIC THUMB

RADIAL LONGITUDINAL DEFICIENCY (Continued)

Nonoperative management is the definitive treatment for children with minimal deformity and stable joints as well as in children with severe deformity and/or associated anomalies precluding safe surgical intervention. Absolute contraindications to operative reconstruction include (1) adults and older children with established patterns of functional compensation, (2) mild deformities with good function and cosmesis, (3) associated medical anomalies precluding safe operative reconstruction, and/or (4) severe, bilateral elbow extension contractures that rely on wrist flexion and radial deviation for placement of the hand to the face.

The goals for operative reconstruction are to optimize upper limb length, straighten the forearm axis, and either reconstruct or ablate the thumb and pollicize the index finger. The forearm and thumb are addressed in staged procedures. The initial surgery is undertaken at 6 to 12 months of age and involves realigning and stabilizing the hand/carpus on the distal ulna. Thumb reconstruction/ablation begins 6 months after wrist realignment with the overall goal of completing all reconstructions by 18 months of age, thus allowing the child to achieve usual developmental milestones.

Forearm

Current techniques attempt to achieve and maintain deformity correction and stability while optimizing growth, improving digital and wrist range of motion, and enhancing function. Maintaining the bony carpus and distal ulnar physis is critical to optimizing upper limb length, wrist motion, and future growth potential, which are prerequisites for a successful surgical outcome. Recently, soft tissue distraction devices have been used as a staged procedure to achieve passive reduction of the hand/carpus in recalcitrant cases.

Thumb

Anatomic reconstruction is appropriate in children demonstrating functional incorporation of their thumbs. The objective is to obtain a stable digit for pinch, grip, and prehension. Reconstruction has the advantages of maintaining a five-digit hand with the potential for polyaxial rotation at the thumb's basilar joint—surgical impossibilities with ablation and index finger pollicization.

Children with Blauth types IIIB, IV, and V have poor cerebrocortical representation of their thumbs. Reconstruction may improve cosmesis but will not restore functional use of an ignored digit. With time, the functionally excluded thumb will become a liability. The surgical details of ablation and index finger pollicization have been well documented. The goals of pollicization are to (1) preserve the neurovascular anatomy, (2) shorten the index metacarpal via diaphyseal deletion, (3) rotate and stabilize the index finger (in 120 degrees pronation, 40 degrees abduction, and 15 degrees

extension), and (4) reattach and balance the musculotendinous units.

SUMMARY

Management of radial longitudinal deficiency challenges even the most experienced orthopedic surgeon. Cooperative effort between the orthopedist, pediatrician, geneticist, and medical specialists ensures optimal medical evaluation and treatment of these children.

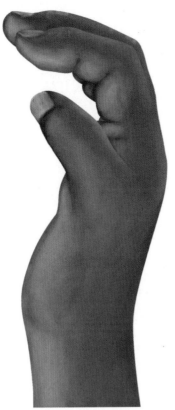

Opponensplasty. Note the tendon going across is the harvested flexor digitorum superficialis from the ring finger. The incision at the wrist demonstrates the tendon going through a loop in the flexor carpi ulnaris tendon (i.e., acting as a sling for the transfer).

Clinical appearance of hypoplastic thumb. Note the diminished thenar musculature and instability of the thumb metacarpophalangeal joint (i.e., deficient ulnar collateral ligament).

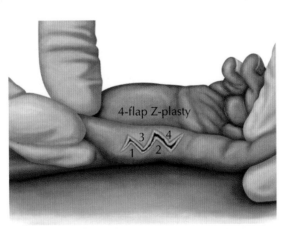

4-flap Z-plasty

3 4
1 2

Four-flap Z-plasty of the first web space to both deepen and lengthen the space

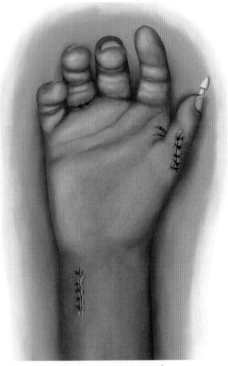

Complete reconstruction for type II hypoplastic thumb

Surgical reconstruction aims to realign and stabilize the forearm, wrist, and hand while providing a functional thumb for strong pinch and grasp. Current and future research strives to identify the underlying developmental insults responsible for deformity and to enhance operative management to optimize forearm length, minimize recurrence, improve both wrist stability and motion, and further advance thumb reconstruction/ablation-pollicization.

HAND AND FINGER

Plate 4.1

Upper Limb: PART I

TOPOGRAPHIC ANATOMY, BONES, AND ORIGINS AND INSERTIONS OF THE HAND (ANTERIOR VIEW)

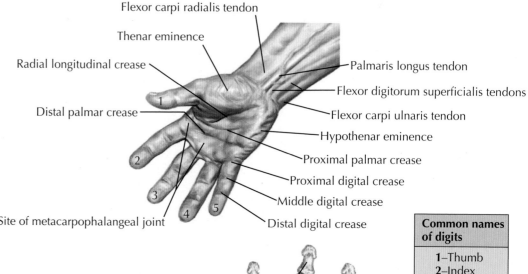

Anterior view

Flexor carpi radialis tendon

Thenar eminence

Radial longitudinal crease

Palmaris longus tendon

Flexor digitorum superficialis tendons

Flexor carpi ulnaris tendon

Distal palmar crease

Hypothenar eminence

Proximal palmar crease

Proximal digital crease

Middle digital crease

Site of metacarpophalangeal joint

Distal digital crease

Common names of digits
1–Thumb
2–Index
3–Long
4–Ring
5–Small

BONES OF THE HAND

METACARPAL BONES

Five metacarpals form the skeleton of the hand. They are miniature "long" bones, comprising a shaft, head, and base. They are palpable on the dorsum of the hand and terminate distally in the knuckles, which are their heads (see Plates 4.1 and 4.2).

The *shaft* is curved longitudinally to be convex dorsally and concave on its palmar aspect. The *head,* the distal extremity, has a rounded smooth surface for articulation with the base of the proximal phalanx. The sides of the head exhibit pits, or tubercles, for the attachment of ligaments. The articular surface of the head is also convex transversely, although less so than dorsopalmarly so that the head fails to be a sphere; however, flexion and extension and abduction and adduction are permitted. The *base* is cuboidal and broader dorsally than palmarward. Its ends and sides are articular, and the dorsal and palmar surfaces are rough for ligamentous attachments.

The *first (thumb) metacarpal* is shorter and stouter than the others, and its palmar surface faces toward the center of the palm. It has a proximal saddle-shaped articular surface for contact with the trapezium. Apart from its regular head configuration, it has two palmar articular eminences for the sesamoids of the thumb.

The *second (index finger) metacarpal* is the longest, and its base is the largest of the metacarpals. There is a deep dorsopalmar groove in the base, which accepts the trapezoid, and the ridges bounding the groove make contact with the trapezium and the capitate. On the ulnar side of the base, there is an incompletely divided facet for the base of the third metacarpal. This complex articulation at the base makes it relatively immobile for power pinch and grip activities.

The *third (long finger) metacarpal* is distinguished by its styloid process, a dorsally and radially placed proximal eminence. The carpal surface of the bone is concave for the capitate. Subdivided facets exist on the sides of the base for articulation with the bases of the second and fourth metacarpals, also making it relatively immobile.

The *fourth (ring finger) metacarpal* has a square base that, proximally, has a large facet for the hamate and, laterally, a small facet for the capitate. Two facets on the lateral side of the base make contact with the base of the third metacarpal, and a single, oval facet on the other side faces the fifth metacarpal, allowing for significant motion during power grip.

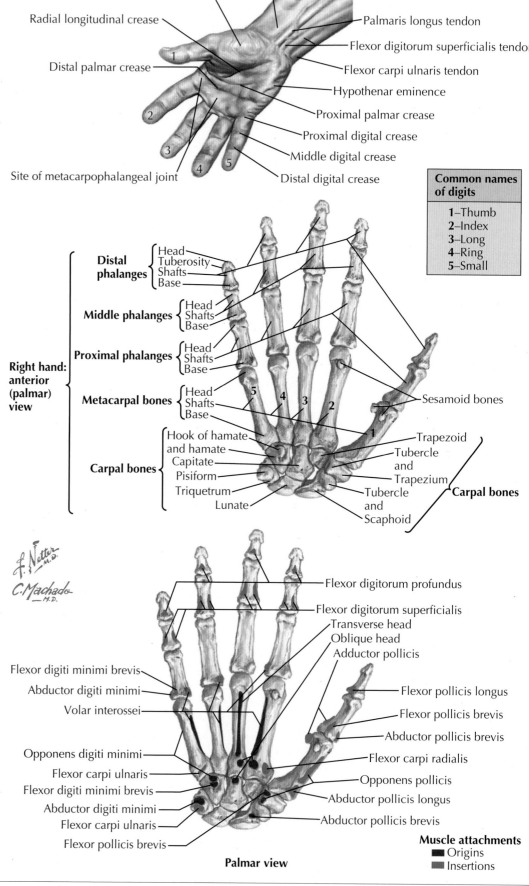

Right hand: anterior (palmar) view

Distal phalanges { Head / Tuberosity / Shafts / Base

Middle phalanges { Head / Shafts / Base

Proximal phalanges { Head / Shafts / Base

Metacarpal bones { Head / Shafts / Base

Sesamoid bones

Carpal bones { Hook of hamate / and hamate / Capitate / Pisiform / Triquetrum / Lunate

Trapezoid

Tubercle and Trapezium

Tubercle and Scaphoid

Carpal bones

Flexor digitorum profundus

Flexor digitorum superficialis

Transverse head

Oblique head

Adductor pollicis

Flexor digiti minimi brevis

Abductor digiti minimi

Volar interossei

Flexor pollicis longus

Flexor pollicis brevis

Abductor pollicis brevis

Flexor carpi radialis

Opponens digiti minimi

Flexor carpi ulnaris

Flexor digiti minimi brevis

Abductor digiti minimi

Flexor carpi ulnaris

Flexor pollicis brevis

Opponens pollicis

Abductor pollicis longus

Abductor pollicis brevis

Muscle attachments
■ Origins
■ Insertions

Palmar view

Plate 4.2

Hand and Finger

TOPOGRAPHIC ANATOMY, BONES, AND ORIGINS AND INSERTIONS OF THE HAND (POSTERIOR VIEW)

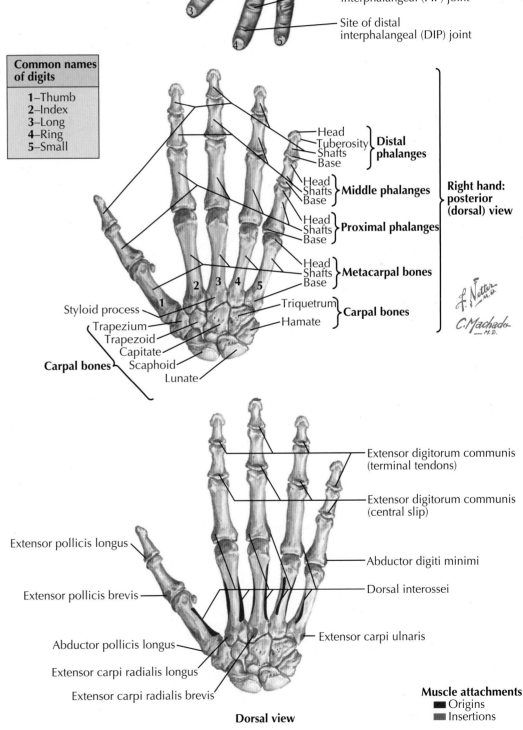

BONES OF THE HAND (Continued)

The *fifth (small finger) metacarpal* has a single, concavoconvex facet on the proximal surface of its base for articulation with the hamate. A slightly convex facet on the radial side is received into the matching oval facet of the fourth metacarpal that allows for the most movement at the carpometacarpal joint of all the lesser fingers. On the ulnar side of the base there is a prominent tubercle for the attachment of the tendon of the extensor carpi ulnaris muscle.

Ossification of the metacarpals proceeds from two centers—one for the body of the bone and one for the distal extremity in each of the four fingers, except for the proximal extremity in the thumb. Ossification begins in the shafts in the eighth or ninth week of fetal life. The centers for the extremity epiphyses appear during the second year, and fusion takes place between ages 16 and 18 years.

PHALANGES

The phalanges number 14, including the thumb (see Plates 4.1 and 4.2). These, too, are miniature long bones, with a shaft and two extremities. The dorsum of the shaft is markedly convex from side to side; its palmar surface is nearly flat. The margins of the palmar surfaces are ridged for attachment of the fibrous flexor sheaths of the digits. The proximal extremity of the first phalanx of each digit is concave and oval and broader from side to side for articulation with the head of the metacarpal. Distally, the proximal extremities of the middle and distal phalanges have two shallow concavities separated by an intervening ridge that articulates with the pulley-like surfaces on the distal ends of the middle and distal phalanges. The distal phalanges exhibit terminal elevated roughened surfaces, which support the pulp of the fingers. The sides of the bases of the phalanges show tubercles for ligaments; the sides of the heads (except on the distal phalanx) exhibit shallow pits for ligamentous attachments.

Ossification of the phalanges proceeds from two centers—one for the body and one for the proximal extremity. Ossification in the shaft begins about the eighth week of fetal life and in the epiphysis occurs during the second and third years, with fusion taking place between 14 and 18 years of age.

Plate 4.3

Upper Limb: PART I

METACARPOPHALANGEAL AND INTERPHALANGEAL LIGAMENTS

Anterior (palmar) view

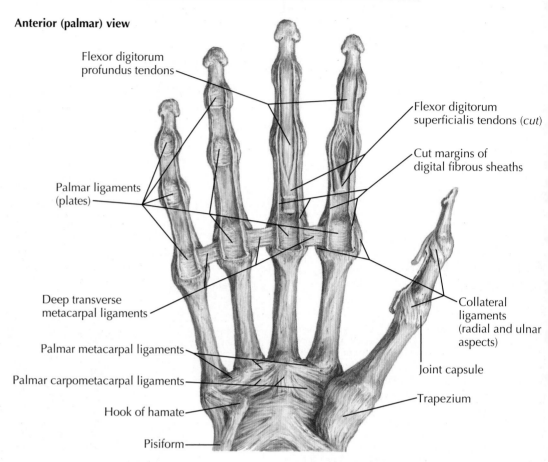

Flexor digitorum profundus tendons

Flexor digitorum superficialis tendons (*cut*)

Cut margins of digital fibrous sheaths

Palmar ligaments (plates)

Deep transverse metacarpal ligaments

Collateral ligaments (radial and ulnar aspects)

Palmar metacarpal ligaments

Palmar carpometacarpal ligaments

Joint capsule

Hook of hamate

Trapezium

Pisiform

JOINTS OF THE HAND

CARPOMETACARPAL JOINT

The carpometacarpal joint of the thumb is the independent joint between the trapezium and the base of the index metacarpal. The articular surfaces are reciprocally concavoconvex, and a loose but strong articular capsule joins the bones. The biaxial nature of this joint provides for flexion and extension and abduction and adduction, and the looseness of its capsule allows opposition of the thumb that involves a small amount of rotary movement (circumduction).

The carpometacarpal joints of the four fingers participate with the intercarpal and intermetacarpal joints in a common synovial cavity. Dorsal and palmar carpometacarpal ligaments run from the carpals of the second row to the various metacarpals. Short interosseous ligaments are usually present between contiguous angles of the capitate and the hamate and the ring and long finger metacarpals.

INTERMETACARPAL JOINTS

These joints occur between the adjacent sides of the bases of the metacarpals of the four fingers. Here, also, there are dorsal and palmar ligaments, and interosseous ligaments close off the common synovial cavity by connecting the bones just distal to their articular facets. Only slight gliding movements occur between the metacarpals and between them and the carpals to which they are related. However, the articulation between the hamate and the small finger metacarpal allows that bone to flex appreciably during a tight grasp

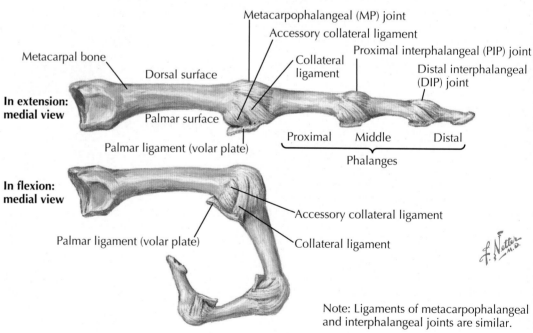

Metacarpophalangeal (MP) joint

Accessory collateral ligament

Metacarpal bone

Dorsal surface

Collateral ligament

Proximal interphalangeal (PIP) joint

Distal interphalangeal (DIP) joint

In extension: medial view

Palmar surface

Palmar ligament (volar plate)

Proximal   Middle   Distal

Phalanges

In flexion: medial view

Accessory collateral ligament

Palmar ligament (volar plate)

Collateral ligament

f. Netter M.D.

Note: Ligaments of metacarpophalangeal and interphalangeal joints are similar.

and also to rotate slightly under the traction of the opponens digiti minimi muscle.

The *deep transverse metacarpal ligaments* are short and connect the palmar surfaces of the heads of the index, long, ring, and small metacarpals. They are continuous with the palmar interosseous fascia and blend with the palmar ligaments of the metacarpophalangeal joints and the fibrous sheaths of the digits. They limit

the spread of the metacarpals, and the tendons of the interosseous and lumbrical muscles pass on either side of them.

METACARPOPHALANGEAL JOINTS

These joints are condyloid, and both the rounded head of the metacarpal and the oval concavity of the

Plate 4.4

Hand and Finger

DEFINITIONS OF HAND MOTION

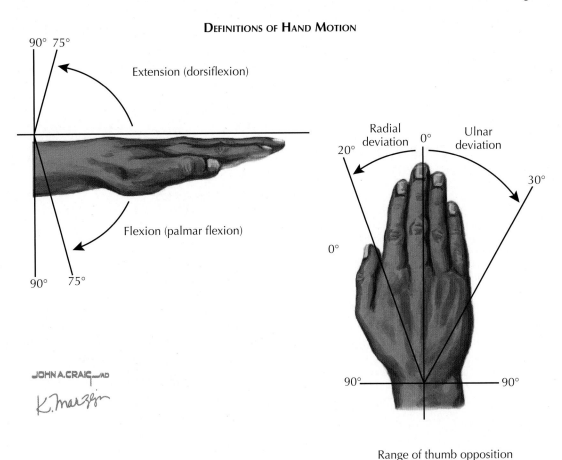

90° 75°

Extension (dorsiflexion)

Flexion (palmar flexion)

90° 75°

JOHN A. CRAIG—AD

K. marzejon

Radial deviation

20°

0°

Ulnar deviation

30°

0°

90°

90°

Range of thumb opposition

JOINTS OF THE HAND (Continued)

proximal end of the phalanx have unequal curvatures along their transverse and vertical axes. An articular capsule and collateral and palmar ligaments unite the bones. The articular capsule is rather loose. Dorsally, it is reinforced by the expansion of the digital extensor tendon.

The *palmar ligament* is a dense, fibrocartilaginous plate, which, by means of its firm attachment to the proximal palmar edge of the phalanx, extends and deepens the phalangeal articular surface. It is loosely attached to the neck of the metacarpal; in flexion, it passes under the head of the metacarpal and serves as part of the articular contact of the bones. At its sides, the palmar ligament is continuous with the deep transverse metacarpal ligaments and the collateral ligaments. The *collateral ligaments* are strong, cord-like bands attached proximally to the tubercle and adjacent pit of the head of the metacarpals and distally to the palmar surface of the side of the phalanx. Their fibers spread fan-like to attach to the palmar ligaments. Movements of flexion and extension, abduction and adduction, and circumduction are permitted at these joints. With extension is associated abduction, as in fanning the fingers; with flexion is associated adduction, as in making a fist. The metacarpophalangeal joint of the thumb is limited in abduction and adduction; its special freedom of motion derives from its carpometacarpal joint.

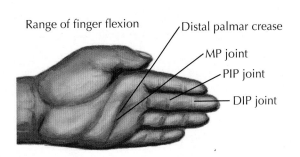

Range of finger flexion

Distal palmar crease

MP joint

PIP joint

DIP joint

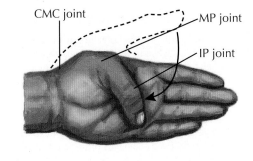

CMC joint

MP joint

IP joint

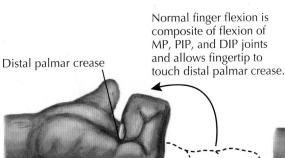

Distal palmar crease

Normal finger flexion is composite of flexion of MP, PIP, and DIP joints and allows fingertip to touch distal palmar crease.

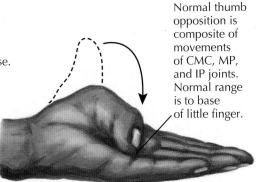

Normal thumb opposition is composite of movements of CMC, MP, and IP joints. Normal range is to base of little finger.

INTERPHALANGEAL JOINTS

Structurally similar to the metacarpophalangeal series, the interphalangeal (IP) joints have the same loose capsule, palmar and collateral ligaments, and dorsal reinforcement from the extensor expansion. However, owing to the pulley-like form of their articular surfaces, action here is limited to flexion and extension. Flexion is freer than extension and may reach 115 degrees at the proximal interphalangeal joint. Arteries and nerves serving these joints are twigs of adjacent proper digital branches.

MOVEMENT OF THE HAND

The unique bony and articular anatomy of the hand allows for a myriad of movements, and the cumulative movement of each joint in series increases the total active motion. By convention, movement toward the palm is described as palmar or volar or anterior and movement toward the back of the hand is described as dorsal or posterior. Movement of the hand toward the thumb side of the arm is described as radial or lateral and toward the small finger as ulnar or medial.

Plate 4.5

Upper Limb: PART I

FLEXOR AND EXTENSOR TENDONS OF THE HAND

As the flexor and extensor tendons pass from the wrist to the hand, clinical zones have been described that help physicians articulate more precisely the significant anatomic differences that exist in each zone that affect finger function after injury (see Plates 4.5 and 4.6). As the extensor digitorum tendons diverge over the dorsum of the hand, they are interconnected by *intertendinous connections (juncturae tendinum)*. These prominently interconnect the tendons for the long, ring, and small fingers and severely limit the independent action of these digits, especially the ring finger. Independent extensor action is retained for the index finger. The convergence of the tendon of the extensor pollicis longus muscle toward the tendons of the abductor pollicis longus and extensor pollicis brevis muscles defines a hollow known as the *anatomic snuffbox* (see Plate 4.14). In the floor of this hollow, the radial artery passes toward the dorsum of the hand and gives off its dorsal carpal branch.

FLEXOR TENDONS AND ACCESSORIES

Digital synovial sheaths, after a gap in the midpalm, pick up over the heads of the metacarpals and continue over the pairs of tendons to the base of the distal phalanges of the index to small finger. Except for about 5 mm of their proximal ends, these synovial sheaths (and the tendons) are contained within the fibrous sheaths of the digits of the hand. The *fibrous sheaths of the digits* are strong coverings of the flexor tendons, which extend from the heads of the metacarpals to the base of the distal phalanges and serve to prevent "bow-stringing" of the tendon away from the bones during flexion. They attach along the borders of the proximal and middle phalanges, the capsules of the interphalangeal joints, and the palmar surface of the distal phalanx. They form strong semicylindrical sheaths that, with the bones, produce fibro-osseous tunnels through which the flexor tendons pass to their insertions. Over the shafts of the proximal and middle phalanges, the sheaths exhibit thick accumulations of transversely running fibers (sometimes called annular ligaments, or pulleys), whereas opposite the joints, an obliquely criss-crossing arrangement is characteristic (cruciate ligaments). These latter portions of the fibrous sheaths are thin and do not interfere with flexion at the joints. Proximally, the digital slips of the palmar aponeurosis attach to the fibrous digital sheaths.

The tendons of the flexor digitorum profundus muscle insert on the bases of the distal phalanges of digits 2 to 5, while the tendons of the flexor digitorum superficialis muscle end on the shafts of the middle phalanges of these digits. It is thus necessary for the tendons of the flexor digitorum profundus muscle to pass those of the flexor digitorum superficialis muscle, and this is accomplished by a splitting of the tendon of the superficialis to allow that of the profundus to pass distalward. The division of the flexor digitorum superficialis

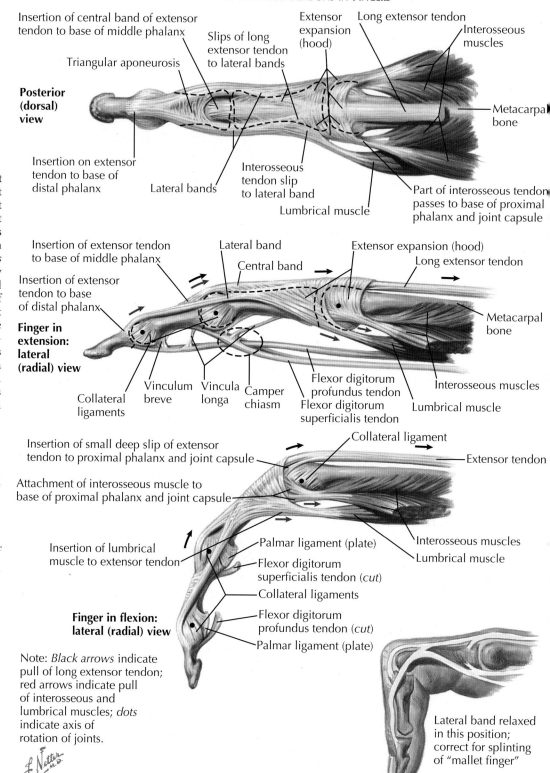

FLEXOR AND EXTENSOR TENDONS IN FINGERS

Insertion of central band of extensor tendon to base of middle phalanx

Triangular aponeurosis

Slips of long extensor tendon to lateral bands

Extensor expansion (hood)

Long extensor tendon

Interosseous muscles

Posterior (dorsal) view

Insertion on extensor tendon to base of distal phalanx

Lateral bands

Interosseous tendon slip to lateral band

Lumbrical muscle

Metacarpal bone

Part of interosseous tendon passes to base of proximal phalanx and joint capsule

Insertion of extensor tendon to base of middle phalanx

Insertion of extensor tendon to base of distal phalanx

Finger in extension: lateral (radial) view

Lateral band

Central band

Extensor expansion (hood)

Long extensor tendon

Metacarpal bone

Collateral ligaments

Vinculum breve

Vincula longa

Camper chiasm

Flexor digitorum profundus tendon

Flexor digitorum superficialis tendon

Interosseous muscles

Lumbrical muscle

Insertion of small deep slip of extensor tendon to proximal phalanx and joint capsule

Attachment of interosseous muscle to base of proximal phalanx and joint capsule

Collateral ligament

Extensor tendon

Insertion of lumbrical muscle to extensor tendon

Palmar ligament (plate)

Flexor digitorum superficialis tendon (cut)

Collateral ligaments

Flexor digitorum profundus tendon (cut)

Palmar ligament (plate)

Interosseous muscles

Lumbrical muscle

Finger in flexion: lateral (radial) view

Note: *Black arrows* indicate pull of long extensor tendon; red arrows indicate pull of interosseous and lumbrical muscles; *dots* indicate axis of rotation of joints.

Lateral band relaxed in this position; correct for splinting of "mallet finger"

tendon takes place over the proximal phalanx, and the two halves separate and roll in under the flexor digitorum profundus tendon to reach the bone of the middle phalanx, their fibers crisscrossing as they attach to that phalanx.

The *vincula tendinum* spring from the internal surface of the digital sheaths of these muscles. They are folds of synovial membrane strengthened by some fibrous tissue that conduct blood vessels to the tendons.

The smaller *vinculum breve* is at the distal end of the sheath; the *vincula longa* are narrow strands that reach the tendons more proximally.

The *lumbrical muscles* are four small, cylindrical muscles associated with the tendons of the flexor digitorum profundus muscle. The two lateral muscles arise distal to the flexor retinaculum from the radial sides and palmar surfaces of the flexor digitorum profundus muscle destined for the index and long fingers. These

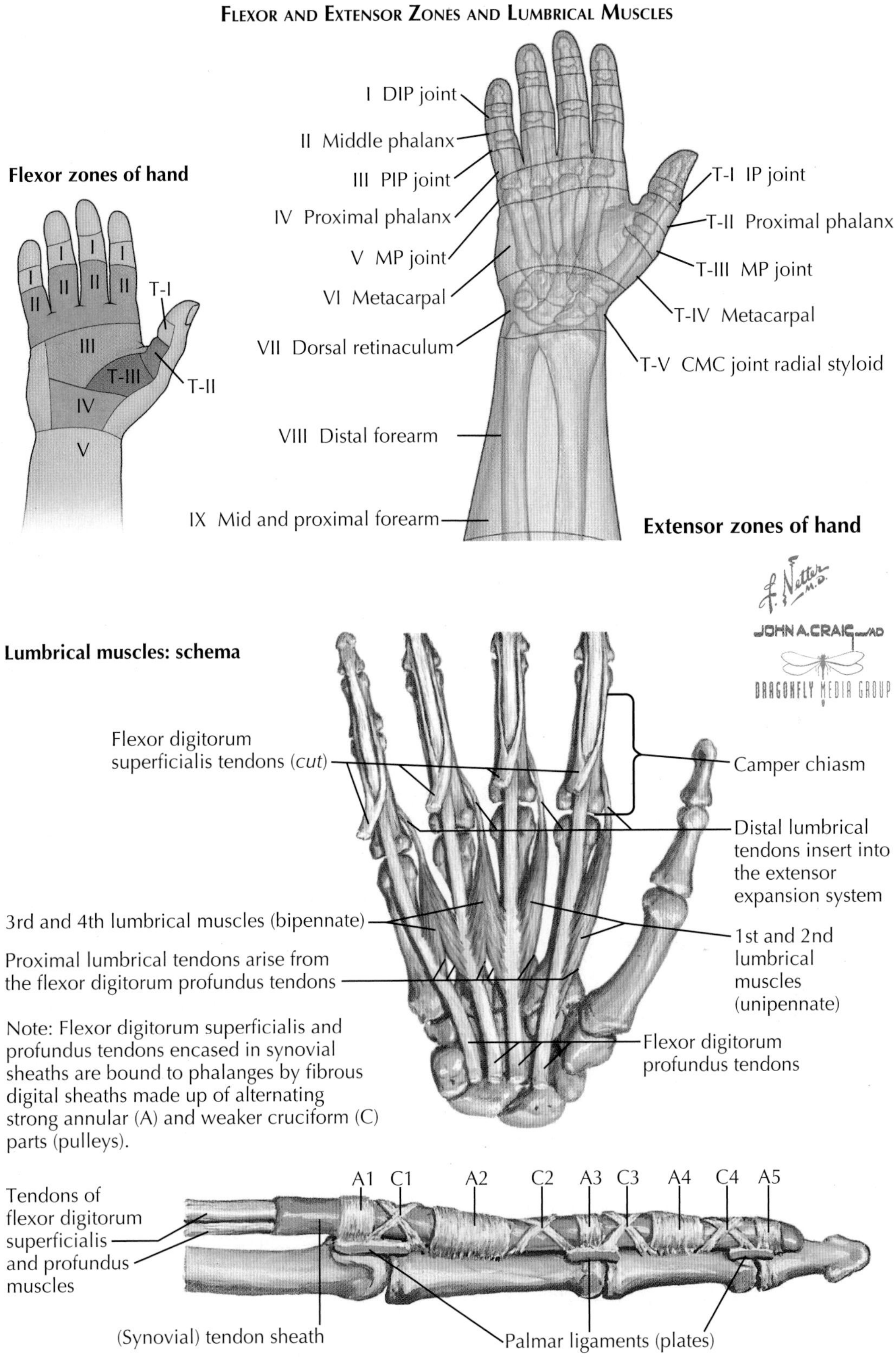

Plate 4.6   Hand and Finger

FLEXOR AND EXTENSOR TENDONS OF THE HAND (Continued)

are supplied by the median nerve. The two medial muscles are bipennate, with the ring finger arising from the long and ring profundus and the small finger arising from the ring and small profundus. These are innervated by the deep branch of the ulnar nerve. Each lumbrical tendon passes distalward on the palmar side of the deep transverse metacarpal ligament and then shifts toward the dorsum. It inserts, at the level of the proximal phalanx, into the radial border of the expansion of the extensor digitorum muscle.

EXTENSOR MECHANISM OF FINGERS

The four tendons of the extensor digitorum muscle of the forearm pass across the metacarpophalangeal joints, become flattened and closely attached to the joint capsules, and substitute as dorsal ligaments for these capsules. At the metacarpophalangeal joint and over the proximal two phalanges, an extensor expansion is formed for each tendon by the participation of the tendons of the lumbrical and interosseous muscles of the hand. Opposite the metacarpophalangeal joints, a band of fibers passes from each side of the digital extensor tendon anteriorly on both sides of the joint and attaches to the palmar ligament of the joint. This proximal spreading of the extensor expansion appears like a hood of fibers over the metacarpophalangeal joint.

Over the dorsum of the proximal phalanx, the digital extensor tendon divides into three slips. Of these, the central, broader slip passes directly forward and inserts on the dorsum of the middle phalanx. The diverging bundles on either side, the lateral bands, receive and combine with the broadening tendon of a lumbrical muscle on the radial side of the digit and with interosseous tendons on both sides of the digit. These tendons unite into a common band that proceeds distalward, the bands of the two sides forming a triangular aponeurosis over the distal end of the middle phalanx. The apex of this aponeurosis attaches to the base of the distal phalanx.

Muscle Actions in Digital Movement

Certain forearm muscles participate in movements of the digits. The tendons of the flexor digitorum superficialis and flexor digitorum profundus muscles emerge from the wrist at the distal border of the flexor retinaculum and enter the central compartment of the palm (see Plate 4.9). Here, they fan out toward their respective digits, arranged in pairs, superficial and deep. They are invested by the ulnar bursa through the upper part of the palm, except that the extension of the bursa along the tendons for the small finger continues to the base of its distal phalanx.

The *flexor digitorum superficialis muscle* is a flexor of the proximal interphalangeal and metacarpophalangeal joints of the medial four fingers and is the principal flexor of the wrist. The *flexor digitorum profundus muscle* primarily flexes the terminal phalanx but,

Flexor zones of hand

Extensor zones of hand

I DIP joint
II Middle phalanx
III PIP joint
IV Proximal phalanx
V MP joint
VI Metacarpal
VII Dorsal retinaculum
VIII Distal forearm
IX Mid and proximal forearm

T-I IP joint
T-II Proximal phalanx
T-III MP joint
T-IV Metacarpal
T-V CMC joint radial styloid

Lumbrical muscles: schema

Flexor digitorum superficialis tendons (*cut*)

3rd and 4th lumbrical muscles (bipennate)

Proximal lumbrical tendons arise from the flexor digitorum profundus tendons

Note: Flexor digitorum superficialis and profundus tendons encased in synovial sheaths are bound to phalanges by fibrous digital sheaths made up of alternating strong annular (A) and weaker cruciform (C) parts (pulleys).

Camper chiasm

Distal lumbrical tendons insert into the extensor expansion system

1st and 2nd lumbrical muscles (unipennate)

Flexor digitorum profundus tendons

Tendons of flexor digitorum superficialis and profundus muscles

A1 C1 A2 C2 A3 C3 A4 C4 A5

(Synovial) tendon sheath

Palmar ligaments (plates)

continuing to act, also flexes the middle and proximal phalanges. This muscle flexes the digits in slow action, the flexor digitorum superficialis muscle being recruited for speed and against resistance. The *extensor digitorum muscle,* assisted by the extensors of the index and small fingers, is the extensor of the fingers. Interconnecting tendinous bands between the tendons (juncturae) of the long to small fingers prevent completely independent extension of these digits, but the index finger can be moved quite separately.

The interosseous and lumbrical muscles of the hand are essential for full extension of the digits. The *interosseous muscles* act most effectively when there is combined metacarpophalangeal flexion and interphalangeal extension, principally producing interphalangeal extension. The *lumbrical muscles* are silent during total flexion but are very active in extension of the proximal or distal interphalangeal joints and also when these joints are being maintained in extension during metacarpophalangeal flexion.

Plate 4.7

Upper Limb: PART I

WRIST AND HAND: DEEP DORSAL DISSECTION

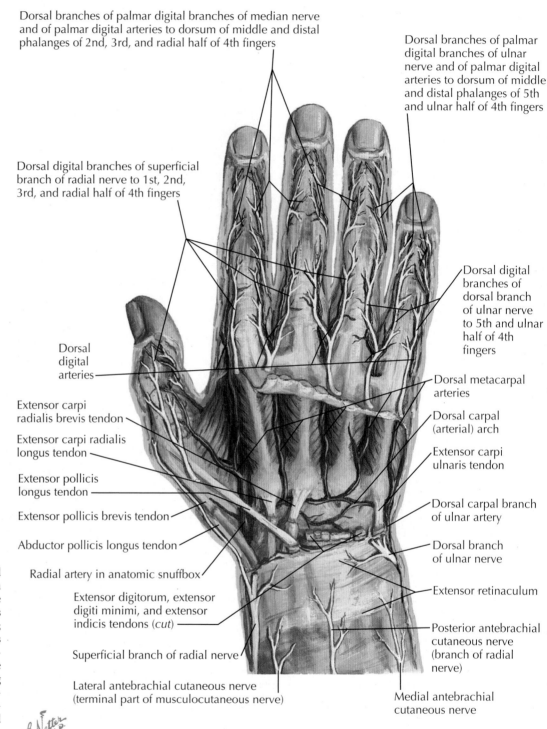

Dorsal branches of palmar digital branches of median nerve and of palmar digital arteries to dorsum of middle and distal phalanges of 2nd, 3rd, and radial half of 4th fingers

Dorsal branches of palmar digital branches of ulnar nerve and of palmar digital arteries to dorsum of middle and distal phalanges of 5th and ulnar half of 4th fingers

Dorsal digital branches of superficial branch of radial nerve to 1st, 2nd, 3rd, and radial half of 4th fingers

Dorsal digital branches of dorsal branch of ulnar nerve to 5th and ulnar half of 4th fingers

Dorsal digital arteries

Dorsal metacarpal arteries

Extensor carpi radialis brevis tendon

Dorsal carpal (arterial) arch

Extensor carpi radialis longus tendon

Extensor carpi ulnaris tendon

Extensor pollicis longus tendon

Dorsal carpal branch of ulnar artery

Extensor pollicis brevis tendon

Dorsal branch of ulnar nerve

Abductor pollicis longus tendon

Extensor retinaculum

Radial artery in anatomic snuffbox

Extensor digitorum, extensor digiti minimi, and extensor indicis tendons (cut)

Posterior antebrachial cutaneous nerve (branch of radial nerve)

Superficial branch of radial nerve

Lateral antebrachial cutaneous nerve (terminal part of musculocutaneous nerve)

Medial antebrachial cutaneous nerve

Posterior (dorsal) view

MUSCLES OF THE HAND

INTRINSIC MUSCLES

The *interosseous muscles* occupy the intermetacarpal intervals and are of two types: dorsal and palmar. Each intermetacarpal space contains one palmar and one dorsal interosseous muscle. The four dorsal interosseous muscles are abductors of the digits and are bipennate; the three palmar interosseous muscles are adductors and are unipennate. The plane of reference for abduction and adduction of the fingers is the midplane of the long finger. This is evident on simultaneously spreading and then approximating the extended digits. The placement of these muscles follows from the above considerations of actions and reference plane for abduction and adduction.

A *dorsal interosseous muscle* lies on either side of the long finger metacarpal, and any movement from its plane of reference is abduction. The second and third dorsal interosseous muscles have the other half of their muscle arising from the index and ring finger metacarpal, respectively. The other two dorsal interosseous muscles occupy the space between the thumb-index metacarpals for the first dorsal muscle and between the ring and small metacarpals for the fourth dorsal muscle. These latter two muscles abduct the index and ring fingers. The bipennate dorsal interosseous muscles arise by two heads from the adjacent sides of the metacarpals between which they lie. The first dorsal interosseous

muscle is considerably larger than the others; the radial artery also passes into the palm between its heads. Dorsal perforating arteries pass between the heads of the other muscles.

The smaller *palmar interosseous muscles* adduct the same digit from whose metacarpal bone they arise and thus take origin from the palmar surfaces of the second, fourth, and fifth metacarpals. The tendons of both the

dorsal and the palmar interosseous muscles pass dorsal to the deep transverse metacarpal ligaments between the heads of the metacarpals, and they have two insertions. The first insertion is to the base of the proximal phalanx; it is concerned with the abduction-adduction function. The second insertion is into the extensor expansion of the tendon of the extensor digitorum muscle; it produces flexion at the metacarpophalangeal

Plate 4.8

Hand and Finger

INTRINSIC MUSCLES OF HAND

Anterior (palmar) view

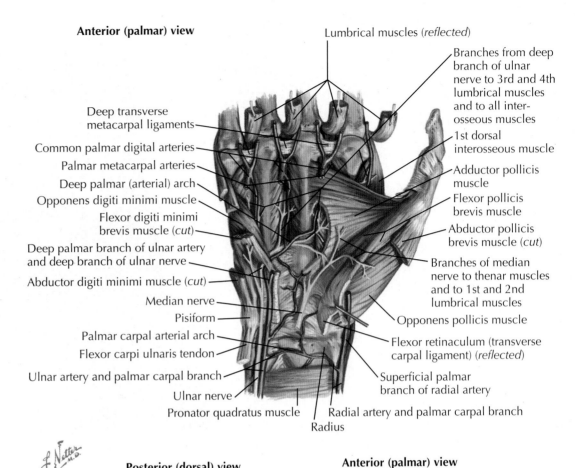

Lumbrical muscles (*reflected*)

Branches from deep branch of ulnar nerve to 3rd and 4th lumbrical muscles and to all inter-osseous muscles

Deep transverse metacarpal ligaments

1st dorsal interosseous muscle

Common palmar digital arteries

Adductor pollicis muscle

Palmar metacarpal arteries

Deep palmar (arterial) arch

Flexor pollicis brevis muscle

Opponens digiti minimi muscle

Abductor pollicis brevis muscle (*cut*)

Flexor digiti minimi brevis muscle (*cut*)

Deep palmar branch of ulnar artery and deep branch of ulnar nerve

Branches of median nerve to thenar muscles and to 1st and 2nd lumbrical muscles

Abductor digiti minimi muscle (*cut*)

Opponens pollicis muscle

Median nerve

Pisiform

Flexor retinaculum (transverse carpal ligament) (*reflected*)

Palmar carpal arterial arch

Flexor carpi ulnaris tendon

Superficial palmar branch of radial artery

Ulnar artery and palmar carpal branch

Ulnar nerve

Radial artery and palmar carpal branch

Pronator quadratus muscle

Radius

Posterior (dorsal) view

Anterior (palmar) view

Tendinous slips to extensor expansions (hoods)

Dorsal interosseous muscles (bipennate)

Deep transverse metacarpal ligaments

Abductor pollicis brevis muscle

Abductor digiti minimi muscle

Palmar interosseous muscles (unipennate)

Radial artery

Radius

Radius

Ulna

Ulna

Note: Arrows indicate action of muscles.

MUSCLES OF THE HAND (Continued)

joints and extension of the middle and distal phalanges at the interphalangeal joints. All the interosseous muscles are innervated by the deep branch of the ulnar nerve.

Free movement of the thumb is most important in the more precise activities of the hand. The *flexor pollicis longus muscle* flexes the thumb, and the *extensor pollicis longus* and *extensor pollicis brevis muscles* extend it. The *abductor pollicis longus muscle* is an accessory flexor of the wrist; it abducts and extends its metacarpal. The short muscles of the thumb provide flexion, abduction, adduction, and opposition. Abduction of the thumb carries it anteriorly out of the plane of the palm because of the rotated position of the first metacarpal, which directs its palmar surface medially. The abductor pollicis brevis muscle also assists in flexion. The *opponens pollicis muscle* acts solely on the metacarpal of the thumb, drawing the digit across the palm and rotating it medially.

The components of opposition are abduction, flexion, and medial rotation, the tip of the thumb reaching contact with the pads of the other slightly flexed digits. In firm grasp, the *flexor pollicis brevis muscle* is especially active. The motor, or recurrent, branch of the median nerve innervates the three muscles involved. The *adductor pollicis muscle* adducts the thumb. The

abductor digiti minimi and the *flexor digiti minimi brevis muscles* produce their characteristic movements. The *opponens digiti minimi muscle* rotates the fifth metacarpal medially and deepens the hollow of the hand.

The intrinsic muscles of the hand are innervated palmarly by either the median or the ulnar nerve. Specific sets of muscles of the thumb and small finger,

respectively, occupy the thenar and hypothenar compartments.

Each compartment contains an *abductor,* an *opponens,* and a *flexor* muscle for its specific digit (abductor pollicis brevis, flexor pollicis brevis, opponens pollicis, abductor digiti minimi, flexor digiti minimi brevis, and opponens digiti minimi muscles). In each compartment, the positions and attachments of these muscles

Plate 4.9

Upper Limb: PART I

SPACES, BURSAE, AND TENDON AND LUMBRICAL SHEATHS OF HAND

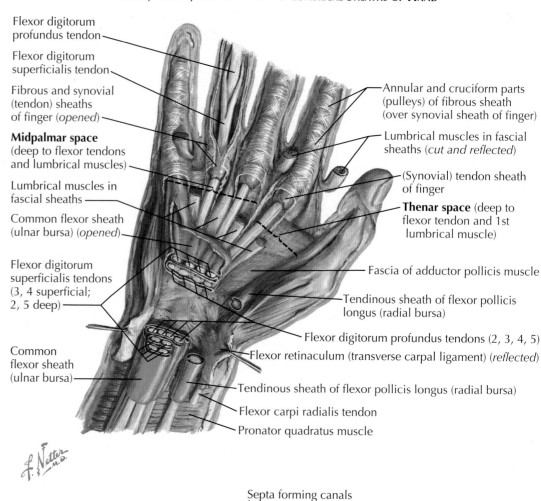

Flexor digitorum profundus tendon

Flexor digitorum superficialis tendon

Fibrous and synovial (tendon) sheaths of finger (*opened*)

Midpalmar space (deep to flexor tendons and lumbrical muscles)

Lumbrical muscles in fascial sheaths

Common flexor sheath (ulnar bursa) (*opened*)

Flexor digitorum superficialis tendons (3, 4 superficial; 2, 5 deep)

Common flexor sheath (ulnar bursa)

Annular and cruciform parts (pulleys) of fibrous sheath (over synovial sheath of finger)

Lumbrical muscles in fascial sheaths (*cut and reflected*)

(Synovial) tendon sheath of finger

Thenar space (deep to flexor tendon and 1st lumbrical muscle)

Fascia of adductor pollicis muscle

Tendinous sheath of flexor pollicis longus (radial bursa)

Flexor digitorum profundus tendons (2, 3, 4, 5)

Flexor retinaculum (transverse carpal ligament) (*reflected*)

Tendinous sheath of flexor pollicis longus (radial bursa)

Flexor carpi radialis tendon

Pronator quadratus muscle

Septa forming canals

Midpalmar space

Profundus and superficialis flexor tendons to 3rd digit

Palmar aponeurosis

Septum between midpalmar and thenar spaces

Common palmar digital artery and nerve

Thenar space

Flexor pollicis longus tendon in tendon sheath (radial bursa)

Lumbrical muscle in its fascial sheath

Flexor tendons to 5th digit in common flexor sheath (ulnar bursa)

Extensor pollicis longus tendon

Hypothenar muscles

Adductor pollicis muscle

Dorsal interosseous fascia

Palmar interosseous fascia

Dorsal subaponeurotic space

Palmar interosseous muscles

Dorsal fascia of hand

Dorsal interosseous muscles

Extensor tendons

Dorsal subcutaneous space

MUSCLES OF THE HAND (Continued)

are similar. The flexor retinaculum and the bones to which it attaches (the scaphoid and trapezium radially and the hamate and pisiform on the ulnar side) provide the sites of origin for these muscles. The insertions of comparable muscles on the two sides are also the same: the base of the proximal phalanx for the abductor and flexor muscles and the shaft of the metacarpal for the opponens muscles.

The central compartment contains four slender *lumbrical muscles* associated with the flexor digitorum profundus tendon. The *interosseous muscles* located in the intervals between the metacarpals occupy, with the *adductor pollicis muscle*, a deeply placed interosseous-adductor compartment that is bound by the dorsal and palmar interosseous fasciae. To complete these generalizations, the rule of nervous innervation may also be stated: the *median nerve* supplies the abductor pollicis brevis, opponens pollicis, flexor pollicis brevis, and the most radial two lumbrical muscles; the *ulnar nerve* supplies all the other intrinsic muscles of the hand.

The *adductor pollicis muscle* has two heads of origin, separated by a gap through which the radial artery enters the palm. The oblique head arises from the capitate and from the bases of the index and long finger metacarpals. The transverse head arises from the palmar ridge (shaft) of the long finger metacarpal. The two

heads insert together by a tendon that ends in the ulnar side of the base of the proximal phalanx of the thumb.

This tendon usually contains a sesamoid that together with the sesamoid in the tendon of the flexor pollicis brevis muscle forms a pair of small sesamoids on either side of the tendon of the flexor pollicis longus muscle. The adductor pollicis muscle overlies the interosseous muscles on the radial side of the long finger

metacarpal. This muscle is supplied by the deep branch of the ulnar nerve.

SPACES, BURSAE, AND TENDON SHEATHS OF THE HAND

Friction between tendons and compartments or bony surfaces is reduced by synovial sheaths. A sheath is

Plate 4.10

Hand and Finger

WRIST AND HAND: PALMAR DISSECTIONS

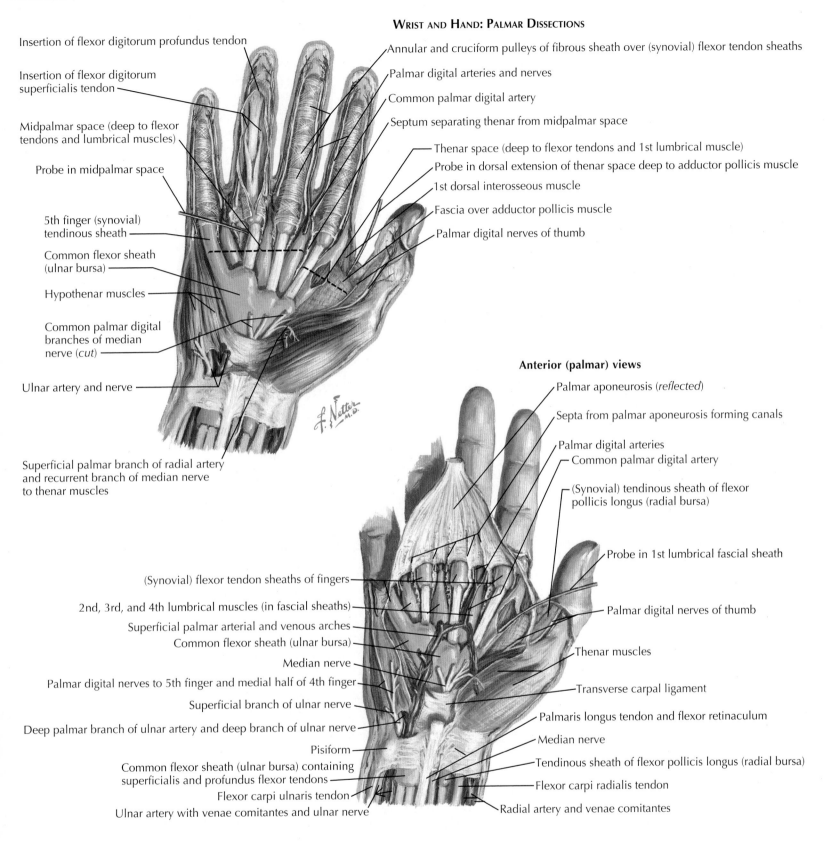

Insertion of flexor digitorum profundus tendon

Insertion of flexor digitorum superficialis tendon

Midpalmar space (deep to flexor tendons and lumbrical muscles)

Probe in midpalmar space

5th finger (synovial) tendinous sheath

Common flexor sheath (ulnar bursa)

Hypothenar muscles

Common palmar digital branches of median nerve (cut)

Ulnar artery and nerve

Superficial palmar branch of radial artery and recurrent branch of median nerve to thenar muscles

Annular and cruciform pulleys of fibrous sheath over (synovial) flexor tendon sheaths

Palmar digital arteries and nerves

Common palmar digital artery

Septum separating thenar from midpalmar space

Thenar space (deep to flexor tendons and 1st lumbrical muscle)

Probe in dorsal extension of thenar space deep to adductor pollicis muscle

1st dorsal interosseous muscle

Fascia over adductor pollicis muscle

Palmar digital nerves of thumb

Anterior (palmar) views

Palmar aponeurosis (reflected)

Septa from palmar aponeurosis forming canals

Palmar digital arteries

Common palmar digital artery

(Synovial) tendinous sheath of flexor pollicis longus (radial bursa)

Probe in 1st lumbrical fascial sheath

Palmar digital nerves of thumb

Thenar muscles

Transverse carpal ligament

Palmaris longus tendon and flexor retinaculum

Median nerve

Tendinous sheath of flexor pollicis longus (radial bursa)

Flexor carpi radialis tendon

Radial artery and venae comitantes

(Synovial) flexor tendon sheaths of fingers

2nd, 3rd, and 4th lumbrical muscles (in fascial sheaths)

Superficial palmar arterial and venous arches

Common flexor sheath (ulnar bursa)

Median nerve

Palmar digital nerves to 5th finger and medial half of 4th finger

Superficial branch of ulnar nerve

Deep palmar branch of ulnar artery and deep branch of ulnar nerve

Pisiform

Common flexor sheath (ulnar bursa) containing superficialis and profundus flexor tendons

Flexor carpi ulnaris tendon

Ulnar artery with venae comitantes and ulnar nerve

MUSCLES OF THE HAND (Continued)

formed like a double-walled tube: the delicate inner wall is closely applied to the tendon, and the outer wall is the lining of the compartment in which the tendon lies. The layers are continuous with each other at the ends of the tube (as elsewhere); their facing surfaces are

smooth and separated by a small amount of synovial fluid.

In the hand, the flexor tendons have significant excursion, which causes friction between the tendons and the carpal ligament and in each finger against the fibro-osseous pulley system during gripping activities. Accordingly, the tendons to the thumb and fingers are protected and lubricated for optimal movement. Variations in the anatomy of the synovial

sheaths (bursae) exist and have an effect on the pattern of presentation of infections when they occur (see Plates 4.37 and 4.38). Similarly, several potential spaces exist in the palm and can become sites of infection. The thenar space exists just anterior to the adductor pollicis muscle. The midpalmar space exists posterior (deep) to the central compartment that contains the extrinsic flexor tendons and lumbrical muscles.

Plate 4.11

Upper Limb: PART I

ARTERIES AND NERVES OF HAND: PALMAR VIEWS

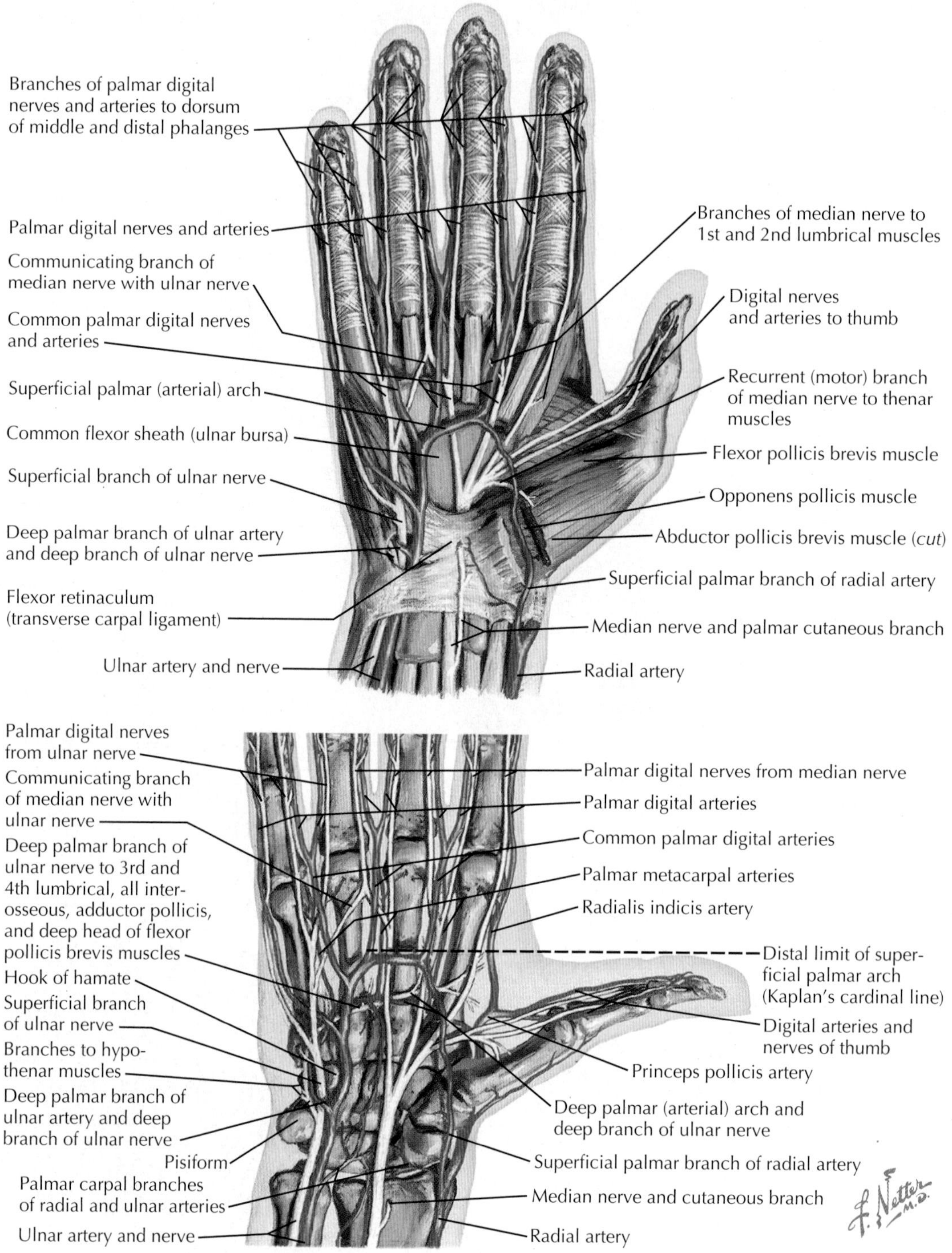

Branches of palmar digital nerves and arteries to dorsum of middle and distal phalanges

Palmar digital nerves and arteries

Communicating branch of median nerve with ulnar nerve

Common palmar digital nerves and arteries

Superficial palmar (arterial) arch

Common flexor sheath (ulnar bursa)

Superficial branch of ulnar nerve

Deep palmar branch of ulnar artery and deep branch of ulnar nerve

Flexor retinaculum (transverse carpal ligament)

Ulnar artery and nerve

Branches of median nerve to 1st and 2nd lumbrical muscles

Digital nerves and arteries to thumb

Recurrent (motor) branch of median nerve to thenar muscles

Flexor pollicis brevis muscle

Opponens pollicis muscle

Abductor pollicis brevis muscle (cut)

Superficial palmar branch of radial artery

Median nerve and palmar cutaneous branch

Radial artery

Palmar digital nerves from ulnar nerve

Communicating branch of median nerve with ulnar nerve

Deep palmar branch of ulnar nerve to 3rd and 4th lumbrical, all interosseous, adductor pollicis, and deep head of flexor pollicis brevis muscles

Hook of hamate

Superficial branch of ulnar nerve

Branches to hypothenar muscles

Deep palmar branch of ulnar artery and deep branch of ulnar nerve

Pisiform

Palmar carpal branches of radial and ulnar arteries

Ulnar artery and nerve

Palmar digital nerves from median nerve

Palmar digital arteries

Common palmar digital arteries

Palmar metacarpal arteries

Radialis indicis artery

Distal limit of superficial palmar arch (Kaplan's cardinal line)

Digital arteries and nerves of thumb

Princeps pollicis artery

Deep palmar (arterial) arch and deep branch of ulnar nerve

Superficial palmar branch of radial artery

Median nerve and cutaneous branch

Radial artery

VASCULAR SUPPLY OF THE HAND AND FINGER

The *ulnar artery,* with its accompanying nerve, enters the hand superficial to the flexor retinaculum and to the radial side of the pisiform (see Plates 4.10 and 4.11). It descends, curving radially, to about the midpalm and there anastomoses with the *superficial palmar branch of the radial artery.* This branch passes across or through the muscles of the thenar eminence, supplies this group of muscles, and emerges medial to the eminence to help form the superficial palmar arterial arch. The arch is convex distalward and crosses the palm at the level of the line of the completely abducted thumb.

The branches of the superficial arch supply the ulnar three and one-half digits; the radial one and one-half digits are supplied from the deep palmar arterial arch. The superficial arch gives origin to three *common palmar digital arteries,* which proceed distalward on the flexor tendons and lumbrical muscles and superficial to the digital nerves of the palm. They unite at the webs of the fingers with the palmar metacarpal arteries and with distal perforating branches of the dorsal metacarpal arteries. From the short trunks thus formed spring *proper palmar digital arteries.*

Two proper palmar digital arteries run distalward along the adjacent margins of the index to small fingers. A proper digital branch to the ulnar side of the small finger arises from the ulnar artery in the hypothenar compartment. At the webs of the fingers, the digital nerves cross the arteries to become superficial to them along the margins of the digits. Thus in each digit, the palmar and dorsal digital arteries lie within the span of the corresponding cutaneous nerves. The proper palmar digital arteries anastomose to form terminal plexuses in the fingers. They also give off branches that supply the last two dorsal segments of the digits.

At the wrist, the *radial artery* shifts from the expanded palmar surface of the radius, through the floor of the anatomic snuffbox, to reach the dorsum of the hand at the proximal end of the first dorsal interosseous space. As it passes under the tendon of the abductor pollicis longus muscle, it gives origin to its *dorsal carpal branch;* continuing distally over the first dorsal interosseous space, it gives origin to the *first dorsal metacarpal artery.* (The radial artery then turns deeply into the palm of the hand and participates in forming the deep palmar arterial arch.) The dorsal carpal branch of the radial artery passes ulnarward across the distal row of carpal bones and under the extensor tendons and joins the dorsal carpal branch of the ulnar artery. Thus is formed the *dorsal carpal arterial arch.*

Three *dorsal metacarpal arteries* descend from this arch on the dorsal interosseous muscles of the second, third, and fourth intermetacarpal intervals, respectively. Opposite the heads of the metacarpals, these vessels divide into *proper dorsal digital arteries,* which proceed distally along the dorsal borders of contiguous digits. These vessels are small and fail to reach the distal phalanges of the digits. Anastomoses are formed between the dorsal metacarpal arteries and the palmar arterial system in two locations: by perforating branches at the bases of the metacarpals and at the division into proper dorsal digital arteries.

The *deep palmar arterial arch* is formed by the junction of the terminal portion of the radial artery and the deep branch of the ulnar artery. The radial artery enters the palm at the base of the first intermetacarpal space by penetrating between the two heads of origin of the first dorsal interosseous muscle. Passing then between the transverse and oblique heads of the adductor pollicis muscle, it joins the deep branch of the ulnar artery.

The *princeps pollicis artery* arises from the radial artery as it emerges from the first dorsal interosseous muscle.

At the head of the first metacarpal, it provides two proper palmar digital branches for the thumb. The *radialis indicis artery* arises with the princeps pollicis to run along the radial side of the index finger. It is a proper digital artery to the radial side of the index finger.

From the convexity of the arch arise three *palmar metacarpal arteries.* These descend under the palmar interosseous fascia of the second to fourth intermetacarpal intervals. At the webs of the fingers, they join the common digital arteries from the superficial arch. *Recurrent carpal branches* are small. They ascend to and help form the palmar carpal network. *Perforating branches* anastomose with the dorsal metacarpal arteries on the dorsum of the hand.

Plate 4.12

Hand and Finger

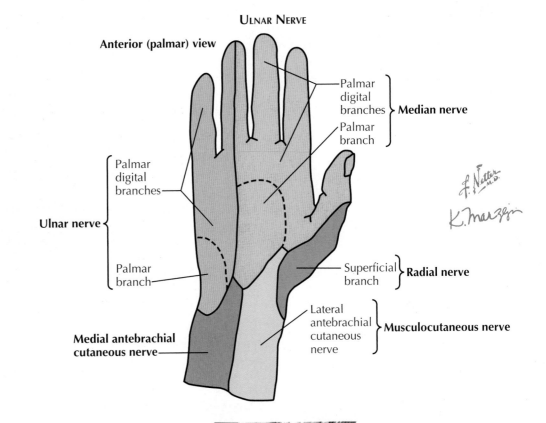

ULNAR NERVE

Anterior (palmar) view

Palmar
digital
branches **Median nerve**

Palmar
branch

Palmar
digital
branches

Ulnar nerve

Superficial **Radial nerve**
branch

Lateral
antebrachial
cutaneous **Musculocutaneous nerve**
nerve

Palmar
branch

**Medial antebrachial
cutaneous nerve**

INNERVATION OF THE HAND

Nerve branches from the ulnar, median, and radial nerves supply motor, sensory, and autonomic vasomotor function in the hand.

ULNAR NERVE

The ulnar nerve (C[7], C8; T1) is the main continuation of the medial cord of the brachial plexus. In the forearm and hand, the ulnar nerve gives off articular, muscular, palmar, dorsal, superficial and deep terminal, and vascular branches. It divides into branches for the areas of skin on the medial side of the back of the hand and fingers. The *ulnar nerve* enters the hand to the radial side of the pisiform between the palmar carpal ligament and the flexor retinaculum. Just distal to the pisiform, the ulnar nerve divides into superficial and deep branches.

The *superficial terminal branch* supplies the palmaris brevis muscle, innervates the skin on the medial side of the palm, and gives off two palmar digital nerves. The first is the *proper palmar digital nerve* for the medial side of the small finger; the second, the *common palmar digital nerve*, communicates with the adjoining common palmar digital branch of the median nerve before dividing into the two *proper palmar digital nerves* for the adjacent sides of the small and ring fingers. Rarely, the ulnar nerve supplies two and one-half rather than one and one-half digits, and the areas supplied by the median and radial nerves are reciprocally reduced.

The *deep terminal branch* of the ulnar nerve, with the deep branch of the ulnar artery, sinks between the origins of the abductor digiti minimi and the flexor digiti minimi brevis muscles and perforates the origin of the opponens digiti minimi muscle. It supplies these muscles and then curves around the hamulus of the hamate into the central part of the palm of the hand in conjunction with the deep palmar arterial arch. As it crosses the hand deep to the flexor tendons to the digits, the nerve gives twigs to the ulnar two lumbrical muscles and to all the interosseous muscles, both dorsal and palmar. It then supplies the adductor pollicis muscle and gives articular twigs to the wrist joint, and it *may* send a

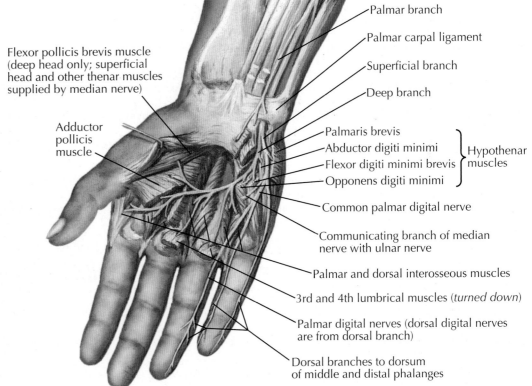

Palmar branch

Palmar carpal ligament

Superficial branch

Deep branch

Flexor pollicis brevis muscle
(deep head only; superficial
head and other thenar muscles
supplied by median nerve)

Palmaris brevis

Abductor digiti minimi

Flexor digiti minimi brevis

Opponens digiti minimi

Hypothenar
muscles

Adductor
pollicis
muscle

Common palmar digital nerve

Communicating branch of median
nerve with ulnar nerve

Palmar and dorsal interosseous muscles

3rd and 4th lumbrical muscles (*turned down*)

Palmar digital nerves (dorsal digital nerves
are from dorsal branch)

Dorsal branches to dorsum
of middle and distal phalanges

terminal branch into the deep head of the flexor pollicis brevis muscle.

Variations in the nerve supplies of the palmar muscles are as common as the variations in the cutaneous distribution; they are due to the variety of interconnections between the ulnar and median nerves.

The *dorsal branch of the ulnar nerve* completes the cutaneous supply of the dorsum of the hand and digits. It arises about 5 cm above the wrist, passes

dorsalward from beneath the flexor carpi ulnaris tendon, and then pierces the forearm fascia. At the ulnar border of the wrist, the nerve divides into three dorsal digital branches. There are usually two or three *dorsal digital nerves*, one supplying the medial side of the small finger, the second splitting into *proper dorsal digital nerves* to supply adjacent sides of the small and ring fingers, and the third (when present) supplying contiguous sides of the ring and long fingers.

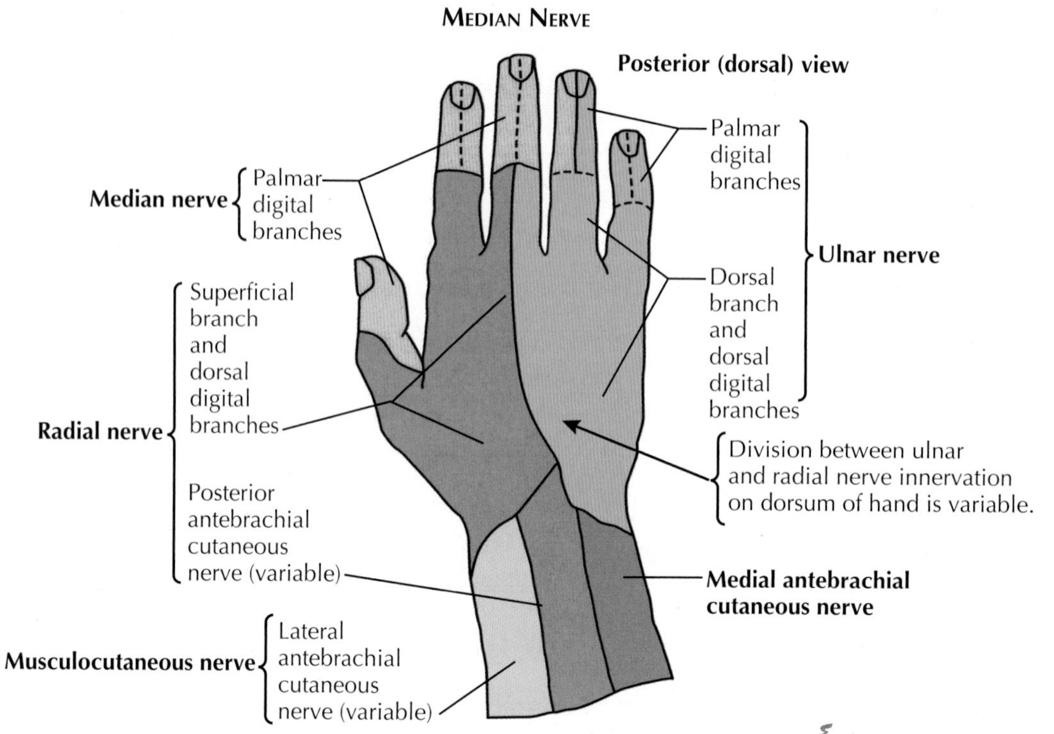

Plate 4.13

Upper Limb: PART I

MEDIAN NERVE

Posterior (dorsal) view

Palmar
digital
branches

Median nerve { Palmar
digital
branches

Ulnar nerve

Dorsal
branch
and
dorsal
digital
branches

Superficial
branch
and
dorsal
digital
branches

Radial nerve {

Division between ulnar
and radial nerve innervation
on dorsum of hand is variable.

Posterior
antebrachial
cutaneous
nerve (variable)

**Medial antebrachial
cutaneous nerve**

Musculocutaneous nerve { Lateral
antebrachial
cutaneous
nerve (variable)

Palmar cutaneous branch of median nerve

Abductor pollicis brevis

Opponens pollicis

Thenar
muscles

Superficial head
of flexor pollicis
brevis (deep head
supplied by
ulnar nerve)

Communicating branch
of median nerve with
ulnar nerve

1st and 2nd lumbrical muscles

Common palmar
digital nerves

Proper palmar digital nerves

Dorsal branches to dorsum of
middle and distal phalanges

INNERVATION OF THE HAND
(Continued)

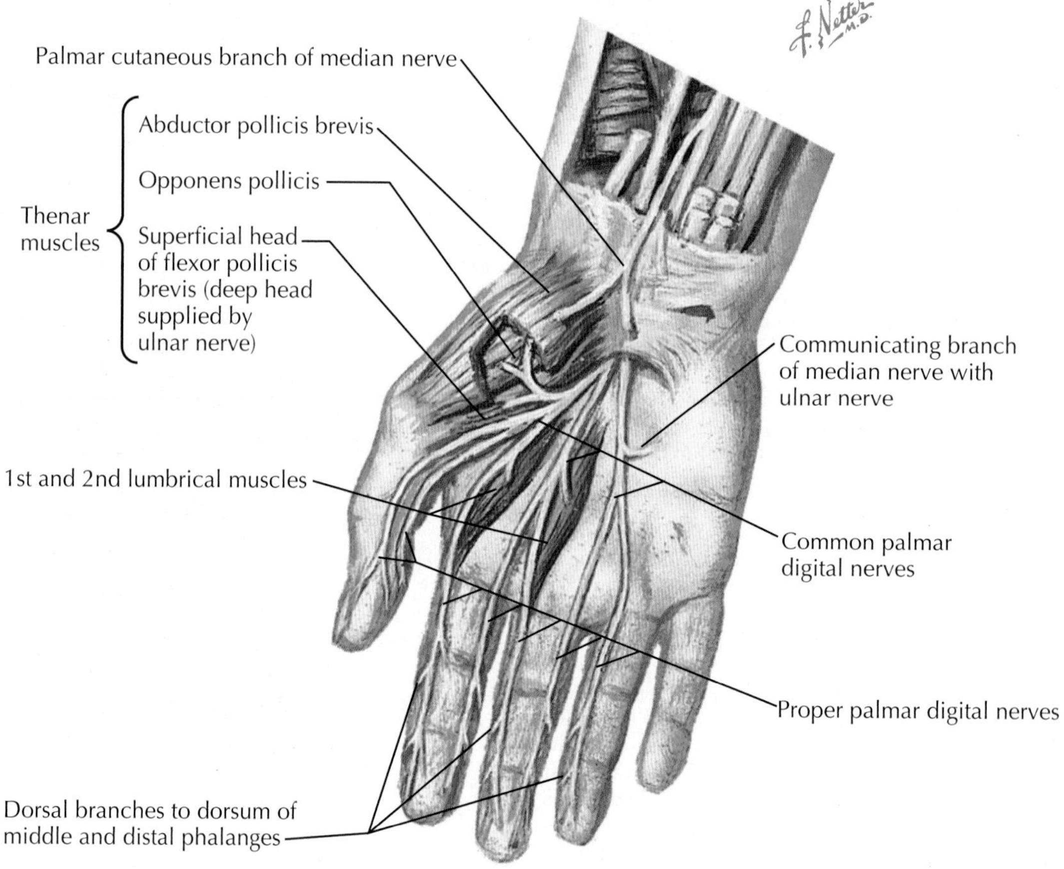

The first branch courses along the ulnar side of the dorsum of the hand and supplies the ulnar side of the small finger as far as the root of the nail. The second branch divides at the cleft between the ring and small fingers and supplies their adjacent sides. The third branch may divide similarly; it may supply the adjacent sides of the long finger and ring finger, or it may simply anastomose with the fourth dorsal digital branch of the superficial branch of the radial nerve. The dorsal branches to the ring finger usually extend only as far as the base of the second phalanx, with the more distal parts of the ring and small finger supplied by palmar digital branches of the ulnar nerve.

The *palmar branch of the ulnar nerve* arises about the middle of the forearm, descending under the antebrachial fascia in front of the ulnar artery. It perforates the fascia just above the wrist and supplies the skin of the hypothenar eminence and the medial part of the palm.

MEDIAN NERVE

The median nerve (C[5], C6, C7, C8; T1) is formed by the union of *medial* and *lateral roots* arising from the corresponding cords of the brachial plexus (see Plate 1.18).

The palmar branch of the median nerve arises just above the wrist. It perforates the palmar carpal ligament between the tendons of the palmaris longus and flexor carpi radialis muscles and distributes to the skin of the central depressed area of the palm and the medial part of the thenar eminence.

The *digital branches of the median nerve,* the proper palmar digital nerves, lie subcutaneously along the margins of each of the digits distal to the webs of the fingers. They arise from common palmar digital nerves, which lie under the dense palmar aponeurosis of the central palm. The first common palmar digital nerve gives rise to the muscular branch to the short muscles of the thumb and then divides into three *proper palmar digital nerves.* Just distal to the flexor retinaculum, its *motor,* or *recurrent, branch* curves sharply into the thenar

eminence and supplies the abductor pollicis brevis, flexor pollicis brevis (sometimes only its superficial head), and opponens pollicis muscles. This branch frequently arises from the median nerve together with its first common digital branch. The first common digital branch then runs to the radial and ulnar sides of the thumb, giving numerous branches to the pad and small, dorsally running branches to the nail bed of the thumb.

The third proper digital branch supplies the radial side of the index finger. The second common palmar digital branch provides two proper palmar digital nerves, which reach the adjacent sides of the index and long fingers. The third common palmar digital nerve communicates with a digital branch of the ulnar nerve in the palm and divides into two proper palmar digital nerves supplying adjacent sides of the long finger and ring fingers.

Plate 4.14

Hand and Finger

RADIAL NERVE

Lateral (radial) view

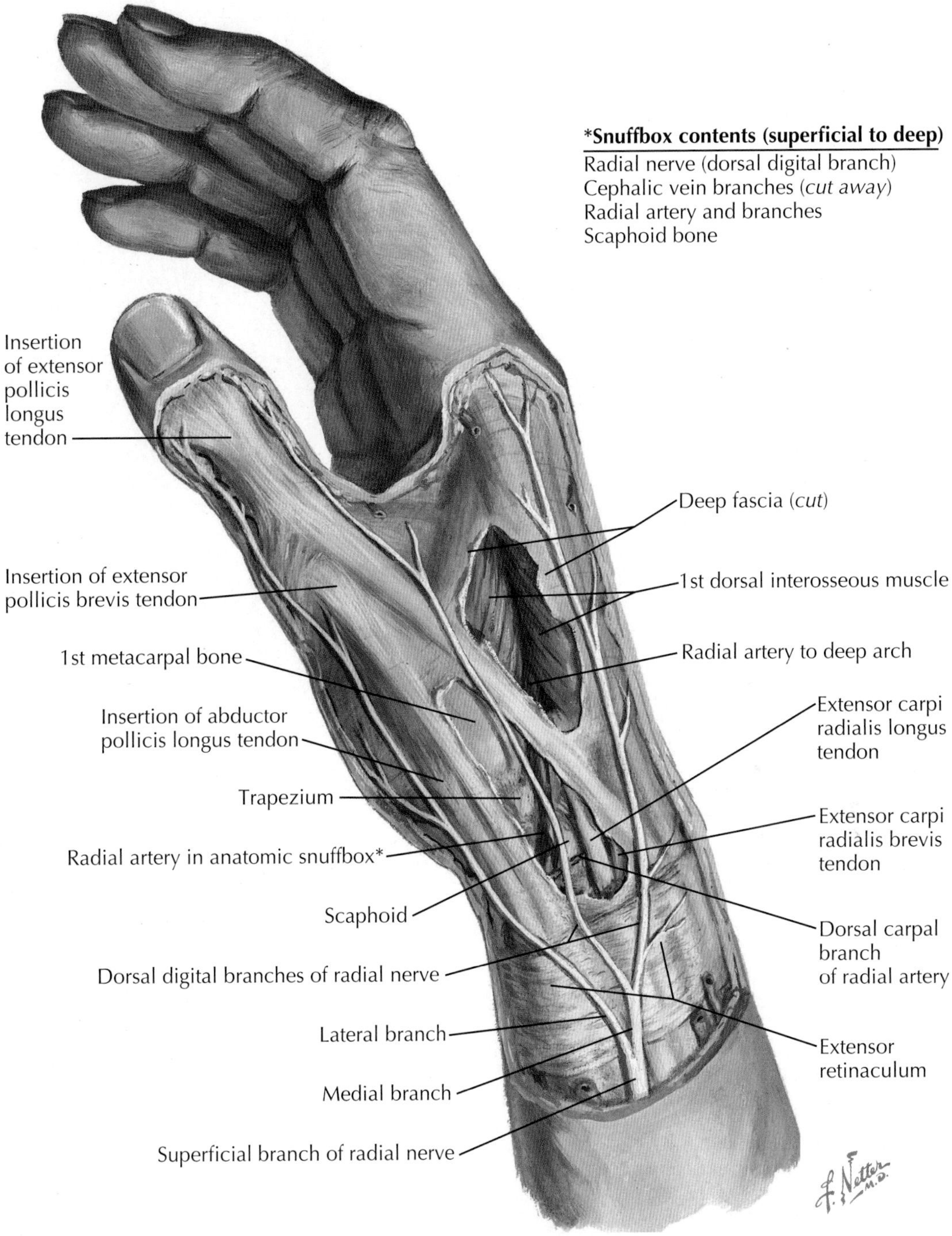

*Snuffbox contents (superficial to deep)
Radial nerve (dorsal digital branch)
Cephalic vein branches (*cut away*)
Radial artery and branches
Scaphoid bone

Insertion of extensor pollicis longus tendon

Insertion of extensor pollicis brevis tendon

1st metacarpal bone

Insertion of abductor pollicis longus tendon

Trapezium

Radial artery in anatomic snuffbox*

Scaphoid

Dorsal digital branches of radial nerve

Lateral branch

Medial branch

Superficial branch of radial nerve

Deep fascia (*cut*)

1st dorsal interosseous muscle

Radial artery to deep arch

Extensor carpi radialis longus tendon

Extensor carpi radialis brevis tendon

Dorsal carpal branch of radial artery

Extensor retinaculum

INNERVATION OF THE HAND (Continued)

Proper palmar digital nerves are large because of the density of nerve endings in the fingers. They lie superficial to the corresponding proper palmar digital arteries and veins. As each nerve passes toward its termination in the pad of the finger, it gives off branches for the innervation of the skin of the dorsum of the digits and the matrices of the fingernails. These dorsal branches innervate the dorsal skin of the distal segment of the index finger, the two terminal segments of the long finger, and the radial side of the ring finger. The *common* and *proper palmar digital nerves* vary in their origins and distributions, but the usual arrangement innervates the skin (including the nail beds) over the distal and dorsal aspects of the lateral three and one-half digits. Occasionally, they supply only two and one-half digits. The proper palmar digital branches to the radial side of the index finger and to the contiguous sides of the index and long fingers also carry motor fibers to supply the first and second lumbrical muscles, respectively. Therefore the digital nerves are not concerned solely with cutaneous sensibility. They contain an admixture of efferent and afferent somatic and autonomic fibers, which transmit impulses to and from sensory endings, vessels, sweat glands, and arrectores pilorum muscles and between fascial, tendinous, osseous, and articular structures in their areas of distribution.

RADIAL NERVE

Dorsally the superficial branch pierces the deep fascia and commonly subdivides into two branches, which usually split into four or five *dorsal digital nerves*. The cutaneous area of supply is shown in Plate 4.14. The smaller *lateral branch* supplies the skin of the radial side and eminence of the thumb and communicates with the lateral antebrachial cutaneous nerve. The larger *medial branch* divides into four dorsal digital nerves. The first dorsal digital nerve supplies the ulnar side of the thumb, the second supplies the radial side of the index finger, the third distributes to the adjoining sides of the index and long fingers, and the fourth supplies the adjacent sides of the long and ring fingers.

There is usually a connection on the back of the hand between the superficial branch of the radial nerve and the dorsal branch of the ulnar nerve, and there is some variability in the apparent source of the last (more median) branch of either nerve. In some such cases, the adjacent sides of the long and ring fingers are in the territory of the ulnar nerve. Dorsal digital nerves fail to reach the extremities of the digits. They reach to the base of the nail of the thumb, to the distal interphalangeal joint of the index finger, and not quite as far as the proximal interphalangeal joints of the long and ring fingers. The distal areas of the dorsum of the digits not supplied by the radial nerve receive branches from the stout palmar digital branches of the median nerve.

The dorsal digital nerves also supply filaments to the adjacent vessels, joints, and bones. (Note that the dorsal digital nerves extend only to the levels of the distal interphalangeal joints and that the first dorsal digital nerve gives off a twig that curves around the radial side of the thumb to supply the skin over the lateral part of the thenar eminence.)

Plate 4.15

Upper Limb: PART I

SKIN AND SUBCUTANEOUS FASCIA OF THE HAND: ANTERIOR (PALMAR) VIEWS

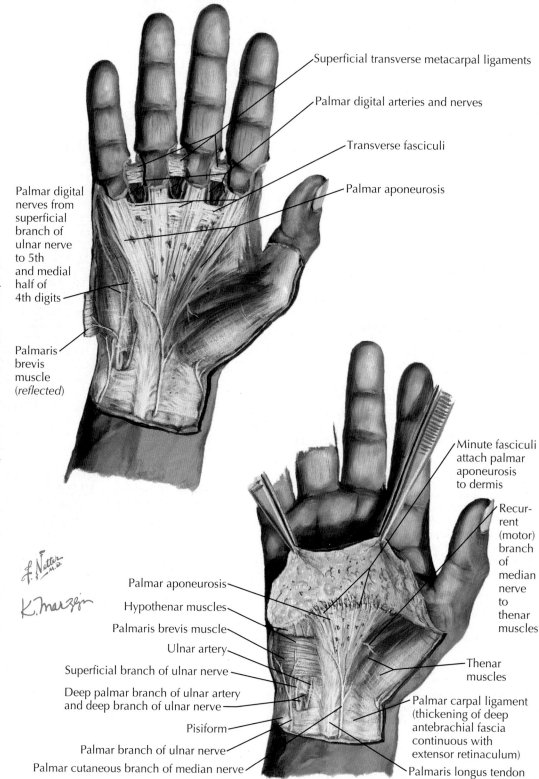

Superficial transverse metacarpal ligaments

Palmar digital arteries and nerves

Transverse fasciculi

Palmar aponeurosis

Palmar digital nerves from superficial branch of ulnar nerve to 5th and medial half of 4th digits

Palmaris brevis muscle (*reflected*)

Minute fasciculi attach palmar aponeurosis to dermis

Recurrent (motor) branch of median nerve to thenar muscles

Palmar aponeurosis

Hypothenar muscles

Palmaris brevis muscle

Ulnar artery

Superficial branch of ulnar nerve

Deep palmar branch of ulnar artery and deep branch of ulnar nerve

Pisiform

Palmar branch of ulnar nerve

Palmar cutaneous branch of median nerve

Thenar muscles

Palmar carpal ligament (thickening of deep antebrachial fascia continuous with extensor retinaculum)

Palmaris longus tendon

FASCIA AND SUPERFICIAL ANATOMY OF THE HAND

DEEP FASCIAE

The *fascia of the palm of the hand* is continuous with the antebrachial fascia of the flexor aspect of the forearm and with the palmar carpal ligament. At the borders of the hand, it is continuous with the fascia of the dorsum at attachments to the index and small finger metacarpals. The *hypothenar fascia* invests the muscles of the small finger and bounds the *hypothenar compartment* of the hand by means of a palmar attachment to the radial side of the small finger metacarpal. In a similar manner, the fascia over the thumb muscles dips deeply to attach to the palmar aspect of the first metacarpal and bounds, with the metacarpal, a *thenar compartment* in the hand. The *central compartment of the palm* is covered by the intervening part of the fascia of the palm, but this portion is reinforced superficially by the *palmar aponeurosis*, an expansion of the tendon of the palmaris longus muscle.

Recognizable in the palmar aponeurosis are a superficial stratum of longitudinally running fibers (which is continuous with the tendon of the palmaris longus muscle) and a deeper layer of transverse fibers. The transverse fibers are continuous with the thenar and hypothenar fasciae; proximally, they are continuous with the flexor retinaculum and the transverse carpal ligament. The palmar aponeurosis broadens distally in the palm and divides into four digital slips, with some of its fibers attaching to the overlying skin at the skin creases of the palm. The central parts of these slips pass into the digits, attaching superficially to the skin of the crease at the base of each digit; deeply, they attach to the fibrous sheath of the digit. The marginal fibers sink deeply between the heads of the metacarpals and attach to the metacarpophalangeal joint capsules, the deep transverse metacarpal ligaments, and the proximal phalanges of the digits. There is usually no digital slip for the thumb, but longitudinal fibers of the aponeurosis usually curve over onto the thenar fascia.

The deep attachments of the margins of the digital slips of the palmar aponeurosis define the entrance to the fibrous sheath of each digit, but they are also continued proximally into the palm for varying distances. They attach to the palmar interosseous fascia and to the shafts of the metacarpals, thus providing communicating subcompartments for each pair of flexor tendons and the associated lumbrical muscles. The septum reaching the third metacarpal is stronger and more constant; it separates a surgical *thenar space* under the aponeurosis to its radial side and a *midpalmar space* to its ulnar side.

Accumulations of the deeper transverse fibers of the aponeurosis appear between the diverging digital slips.

Located at the level of the heads of the metacarpals, these fibers are designated as the *superficial transverse metacarpal ligament*. Distally, the webs of the fingers are reinforced by another accumulation of transverse fibers designated as *transverse fasciculi*.

The *fascia of the dorsum of the hand* is continuous with the antebrachial fascia of the extensor surface of the forearm and with the extensor retinaculum. It encloses the tendons of the extensor muscles as they pass to the digits and continues into the extensor expansions on the dorsum of the digits; deep to it is a *subaponeurotic space*. This interfascial cleft separates the fascia of the dorsum from the deeper *dorsal interosseous fascia* covering the dorsal interosseous muscles and the descending branches of the dorsal carpal arterial arch (see Plate 4.16).

Plate 4.16

Hand and Finger

FASCIA AND SUPERFICIAL ANATOMY OF THE HAND (Continued)

LYMPHATIC DRAINAGE

The superficial lymphatic vessels of the upper limb begin in the hand and pervade the skin and subcutaneous tissues (see Plates 4.16 and 4.17). The dense digital lymphatic plexuses are drained by channels accompanying the digital arteries. At the interdigital clefts (and also more distally), collecting vessels of the palmar surfaces of the fingers pass to join dorsal collecting vessels and empty into the *plexus of the dorsum of the hand.*

Drainage of the thumb, index finger, and radial portion of the long finger is by collecting vessels that ascend along the radial side of the forearm; channels draining the ulnar fingers ascend along the ulnar side. Vessels from the *lymphatic plexus of the palm* radiate to the sides of the hand and also upward through the wrist, coalescing into two or three collecting vessels that ascend in the middle of the anterior surface of the forearm. The radial and ulnar channels turn onto the anterior surface of the forearm, lying parallel to the middle group, and all continue subcutaneously through the forearm and arm to reach the axillary nodes.

Some of the ulnar lymphatic channels are efferent to the *cubital lymph nodes.* This superficial group of one or two nodes is located 3 to 4 cm above the medial epicondyle of the humerus and below the aperture in the brachial fascia for the basilic vein. The afferent vessels of these nodes include channels originating in the ulnar three fingers and the ulnar portion of the forearm. The efferent vessels accompany the basilic vein under the brachial fascia and reach the lateral and central groups of axillary lymph nodes.

Several lymphatic channels collecting from the dorsal surface of the arm follow the upper course of the cephalic vein to the deltopectoral triangle, perforate the costocoracoid membrane with the vein, and terminate in an apical node of the axillary group. In about 10% of cases, this channel is interrupted in the deltopectoral triangle by one or two small *deltopectoral nodes.*

AXILLARY LYMPH NODES

The axillary lymph nodes, usually large and numerous, are arranged in five subgroups, some related to the axillary walls and others to vessels.

A *lateral group* of three to five nodes lies medial and posterior to the distal segment of the axillary vein. These nodes are in the direct line of lymph drainage from the upper limb, except for the drainage lymphatics along the cephalic vein. Efferent vessels from these nodes drain to the central and apical nodes.

A *pectoral group* is located along the lateral thoracic artery adjacent to the axillary border of the pectoralis

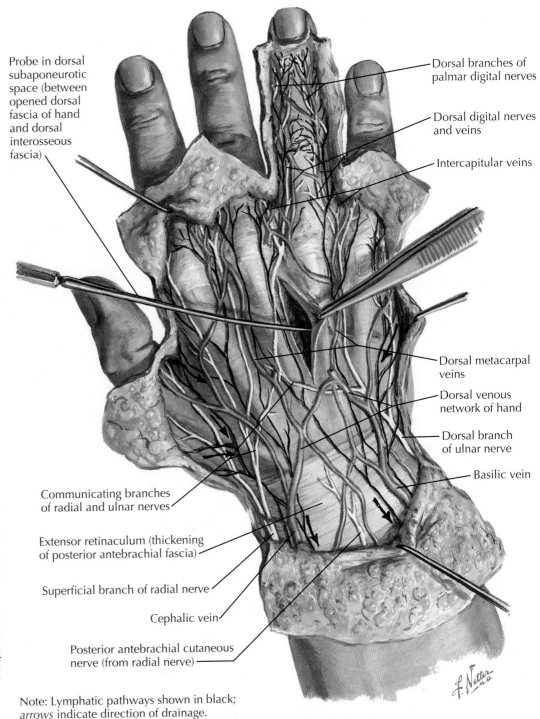

Probe in dorsal subaponeurotic space (between opened dorsal fascia of hand and dorsal interosseous fascia)

Dorsal branches of palmar digital nerves

Dorsal digital nerves and veins

Intercapitular veins

Dorsal metacarpal veins

Dorsal venous network of hand

Dorsal branch of ulnar nerve

Basilic vein

Communicating branches of radial and ulnar nerves

Extensor retinaculum (thickening of posterior antebrachial fascia)

Superficial branch of radial nerve

Cephalic vein

Posterior antebrachial cutaneous nerve (from radial nerve)

Note: Lymphatic pathways shown in black; *arrows* indicate direction of drainage.

minor muscle. These three to five nodes receive the lymphatic drainage of the anterolateral part of the thoracic wall, including most of the lateral drainage from the mammary gland, and of the skin and muscles of the supraumbilical part of the abdominal wall. Efferent lymphatic vessels reach the central and apical groups.

A *subscapular group* of five or six nodes is stretched along the subscapular blood vessels, from their origin in the axillary vessels to their contact with the chest wall. These nodes drain the skin and muscles of the posterior thoracic wall and shoulder region and also the lower part of the back of the neck. Their efferent lymph channels pass to the central axillary nodes.

A *central group* of four or five nodes lies under the axillary fascia, embedded in its fat. Among the largest of the axillary nodes, these nodes receive some lymphatic vessels directly from the arm and mammary regions but, primarily, they receive lymph from the

Plate 4.17

Upper Limb: PART I

FASCIA AND SUPERFICIAL ANATOMY OF THE HAND (Continued)

lateral, pectoral, and subscapular groups. Their efferent channels pass to the apical nodes.

The *apical group,* consisting of 6 to 12 nodes, lies along the axillary vein at the apex of the axilla and adjacent to the superior border of the pectoralis minor muscle. The apical nodes receive efferent vessels of all other axillary groups, lymphatic vessels that accompany the cephalic vein, and lymphatic vessels from the mammary gland. From lymph vessels interconnecting the apical nodes arises a larger common channel, the *subclavian lymphatic trunk.*

Deep Lymphatics

These vessels serve the upper limb, draining joint capsules, periosteum, tendons, nerves, and, to a lesser extent, muscles. Collecting vessels accompany the major arteries, along whose paths lie small intercalated lymph nodes. The deep lymphatics are afferent to the central and lateral axillary nodes.

SUPERFICIAL VEINS

The subcutaneous veins of the limb are interconnected with the deep veins of the limb via perforating veins. Certain prominent veins, unaccompanied by arteries, are found in the subcutaneous tissues of the limbs. The *cephalic* and *basilic veins,* the principal superficial veins of the upper limb, originate in venous radicals in the hand and digits.

Anastomosing longitudinal *palmar digital veins* empty at the webs of the fingers into longitudinally oriented dorsal digital veins. The *dorsal veins* of adjacent digits then unite to form relatively short *dorsal metacarpal veins,* which end in the *dorsal venous arch.* The radial continuation of the dorsal venous arch is the *cephalic vein,* which receives the dorsal veins of the thumb and then ascends at the radial border of the wrist. In the forearm, it tends to ascend at the anterior border of the brachioradialis muscle, with tributaries from the dorsum of the forearm. In the cubital space, the obliquely ascending *median cubital vein* connects the cephalic and basilic veins. Above the cubital fossa, the cephalic vein runs in the lateral bicipital groove and then in the interval between the deltoid and pectoralis major muscles, where it is accompanied by the small deltoid branch of the thoracoacromial artery. At the deltopectoral triangle, the cephalic vein perforates the costocoracoid membrane and empties into the *axillary vein.* An *accessory cephalic vein* passes from the dorsum of the forearm spirally and laterally to join the cephalic vein at the elbow.

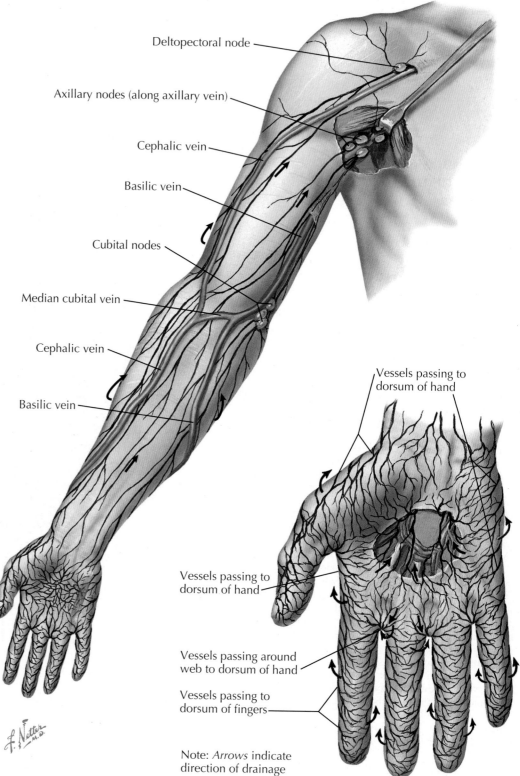

Deltopectoral node

Axillary nodes (along axillary vein)

Cephalic vein

Basilic vein

Cubital nodes

Median cubital vein

Cephalic vein

Basilic vein

Vessels passing to dorsum of hand

Vessels passing to dorsum of hand

Vessels passing around web to dorsum of hand

Vessels passing to dorsum of fingers

Note: *Arrows* indicate direction of drainage

The *basilic vein* continues the ulnar end of the venous arch of the dorsum of the hand. It ascends along the ulnar border of the forearm and enters the cubital fossa anterior to the medial epicondyle of the humerus. After receiving the median cubital vein, the basilic vein continues upward in the medial bicipital groove, pierces the brachial fascia a little below the middle of the arm, and enters the neurovascular compartment of the medial intermuscular septum, where it lies superficial to the brachial artery. In the distal axilla, it joins the brachial veins to form the *axillary vein.*

The *median antebrachial vein* is a frequent collecting vessel of the middle of the anterior surface of the forearm. It terminates in the cubital fossa in the median cubital vein or in the basilic vein. It sometimes divides into a *median basilic vein* and a *median cephalic vein,* which borders the biceps brachii laterally and joins the cephalic vein. The median antebrachial vein may be large or absent.

Plate 4.18

Hand and Finger

SECTIONAL ANATOMY: FINGERS

Sagittal section

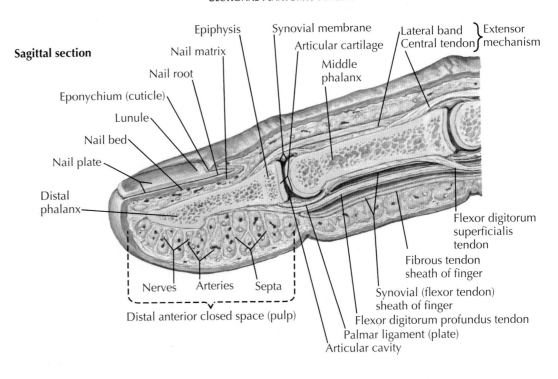

Epiphysis
Synovial membrane
Nail matrix
Articular cartilage
Lateral band
Central tendon } Extensor mechanism
Middle phalanx
Nail root
Eponychium (cuticle)
Lunule
Nail bed
Nail plate
Distal phalanx
Nerves   Arteries   Septa
Distal anterior closed space (pulp)
Flexor digitorum superficialis tendon
Fibrous tendon sheath of finger
Synovial (flexor tendon) sheath of finger
Flexor digitorum profundus tendon
Palmar ligament (plate)
Articular cavity

Cross section through distal phalanx

Subungual space
Minute arteries
Fine nerves
Nail plate
Nail bed
Distal phalanx
Fibrous septa and areolar tissue in anterior closed space (pulp)

Arteries and nerves

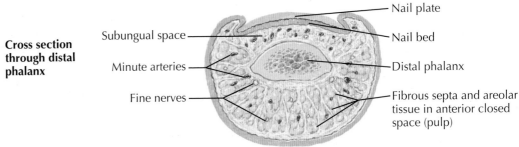

Dorsal branches of palmar digital arteries and nerves to dorsum of middle and terminal phalanges
Dorsal digital artery and nerve
Metacarpal head
Nutrient branch to epiphysis
Nutrient branches to metaphysis
Palmar digital artery and nerve
Palmar digital artery to neighboring digit

DIGITS

The specializations of the fingers frequently have clinical importance. The bones, joints, and tendon attachments of the fingers have already been described. It remains to add other specific items of interest or importance.

NAILS

The fingernail is an approximately rectangular horny plate, the *nail plate*, composed of closely welded, horny scales, or cornified epithelial cells. Its semitransparency allows the pink of the highly vascular *nail bed* to show through. The nail is partially surrounded by a fold of skin, the *nail wall*, and adheres to the subjacent nail bed where strong fibers pass to the periosteum of the distal phalanx, providing the firm attachment necessary for the prying and scratching functions of the nail. The nail is formed from the proximal part of the nail bed, where the epithelium is particularly thick and extends as far distally as the whitened lunula. Developing from this *nail matrix,* the nail moves out over the longitudinal dermal ridges of the nail bed at a growth rate of approximately 1 mm per week. Sensory nerve endings and blood vessels are abundant in the nail bed.

ANTERIOR CLOSED SPACE

To the palmar aspect of the distal phalanx lies the anterior closed space. Areolar tissue of mixed forms lies in this region. Fiber bundles surround fatty collections and support the finer arterial and nerve branching.

More discrete septa of connective tissue fibers pass from the periosteum of the distal phalanx to blend with the underside of the dermis. An especially abundant collection of fibers attaches to form the distal skin crease of the finger and thus serves to bound the anterior closed space of the finger pad. More proximally at the level of the proximal and distal interphalangeal joints the palmar skin is held fast by Cleland and Grayson ligaments during flexion and extension.

SMALL ARTERIES OF DIGITS

The general origin and distribution of the dorsal and palmar digital arteries have been fully discussed, and it has been emphasized that the palmar digital arteries are the major arteries because they send dorsal terminal branches over the distal and middle phalanges to supply the dorsum of the fingers and thumb. The dorsal digital arteries are poorly developed, except in the thumb. The proper palmar arteries are not necessarily

Plate 4.19

Upper Limb: PART I

SECTIONAL ANATOMY: THUMB

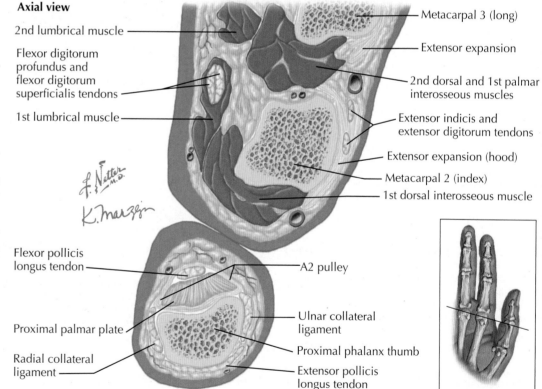

Sagittal view

- Distal phalanx
- Joint capsule
- Proximal phalanx
- Sesamoid
- Joint capsule
- Flexor pollicis longus tendon
- Metacarpal
- Extensor pollicis brevis tendon
- Thenar mass
- Flexor digitorum profundus and flexor digitorum superficialis tendons to index finger
- Trapezium

Axial view

- 2nd lumbrical muscle
- Flexor digitorum profundus and flexor digitorum superficialis tendons
- 1st lumbrical muscle
- Metacarpal 3 (long)
- Extensor expansion
- 2nd dorsal and 1st palmar interosseous muscles
- Extensor indicis and extensor digitorum tendons
- Extensor expansion (hood)
- Metacarpal 2 (index)
- 1st dorsal interosseous muscle
- Flexor pollicis longus tendon
- A2 pulley
- Proximal palmar plate
- Ulnar collateral ligament
- Radial collateral ligament
- Proximal phalanx thumb
- Extensor pollicis longus tendon

DIGITS (Continued)

of equal size on the two sides of the digit, although they are essentially so for the middle and ring fingers. However, in the thumb and the index and small fingers, the larger artery is on the median side of the digit; the more diminutive artery is on the opposite side.

These proper palmar digital arteries have cross-anastomoses or transverse interconnections. There is a pair of proximal transverse digital arteries that anastomoses at the level of the neck of the proximal phalanx; a pair of distal transverse digital arteries also anastomoses at the level of the neck of the middle phalanx. These arteries run close to the bone and deep to the flexor tendons. There is a rich terminal anastomosis of the palmar digital arteries, which forms a profuse tuft of small vessels in each finger pad. The proximal edge of this tuft of vessels lies on the palmar surface of the distal phalanx at about its epiphyseal line.

DIGITAL NERVES

The cutaneous nerves parallel the arteries in course and distribution. In their course along the fingers, the proper digital nerves are outside the arteries; that is, as the digit is viewed from the side, the arteries are within the span of the dorsal and palmar nerves. Cutaneous nerves are of two types. Included are afferent somatic fibers mediating general sensation (pain, touch, pressure, and temperature) and efferent autonomic fibers supplying the smooth muscles, sweat glands, and sebaceous glands.

Both free and encapsulated nerve endings are involved in various sensations. Of the encapsulated endings, the Meissner tactile corpuscles are richly represented in the dermal papillae, and pacinian corpuscles lie in the subcutaneous connective tissue, especially along the sides of the digits, and they are quickly adapting receptors responsible for moving touch (tested by moving two-point discrimination). The slowly adapting receptors (Merkel cell neurite complexes and Ruffini end organs) respond to static touch (measured by static two-point discrimination or with Semmes-Weinstein monofilament testing). The relatively large size of the proper palmar digital nerves suggests the high density of nerve endings in the fingers, especially in the finger pads. The tactile corpuscles are most numerous in the fingertips, less so on the palm, and rare on the dorsum of the fingers or hand.

Plate 4.20

Hand and Finger

HAND INVOLVEMENT IN OSTEOARTHRITIS

Early Heberden nodes with inflammatory changes

Chronic Heberden nodes with 4th and 5th proximal interphalangeal joints also involved in degenerative process

ARTHRITIS IN THE HAND

The term *rheumatic disease* refers to any illness characterized by pain and stiffness in or around the joints. These diseases are divided into two main groups: disorders that involve the joints primarily (the different forms of arthritis) and disorders that, although not directly affecting the joints, involve connective tissue structures around the joints (the periarticular disorders, or nonarticular rheumatism). The many types of arthritis and nonarticular disorders differ from one another in etiology, pathogenesis, pathology, and clinical features.

Rheumatoid arthritis and osteoarthritis (also called degenerative joint disease) are the most common forms of arthritis. Both of these chronic conditions are characterized by pain, stiffness, restricted joint motion, joint deformities, and disability, but their differences in pathogenesis, pathology, and clinical features must be distinguished because the prognosis and treatment of the two diseases differ. Other inflammatory arthritides that are of concern in the hand, especially gout, lupus, and psoriatic arthritis, are frequently seen.

Posttraumatic and postinfectious arthritis and treatment are typically specific to the joint affected by the insult, and the principles of treatment are often similar to those for the more common types of arthritis.

OSTEOARTHRITIS

Some clinical manifestations are unique to particular joints. Heberden nodes, hallmarks of osteoarthritis, develop only at the terminal joints of the fingers. As the cartilage of the distal interphalangeal joint is degenerating, osteophytes grow from the dorsomedial and lateral aspects of the base of the distal phalanx to produce these nodular protuberances. Flexion or lateral deviation deformity usually results when the pathologic changes are severe. Early in their development, the nodes are tender and painful, especially when ganglion (mucoid) cysts

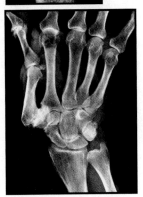

Radiograph of distal interphalangeal joint reveals late-stage degenerative changes. Cartilage destruction and marginal osteophytes (Heberden nodes).

Late-stage degenerative changes in carpometacarpal articulation of thumb

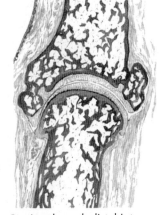

Section through distal interphalangeal joint shows irregular, hyperplastic bony nodules (Heberden nodes) at articular margins of distal phalanx. Cartilage is eroded and joint space narrowed.

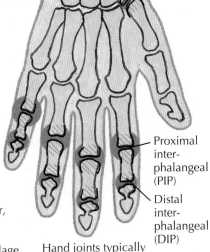

1st carpometacarpal (CMC)

Proximal interphalangeal (PIP)

Distal interphalangeal (DIP)

Hand joints typically involved in osteoarthritis

coexist; when mature, they are asymptomatic and have only cosmetic significance. Heberden nodes are more common in women and are often familial. Bouchard nodes, similar to but less common than Heberden nodes, develop at the proximal interphalangeal finger joints.

At the base of the thumb, the carpometacarpal articulation is the most common joint to undergo the degenerative changes of osteoarthritis. This joint is affected much more often in women and in the nondominant hand. Local tenderness and pain, usually severe, are exacerbated by firm grasping and pinching, and progressive stiffness ensues.

RHEUMATOID ARTHRITIS

Early and Moderate Hand Involvement

The joints of the hands and wrists are among the most frequent sites of involvement. In the fingers, some or all

Plate 4.21

Upper Limb: PART I

HAND INVOLVEMENT IN RHEUMATOID ARTHRITIS AND PSORIATIC ARTHRITIS

Rheumatoid arthritis

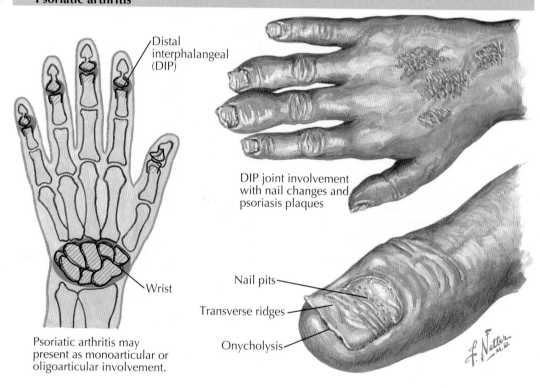

Deformed hand with marked ulnar deviation of fingers and subluxation of metacarpophalangeal joints. Deformities are secondary to rheumatoid arthritis.

Psoriatic arthritis

Distal interphalangeal (DIP)

Wrist

Psoriatic arthritis may present as monoarticular or oligoarticular involvement.

DIP joint involvement with nail changes and psoriasis plaques

Nail pits

Transverse ridges

Onycholysis

ARTHRITIS IN THE HAND (Continued)

of the proximal interphalangeal joints are often bilaterally affected, whereas the distal interphalangeal joints are seldom involved. Because the inflammatory swelling occurs only at the middle joints, the affected fingers become fusiform in the early stages of disease. The metacarpophalangeal and wrist joints may also become inflamed. At first, there is little restriction of motion in the involved joints, but stiffness, swelling, and pain prevent the patient from making a tight fist, thus weakening grip strength. Except for soft tissue swelling, radiographs reveal no abnormalities.

Advanced Hand Involvement

As the disease progresses and the inflammation invades the joints, destroying articular cartilage and bone, joint motion becomes severely limited and joint deformities develop. Flexion deformities frequently occur at the proximal interphalangeal and metacarpophalangeal joints. The patient cannot fully extend or flex the fingers, and the grip becomes progressively weaker. Radiographs reveal cartilage thinning, bone erosions at the joint margins, and metaphyseal osteoporosis. After years of chronic inflammation, joint damage becomes severe; the joint capsule stretches, muscles atrophy and weaken, and tendons stretch, fray, and even rupture. All of these changes result in severe, incapacitating deformities.

A number of hand deformities are seen in the late stages of rheumatoid arthritis. For example, the muscles on the ulnar side of the fingers and wrist may overpower those of the radial group, causing ulnar deviation of the fingers at the metacarpophalangeal joints; the wrists may also be affected. The swan neck deformity of the finger is common, as is the boutonnière deformity of the thumb, which is caused by hyperextension of the proximal interphalangeal joint and flexion at the metacarpophalangeal joint. The long extensor tendon may rupture near the distal interphalangeal joint,

leaving the distal phalanx permanently flexed. Prolonged disease may lead to permanent subluxation or dislocation of the finger joints, and severe cartilage and bone erosion at the wrist may literally destroy the carpus. In this late stage of the disease, radiographs help define the severity of the structural damage and deformities.

PSORIATIC ARTHRITIS

About 10% of persons with psoriasis have some form of inflammatory joint disease. Onset of the skin disease may long precede the arthropathy, but occasionally the reverse is true. The distinguishing features of psoriatic arthritis are (1) a predilection for the distal joints of the fingers and toes, frequently accompanied by psoriatic

Plate 4.22

Hand and Finger

HAND INVOLVEMENT IN GOUTY ARTHRITIS AND REITER SYNDROME

Gouty arthritis

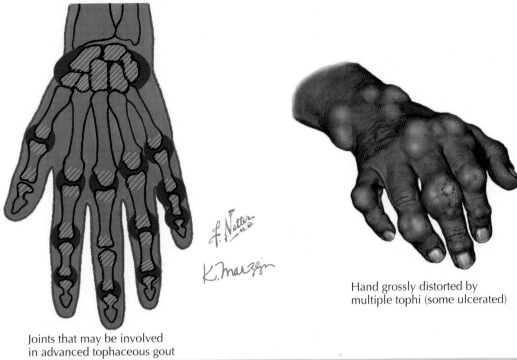

Joints that may be involved
in advanced tophaceous gout

Hand grossly distorted by
multiple tophi (some ulcerated)

Reiter syndrome

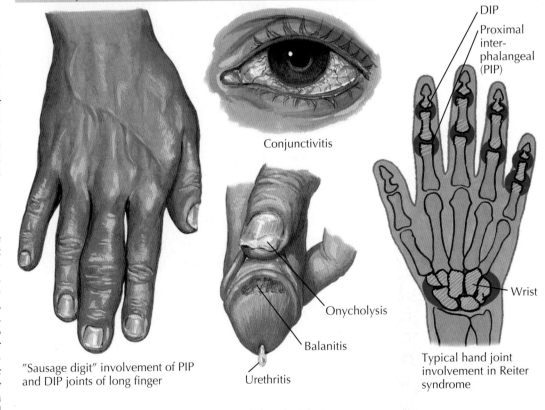

Conjunctivitis

"Sausage digit" involvement of PIP
and DIP joints of long finger

Onycholysis

Balanitis

Urethritis

DIP

Proximal
inter-
phalangeal
(PIP)

Wrist

Typical hand joint
involvement in Reiter
syndrome

ARTHRITIS IN THE HAND
(Continued)

involvement of only a few other joints of the limbs; (2) destructive and mutilating changes of the phalanges adjacent to the inflamed joints, which produce the radiographic appearance of a "whittling" or "pencil point in cup" of the proximal phalanx and a "cupping" of the central portion of the base of the apposing distal phalanx, with bony proliferation of the borders; (3) shortening, angulation, and telescoping of the fingers due to extensive bone resorption in the phalanges; and (4) frequent involvement of the sacroiliac joints and spine, which simulates ankylosing spondylitis.

GOUT AND GOUTY ARTHRITIS

Almost always, the first clinical evidence of gout is acute arthritis in one or a few peripheral joints. A fulminant synovitis begins abruptly, typically during the night, frequently involving the first metatarsophalangeal joint. After several years of recurrent acute arthritis and persistent hyperuricemia, deposits of monosodium urate, called *tophi,* form in joint structures (and other tissues). Tophi are the hallmark of chronic gout, occurring in 50% of patients. They cause structural damage to articular cartilage and adjacent bone, resulting in chronic arthritis. In this late stage of the disease, known as *chronic tophaceous gout,* the affected joints show irregular knobby swelling and signs of chronic inflammation. Joint motion is limited; painful, deformities develop; and sinuses tend to form at the swollen joint, from which a calcific exudate drains from the underlying urate deposits.

Radiographs show marked destruction of bone and cartilage and "punched-out" areas in the bone caused by the urate deposits.

Tophi often form in extraarticular structures as well, especially in the extensor tendons of the fingers and toes, the olecranon and infrapatellar bursae, the calcaneal tendon, the cartilage of the external ear, and the parenchyma of the kidney.

REITER SYNDROME

Reiter syndrome has been considered a clinical triad of urethritis, conjunctivitis, and arthritis. It is now accepted that a specific type of dermatitis is another characteristic of the disease, and diagnosis of complete Reiter syndrome requires the presence of at least three

of these four signs: rarefaction of bone near the inflamed joints visible on radiographs (in chronic disease, articular cartilage destruction and joint deformities are also apparent), sacroiliac involvement (sometimes unilateral), vertebral syndesmophytes in skip distribution, and periosteal new bone formation at the insertion of the calcaneal tendon and calcaneal spurs.

Plate 4.23

Upper Limb: PART I

METACARPOPHALANGEAL DEFORMITIES OF THUMB

Boutonnière deformity

Swan neck deformity

Abductor pollicis longus tendon

Extensor pollicis brevis tendon

Extensor pollicis longus tendon

Hyperextension of carpometacarpal joint with abduction of metacarpal and fixed flexion of metacarpophalangeal joint. Interphalangeal joint usually extended.

Abductor pollicis longus tendon

Extensor pollicis brevis tendon

Extensor and flexor pollicis longus tendons

Adductor pollicis muscle

Adduction of metacarpal with subluxation of base on the trapezium. Metacarpophalangeal joint hyperextended and interphalangeal joint flexed.

DEFORMITIES OF THUMB JOINTS

The thumb is the most important digit of the hand. All three joints of the thumb are important in functional adaptations, and each may be affected primarily or secondarily by imbalances of the other joints (e.g., boutonnière and swan neck deformities). Thus reconstructive surgery of the thumb must consider the entire thumb (radial) ray; the balance of its musculotendinous system; and the position, mobility, and stability of all its joints. The joints of the thumb may be impaired as a result of osteoarthritis, rheumatoid arthritis, or posttraumatic arthritis. Thumb deformities can be classified as (1) postural, including longitudinal collapse (boutonnière, swan neck) and fixed positional (adducted retroposed thumb) deformities; (2) unstable, stiff, or painful interphalangeal, metacarpophalangeal, or carpometacarpal joints; and (3) tendon deformities, including contracture, displacement, or rupture of the flexor pollicis longus, extensor pollicis longus or brevis, abductor pollicis longus, or intrinsic tendons.

POSTURAL DEFORMITIES

The *boutonnière deformity* is caused primarily by arthritic involvement of the metacarpophalangeal joint. Although it is found in 57% of patients with hands affected by rheumatoid arthritis, boutonnière deformity does not usually occur in osteoarthritis. Initially, the capsule and extensor apparatus around the metacarpophalangeal joint are stretched by synovitis. The extensor pollicis longus tendon and adductor expansions are displaced ulnarly, and the lateral thenar expansions are displaced radially. The extensor pollicis brevis tendon attachment to the base of the proximal phalanx is lengthened, and the ability to extend the metacarpophalangeal joint is decreased, causing a flexion deformity of the proximal phalanx. The extensor pollicis longus tendon and extensor insertions of the intrinsic muscles apply all their power to the distal phalanx and produce secondary hyperextension of the interphalangeal joint. Pinch movements further aggravate the deformity. As contractures develop, the deformity becomes fixed. Destructive articular changes compound the deformity, and disorganization and subluxation of the joint may occur.

Swan neck deformity, in contrast, is far more common in osteoarthritis than in rheumatoid arthritis. It is usually initiated by destructive changes at the carpometacarpal joint, followed by stretching of the joint capsule and radial subluxation of the base of the metacarpal. As motion at the trapeziometacarpal joint during abduction becomes painful, the patient avoids abduction, using the distal joints to compensate for lack of motion at the base of the thumb. An increasing adduction

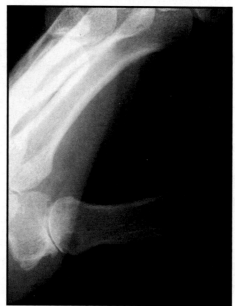

Anteroposterior (AP) radiograph of thumb of 56-year-old male with activity-related pain at base of thumb. Radiograph shows early stages of disease with narrowing of thumb carpometacarpal joint and no mild subluxation.

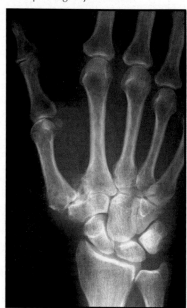

AP radiograph of hand of 73-year-old female with severe pain at base of thumb. Exam showed swelling and tenderness to palpation at the base of the thumb. Radiograph shows subluxation and degenerative changes at the thumb carpometacarpal joint with a large osteophyte between the first and second metacarpal. The joint space between the trapezioscaphoid was preserved.

deformity with contracture of the adductor pollicis muscle develops. Effusion in the joint further loosens the capsule, permitting a proximal radial subluxation of the metacarpal. Subluxation may result in hyperextension of the interphalangeal joint, but more frequently it causes hyperextension of the metacarpophalangeal joint and adduction of the first metacarpal. Further adduction contracture of the metacarpal aggravates the hyperextension of the metacarpophalangeal joint and permits

collapse of the thumb ray. The interphalangeal joint becomes flexed, as in a swan neck deformity of the finger.

In the *adducted retroposed thumb,* the first metacarpal is retropositioned, adducted, and externally rotated. The deformity is probably initiated by synovitis of the carpometacarpal joint and aggravated by awkward positioning of the thumb, as on a flat surface during acute illness. There seems to be a contracture of the extensor

Plate 4.24

Hand and Finger

THUMB CARPOMETACARPAL OSTEOARTHRITIS

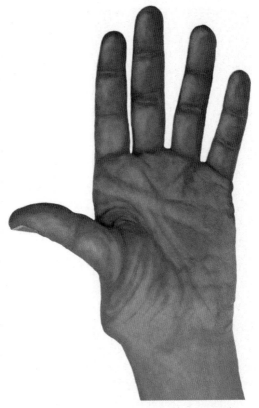

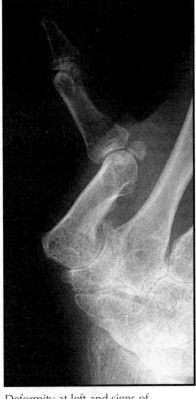

DEFORMITIES OF THUMB JOINTS (Continued)

pollicis longus muscle, with adduction and external rotation of the metacarpal and with palmar and radial subluxation of the metacarpal base off the trapezium.

TENDON DEFORMITIES

In rheumatoid arthritis, tendon deformities are related to muscle contracture, tendon displacement, adhesions, or tendon rupture. Rupture of the extensor pollicis longus tendon is most common, usually occurring within the third extensor compartment in the area of the distal tubercle of the radius. Sudden rupture of the tendon results in a sudden drop of the metacarpophalangeal joint of the thumb and, in some cases, loss of extensor power at the distal phalanx.

Rupture of the flexor pollicis longus tendon usually occurs in the carpal area and must be considered in the diagnosis of hyperextension deformity of the interphalangeal joint of the thumb. Rupture of the abductor pollicis longus and extensor pollicis brevis tendons is rare.

Synovial invasion and stretching of the dorsal hood of the metacarpophalangeal joint may result in displacement and secondary contractures of the tendons of the intrinsic muscles.

SURGERY FOR INTERPHALANGEAL JOINT

Arthrodesis is usually the preferred treatment for instability of the interphalangeal joint of the thumb; bone grafting is necessary if bone resorption is severe.

SURGERY FOR METACARPOPHALANGEAL JOINT

Arthrodesis is indicated in joint destruction and collapse deformities to simplify the articular system of the thumb ray, providing the distal and basal joints have adequate mobility. This can be achieved by a traditional tension band wire technique or more modern intramedullary locked-screw technology that provides a reproducible 25 degrees of flexion and more rapid return to function.

Capsulodesis is the treatment of choice in hyperextension deformities of more than 20 degrees with good flexion, lateral stability, and intact articular surfaces. The palmar aspect of the joint is exposed through a straight volar incision, and the central third of the proximal membranous insertion of the palmar plate is incised (alternatively, all is incised if using a bone anchor). The sesamoids and their tendon attachments are left intact. The periosteum is stripped from the palmar aspect of the metacarpal neck and the joint is pinned at 30 degrees of flexion with a Kirschner wire, which is

Osteoarthritis causes stiff, adduction deformity at the CMC joint resulting in secondary hyperextension of the MP joint and stretching out of the volar plate.

Deformity at left and signs of advanced degenerative change in the CMC and MP joints with joint space narrowing and subchondral sclerosis

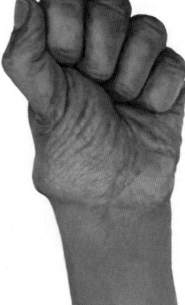

Despite deformity, most patients have adequate function unless their osteoarthritis is painful.

removed 6 weeks after surgery. The central third of the plate is sutured to the radial and ulnar thirds (or the whole plate is sewn to a bone anchor placed in the metacarpal neck).

SURGERY FOR BASAL JOINTS

The problems presented at the basal joints of the thumb differ in osteoarthritis and rheumatoid arthritis. Accurate

diagnosis and evaluation of the location of the arthritic involvement and alignment of adjacent bones are essential in selecting the appropriate treatment. The pathologic changes may involve the trapeziometacarpal joint alone or also affect the peritrapezial or other carpal bone articulations, with or without resorption or displacement of adjacent carpal bones.

Basilar joint surgery is indicated when there is (1) localized pain and crepitation during passive

Plate 4.25

Upper Limb: PART I

LIGAMENT REPLACEMENT AND TENDON INTERPOSITION ARTHROPLASTY FOR CARPOMETACARPAL JOINT ARTHRITIS

DEFORMITIES OF THUMB JOINTS (Continued)

circumduction, with axial compression of the thumb (grind test); (2) loss of motion, with decreased pinch and grip strength; (3) radiographic evidence of arthritic changes of the trapeziometacarpal, trapeziotrapezoid, trapezioscaphoid, and trapezium–second metacarpal joints; and (4) unstable, stiff, or painful distal joints of the thumb or a swan neck deformity. Treatment must be selected from several options, most frequently trapezial resection and, less commonly, trapezial metacarpal arthrodesis. Many variations of suspension and interposition have been used in conjunction with trapezial resection, but no clear indication or superiority of one technique exists.

Surgically, the trapezium is sectioned with an osteotome and removed piecemeal, with care not to injure the underlying flexor carpi radialis tendon. The radial artery must be carefully protected throughout the procedure. Then a tendon (typically the flexor carpi radialis longus either whole or half thickness) is passed through the base of the metacarpal and then sewn back onto itself snugly to re-create the volar beak ligament. The remaining tendon is sewn into a bundle and anchored to the floor trapezial space, thus creating an interposition arthroplasty. The dorsal capsular flaps are closed and secured to the proximal origin at the scaphoid, reducing the metacarpal and restoring natural thumb abduction. The first dorsal compartment is loosely closed over the abductor pollicis longus and extensor pollicis brevis tendons. The extensor pollicis longus tendon is left subcutaneous. The incision is closed, with care to avoid the branches of the superficial radial nerve. A conforming hand dressing, including a thumb spica plaster splint, is applied. The limb is kept elevated, and a thumb spica short-arm cast or thermoplastic splint is applied after 4 to 6 days and worn for 4 to 6 weeks. Guarded motion and pinch and grasp activities using various exercise devices are then started.

Basilar joint arthroplasty avoids tendon harvesting and uses a simple heavy suture suspension between the flexor carpi radialis and the abductor pollicis longus that creates a supportive sling for the metacarpal. Subsequently, capsular contraction and scar interposition occur, which provide pain-free pinch and grip strength activities. Prosthetic implant arthroplasty has also been used with varying success for osteoarthritis but is not used for inflammatory arthritis.

Of special consideration in reconstruction of the basal joint of the thumb is the presence of hyperextension of the metacarpophalangeal joint, which contributes

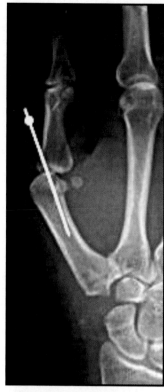

Postoperative demonstration of trapeziectomy and suspension; interposition arthroplasty of CMC joint with correction of MP joint hyperextension to flexion at 30 degrees, which is pinned to allow volar plate capsulodesis to heal.

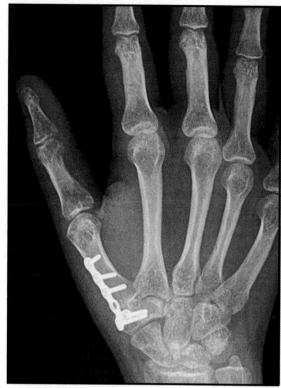

Arthrodesis of the CMC joint with a plate/screw construct in slight hyperextension creates corrective flexion at the MP joint.

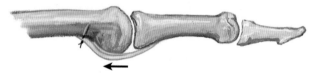

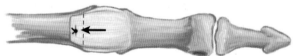

Plication of the stretched volar plate can be done by advancing a central portion and suturing it to the remaining intact portions or by placing a suture anchor in the bone and securing it.

The diseased joint is removed and replaced with a tendon graft taken from the patient's wrist or arm. The patient will have less pain and be able to use the thumb again.

to the metacarpal adduction and swan neck deformity. If hyperextension is less than 10 degrees, a cast is applied postoperatively so that the metacarpal, but not the proximal phalanx, is abducted and the carpometacarpal joint is abducted. If the hyperextension ranges from 10 to 20 degrees, temporary fixation with a Kirschner wire is indicated; if it is between 20 and 45 degrees, stabilization with either palmar capsulodesis or arthrodesis is essential. If the angle is more than 45 degrees, the metacarpophalangeal joint should be arthrodesed, and origin of the adductor pollicis muscle possibly released.

Plate 4.26

Hand and Finger

IMPLANT RESECTION ARTHROPLASTY FOR METACARPOPHALANGEAL JOINTS

DEFORMITIES OF THE METACARPOPHALANGEAL JOINTS

ARTHRITIS OF THE METACARPOPHALANGEAL JOINTS

Arthritic diseases may affect any joint, but their effect on the hands can be especially devastating. The disease process attacks the joints, ligaments, and tendons, causing painful and disabling deformities. Fortunately, developments in joint reconstruction and replacement have made it possible to restore hands deformed by crippling arthritis to a nearly normal appearance and useful function.

Ideally, arthroplasty should produce a joint that is pain free, mobile, stable, durable, and cosmetically pleasing. Four methods of reconstruction for arthritic joints of the hand have emerged: arthrodesis, resection interposition arthroplasty, resurfacing joint replacement, and flexible implant resection arthroplasty.

Arthrodesis works very well for the thumb at the metacarpophalangeal joint level and for the lesser fingers at the proximal and distal interphalangeal joint level, but lack of motion is debilitating in the lesser fingers at the metacarpophalangeal joint level and rarely used.

Resection interposition arthroplasty can improve motion by shortening skeletal structures, lengthening soft parts, providing new gliding surfaces, and allowing the development of a new supportive fibrous joint capsule. The chief disadvantage of the procedure in the metacarpophalangeal joints is the unpredictability of results.

Resurfacing joint replacement has proved successful in knee and hip joints, but early results in finger joints have been mixed because of dislocation, bone resorption, and implant loosening. Newer designs are proving useful in patients with osteoarthritis and early rheumatoid arthritis where the soft tissue balance is still relatively normal.

In *flexible implant resection arthroplasty*, a flexible silicone implant is used as an adjunct to resection arthroplasty. This method was devised in 1962 and has been used successfully in several hundred thousand patients. This discussion emphasizes the techniques of implant resection arthroplasty.

The basic concept of flexible implant resection arthroplasty can be summarized as bone resection + implant + encapsulation = functional joint. The flexible implant acts as a dynamic spacer, maintaining internal alignment and spacing of the reconstructed joint and supporting the capsuloligamentous system that develops around it. The joint is thus rebuilt through a healing phenomenon called the *encapsulation process*.

Because the capsuloligamentous system around a new joint is adaptable, a functional balance of mobility

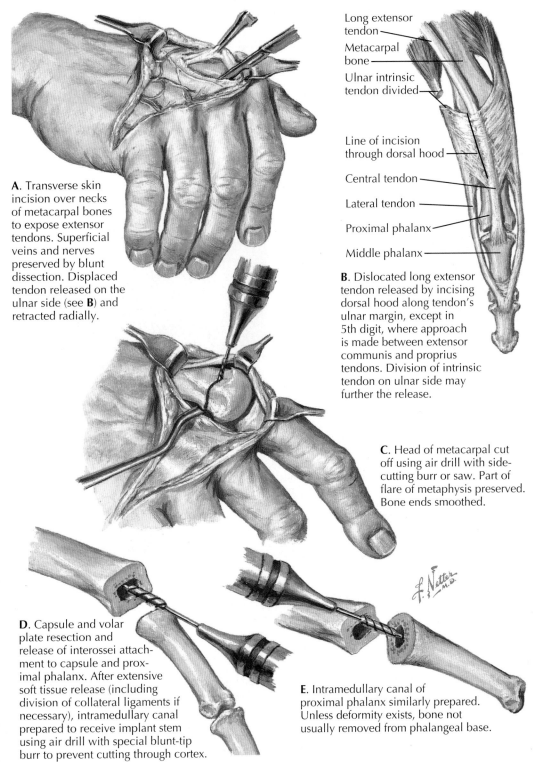

A. Transverse skin incision over necks of metacarpal bones to expose extensor tendons. Superficial veins and nerves preserved by blunt dissection. Displaced tendon released on the ulnar side (see **B**) and retracted radially.

Long extensor tendon

Metacarpal bone

Ulnar intrinsic tendon divided

Line of incision through dorsal hood

Central tendon

Lateral tendon

Proximal phalanx

Middle phalanx

B. Dislocated long extensor tendon released by incising dorsal hood along tendon's ulnar margin, except in 5th digit, where approach is made between extensor communis and proprius tendons. Division of intrinsic tendon on ulnar side may further the release.

C. Head of metacarpal cut off using air drill with side-cutting burr or saw. Part of flare of metaphysis preserved. Bone ends smoothed.

D. Capsule and volar plate resection and release of interossei attachment to capsule and proximal phalanx. After extensive soft tissue release (including division of collateral ligaments if necessary), intramedullary canal prepared to receive implant stem using air drill with special blunt-tip burr to prevent cutting through cortex.

E. Intramedullary canal of proximal phalanx similarly prepared. Unless deformity exists, bone not usually removed from phalangeal base.

and stability can be obtained. This allows for realignment of severely dislocated and angulated joints after the significant bony and soft tissue resection needed in severe rheumatoid deformities. Postoperative mobilization is tailored to the amount of instability present after reconstruction; delay in mobilization increases stability. This is typically acceptable because the flexors greatly overpower the extensors and prolonged immobilization in extension is rapidly overcome, giving a stable, mobile grip. Soft tissue balance at the time of surgery and postoperatively through the use of a tailored hand therapy protocol of rest, splinting, and selective motion is key to preventing the recurrence of deformity and implant breakage, dislocation, and failure.

Plate 4.27

Upper Limb: PART I

IMPLANT RESECTION ARTHROPLASTY FOR METACARPOPHALANGEAL JOINTS (CONTINUED)

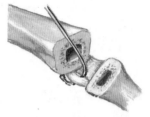

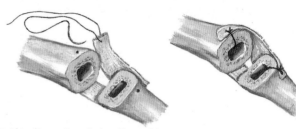

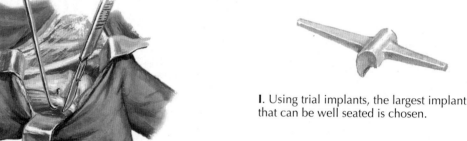

F. Flexor tendon may be drawn up (after incision of its sheath) to determine if partial synovectomy and release of sheath are indicated.

G. If indicated, radial collateral ligament reconstructed with distally based flap composed of collateral ligament and radial half of palmar plate. Two small holes drilled in radial side of dorsum of metacarpal. Flap stitched to metacarpal through drill holes. The radial capsule may be included in this repair.

DEFORMITIES OF THE METACARPOPHALANGEAL JOINTS (Continued)

GENERAL CONSIDERATIONS

The candidate for arthroplasty must be in good general condition. Skin cover and neurovascular status must be adequate. The elements necessary to restore a functioning musculotendinous system and sufficient bone stock to receive and support the implant must be available. In certain patients with progressive rheumatoid arthritis who have insufficient bone stock to support the implant, a simple resection arthroplasty or arthrodesis with a bone graft is preferable. Surgery is also contraindicated if postoperative hand therapy is not available or adequate.

Proper staging of the reconstructive procedures is important in planning the treatment program. Procedures in the upper limbs should be delayed in patients who also need lower limb reconstruction that will necessitate the use of crutches. After hand reconstruction, patients should avoid excessive manual labor and awkward hand weight-bearing when using crutches. The special platform type of crutch is recommended.

In deformities of the metacarpophalangeal joint associated with severe wrist involvement, the wrist should be treated first to correct the supination and radial deviation deformity of the wrist. In the patient with rheumatoid arthritis, tendon repair and synovectomy of tendon sheaths must precede arthroplasty of the metacarpophalangeal joints by 6 to 8 weeks. If both metacarpophalangeal and proximal interphalangeal joints are involved, the metacarpophalangeal joint is usually treated first or simultaneously if only operating on one or two metacarpophalangeal joints. In swan neck deformity, the metacarpophalangeal and proximal interphalangeal joints are reconstructed at the same stage. In boutonnière deformity, the proximal interphalangeal joint is reconstructed first. Tendon imbalances and joint misalignment must be corrected. Implant arthroplasty for both the metacarpophalangeal and proximal interphalangeal joints of the same digit is usually avoided if possible.

Several procedures can be performed during one operation, depending on the time available. Surgery for the thumb, proximal interphalangeal and distal interphalangeal joints, wrist, and, occasionally, the elbow joint can often be combined. A limb procedure should be limited to no more than 2 to 2.5 hours, and an axillary or supraclavicular block is recommended if the tourniquet time exceeds 1.5 hours. Small joints may also be injected with corticosteroids or other agents during surgery.

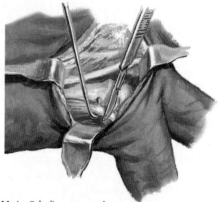

H. In 5th finger, tendon of abductor digiti minimi is divided. Flexor digiti minimi tendon is preserved.

I. Using trial implants, the largest implant that can be well seated is chosen.

J. Implant is inserted into metacarpal using "no touch," atraumatic technique.

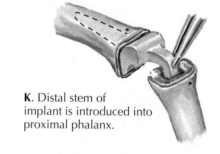

K. Distal stem of implant is introduced into proximal phalanx.

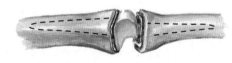

L. With joint in extension, neither metacarpal nor proximal phalanx should impinge on implant. More soft tissue release or bone removal is indicated if fit is not optimal. Wound is irrigated with saline solution before inserting implant.

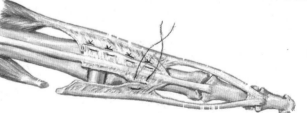

M. Sagittal fibers of dorsal hood are reefed in overlapping fashion on radial side to centralize long extensor tendon and maintain correction.

DEFORMITIES OF FINGER JOINTS

In the normal hand, a delicate balance exists among the muscles and tendons and the bones and joints through which they interact. The hand has three functional arches, one longitudinal and two transverse. The proximal transverse arch crosses the carpal area, with its center at the capitate. The distal transverse arch is formed by the metacarpal heads and is centered on the head of the third metacarpal. The digits make up the longitudinal arches, each with its apex at the metacarpophalangeal joint.

Plate 4.28

Hand and Finger

DEFORMITIES OF THE METACARPOPHALANGEAL JOINTS (Continued)

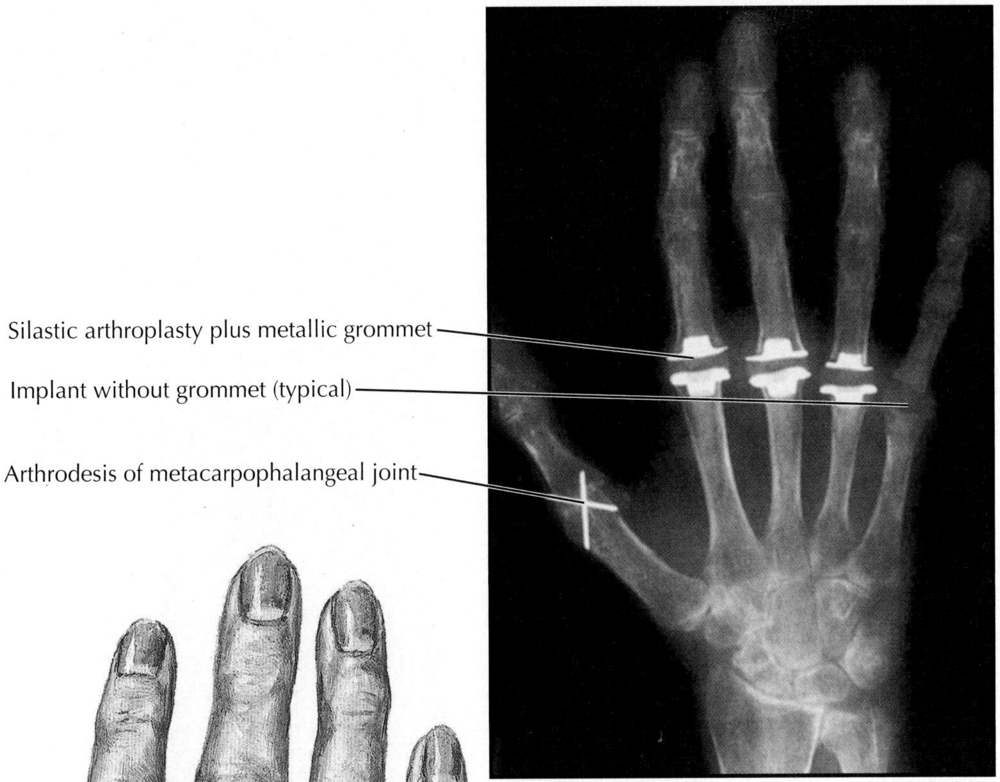

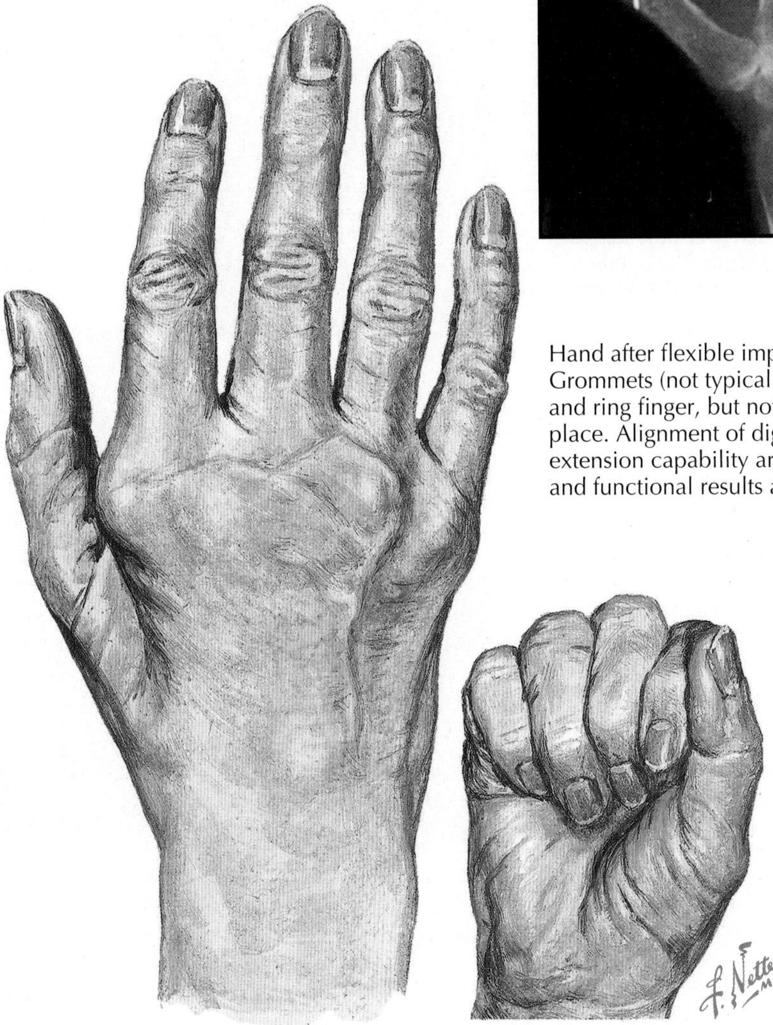

In rheumatoid arthritis, this balance among the muscles, tendons, and bones is compromised as the inflammatory synovial membrane grows over the surface of the cartilage, into the ligamentous attachments, and into and around the tendons. The result is capsular distention, destruction of cartilage, subchondral erosions, loosening of ligamentous insertions, impaired tendon function, and, finally, joint disorganization, subluxation, and dislocation. A break in the longitudinal arch system causes collapse deformities of the multiarticular structure of the hand, disturbing the stability and balance necessary for prehension. Use of the hand in daily activities (functional adaptation) causes further deformity.

DEFORMITIES OF METACARPOPHALANGEAL JOINT

The metacarpophalangeal joint is a key element in finger function. This joint not only flexes and extends but also abducts and adducts; it also has some passive axial rotation. The index finger can pronate up to 45 degrees.

Rheumatoid arthritis commonly involves the metacarpophalangeal joints, resulting in increased ulnar deviation of the fingers, subluxation of extensor tendons, and palmar subluxation of joints (see Plate 4.21). The flexor tendons enter the fibrous sheath at an angle, exerting an ulnar and palmar pull that is resisted in the normal hand. When the rheumatoid process distends and weakens the capsule and ligaments of the metacarpophalangeal joint, the forces generated by the long flexor tendons across the sheath during flexion may elongate these supporting structures. Resistance to the deforming pull of the tendons is gradually lost, and the sheath inlet and tendons are displaced in distal, ulnar, and palmar directions. Eventually, the base of the proximal phalanx moves ulnarly and palmarly. The intrinsic muscles, which normally form a bridge between the extensor and flexor systems and provide direct flexor power across the metacarpophalangeal joint, can also become deforming elements once the disease has lengthened the restraining structures of the metacarpophalangeal joint.

Increased mobility of the fourth and fifth metacarpals, common in rheumatoid arthritis, results from loosening of ligaments at the carpometacarpal joints and dysfunction of the extensor carpi ulnaris tendon (ulnar head syndrome). Flexion of the metacarpophalangeal joints

Silastic arthroplasty plus metallic grommet

Implant without grommet (typical)

Arthrodesis of metacarpophalangeal joint

Hand after flexible implant resection arthroplasty. Grommets (not typically used) in index, long, and ring finger, but not in small finger, are in place. Alignment of digits and flexion and extension capability are restored. Good cosmetic and functional results are achieved.

increases the breadth of the transverse arch of the hand, which pulls the extensor tendons in an ulnar direction through the juncture tendons. The extensor tendon expansions (hoods) are loosely fixed and vulnerable to disruption. Ulnar subluxation of the extrinsic extensor tendons compromises the balance of the intrinsic extensor tendons, which in turn increases the tendency for palmar subluxation and ulnar deviation.

Factors that exacerbate ulnar deviation include (1) the normal mechanical advantage of the ulnar intrinsic muscles, (2) the asymmetry and ulnar slope of the metacarpal heads of the index and middle fingers, (3) the asymmetry of the collateral ligaments, (4) the ulnar

Plate 4.29

Upper Limb: PART I

MODULAR VERSUS IMPLANT RESECTION ARTHROPLASTY

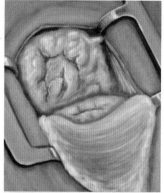

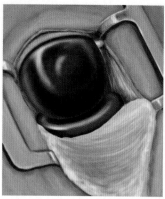

Advanced osteoarthritis of the meta-carpophalangeal (MCP) joint secondary to avascular necrosis and collapse of the metacarpal head. The joint capsule is reflected distally.

Pyrolytic carbon-coated implant arthroplasty of the MCP joint. This type of arthroplasty replaces the articular surfaces but is modular without a connecting hinge between components, thus requiring a stable aligned joint.

DEFORMITIES OF THE METACARPOPHALANGEAL JOINTS (Continued)

forces applied on pinch and grasp, and (5) the postural forces of gravity. Wrist deformities and rupture of the extensor tendons play a secondary role in aggravating the joint disturbances.

Pronation deformity of the index finger is common in the rheumatoid hand. In the normal hand, pinch between the thumb and index finger requires a slight supination of the index finger so that the palmar surfaces can meet. In pronation deformity, the less useful lateral surfaces are opposed. During pinch, pronation deformity is seen in all three digital joints, but it is more pronounced in the metacarpophalangeal joint. Arthroplasty of this joint should include reconstruction of the capsuloligamentous and musculotendinous systems.

MCP arthroplasties are either modular (*left*) for stable aligned joints or hinged (*right*) for joints that have severe destruction and/or instability.

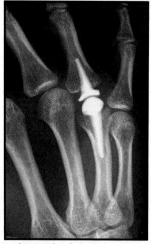

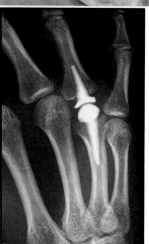

Radiograph of modular arthroplasty of ring finger MCP joint

SURGERY FOR METACARPOPHALANGEAL JOINT

Flexible implant resection arthroplasty of the metacarpophalangeal joints is carried out for deformities due to rheumatoid arthritis and trauma, with radiographic evidence of joint destruction too great to support resurfacing implants or subluxation greater than 25%, ulnar deviation not correctable with soft tissue surgery alone, and contraction of the intrinsic and extrinsic musculature and ligamentous system.

The surgical technique for implant resection arthroplasty for the metacarpophalangeal joint is shown in Plates 4.26 to 4.28. Soft tissue release must be complete to obtain an appropriate joint space. The ulnar collateral ligament is incised at its phalangeal insertion in all fingers; if severely contracted, it is excised with the palmar ligament (plate). The ulnar intrinsic tendon, if tight, is sectioned at its myotendinous junction and the abductor digiti minimi is released.

Reconstruction of the radial collateral ligament is done for index and middle fingers. The radial collateral ligament and related structures are reattached proximally to the metacarpal neck and distally to the proximal phalanx through small drill holes. The radial half of the palmar plate and the preserved radial capsule are included in this repair. The ulnar edge of the capsule is sutured to the distally released ulnar collateral ligament. Sutures are placed before the implant is inserted and tied with the finger held in supination and radial deviation. Although the procedure seems to slightly limit flexion of the metacarpophalangeal joint, this is outweighed by increased lateral and vertical stability and better correction of the pronation deformity.

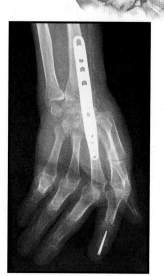

This patient has severe lack of motion of MCP joints due to rheumatoid arthritis causing joint dislocation and ulnar drift of fingers.

Radiograph of patient demonstrating dislocation of MCP joints and ulnar deviation of fingers. Previous wrist fusion by plate fixation and index finger arthrodesis with an intramedullary screw is seen.

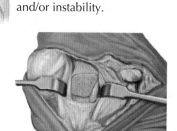

Operative image of patient demonstrating MCP joint space after metacarpal head resection. Collateral ligaments can be seen intact.

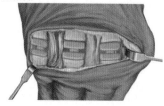

Operative image demonstrating Silastic hinged MCP arthroplasties of the long, ring, and small fingers in place.

After the procedure, a voluminous conforming dressing, including a palmar splint, is applied with the metacarpophalangeal joints in 30 degrees of flexion and slight radial deviation. During the postoperative period, the limb must be elevated. A meticulous postoperative therapy program is usually started 3 to 5 days after surgery and consists of static splinting of the metacarpophalangeal joints for 4 weeks with free movement of the proximal and distal interphalangeal joints followed by mobilization of the metacarpophalangeal joints in a radial deviation support brace. Full hand night splinting in a slightly overcorrected position is used for 6 months.

Plate 4.30

Hand and Finger

DEFORMITIES OF INTERPHALANGEAL JOINT: RADIOGRAPHIC FINDINGS

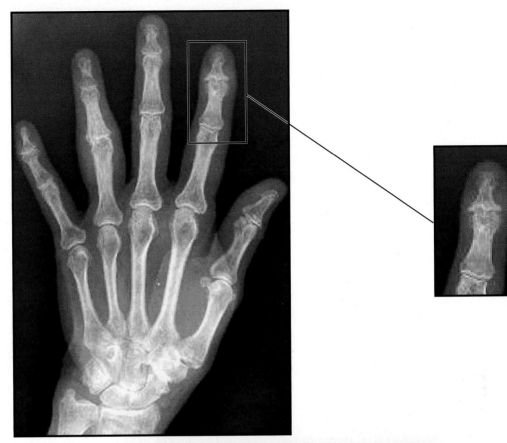

DEFORMITIES OF INTERPHALANGEAL JOINT

The collateral ligament system and the flexor and extensor tendons play an important role in maintaining the normal configuration of the proximal interphalangeal joint. The distal interphalangeal joint acts as a simple hinge but is very important for balancing the proximal interphalangeal joint, and hyperextension or flexion (mallet) deformity can cause boutonnière or swan neck deformities, respectively. The rheumatoid process compromises the normal anatomy of the joint and may lead to joint stiffness, with or without lateral deviation, or to collapse deformities, most notably boutonnière and swan neck deformities. Mallet finger is not common in rheumatoid arthritis but is common in osteoarthritis. Limited joint movement may result from articular factors (adhesions and disorganization of the joint), periarticular factors (adhesions or laxity of ligaments), or tendinous factors (synovial invasion of the flexor tendons and adhesions).

Collapse deformities of the three-joint system of the digit are characterized by hyperextension of one joint and reciprocal flexion of adjacent joints. The deformity occurs when the balance between the tendon and ligament systems is compromised. Axially applied forces further aggravate the deformity, establishing a cycle of deforming forces.

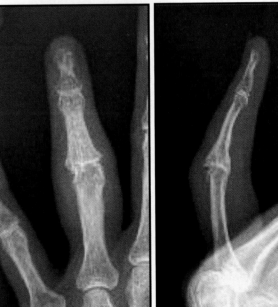

Advanced ring finger proximal interphalangeal joint and index finger distal interphalangeal joint arthritis

BOUTONNIÈRE DEFORMITY

This condition is characterized by flexion of the proximal interphalangeal joint and hyperextension of the distal interphalangeal joint (see Plate 4.31). In rheumatoid arthritis, causes of boutonnière deformity include (1) capsular distention of the proximal interphalangeal joint; (2) lengthening of the central long extensor tendon, with lack of extension in the middle phalanx; (3) lengthening of the transverse fibers; (4) palmar subluxation of the lateral bands, which become flexors of the proximal interphalangeal joint; (5) increased extensor pull on the distal phalanx; (6) self-perpetuating collapse deformity; and (7) soft tissue contracture, joint stiffness, and disorganization.

SWAN NECK DEFORMITY

The term *swan neck deformity* refers to hyperextension of the proximal interphalangeal joint and flexion of the distal interphalangeal joint (see Plate 4.31). In rheumatoid arthritis, the deformity may result from (1) synovitis of the flexor tendon sheath, which causes difficulty in initiating or completing flexion of the interphalangeal joint; (2) increased flexor pull at the metacarpophalangeal joint; (3) increased pull of the intrinsic muscles to the central tendon; (4) loosened attachments of the palmar ligament and accessory collateral ligaments of

Plate 4.31

Upper Limb: PART I

RECONSTRUCTIVE SURGERY FOR SWAN NECK AND BOUTONNIÈRE DEFORMITIES

Reconstruction of swan neck deformity

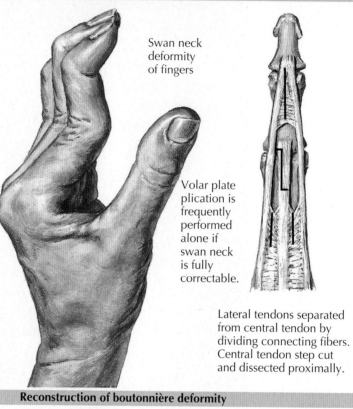

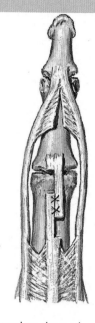

Swan neck deformity of fingers

Volar plate plication is frequently performed alone if swan neck is fully correctable.

Lateral tendons separated from central tendon by dividing connecting fibers. Central tendon step cut and dissected proximally.

Lateral tendons relocated palmarly. Central tendon sutured in lengthened position with buried knots, maintaining 10 to 15 degrees of flexion.

Reconstruction of boutonnière deformity

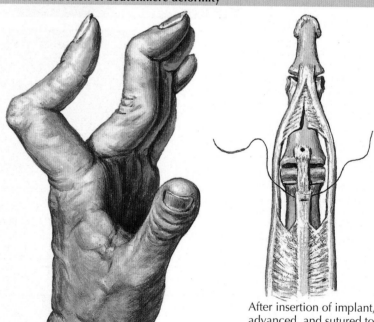

Boutonnière deformity of index finger with swan neck deformity of other fingers

After insertion of implant, central tendon released, advanced, and sutured to base of middle phalanx through drill hole. Lateral tendons released and relocated dorsally by suturing connecting fibers or overlapping fibers if redundant.

DEFORMITIES OF INTERPHALANGEAL JOINT (Continued)

the proximal interphalangeal joint; (5) hyperextension of the proximal interphalangeal joint; (6) stretching of the oblique retinacular ligaments; (7) dorsal subluxation of the lateral bands, which become extensors of the proximal interphalangeal joint; (8) pull of the flexor digitorum profundus tendon, which flexes the distal interphalangeal joint; and (9) joint disorganization and subluxation. Other factors that increase the mechanical advantage of the extensor pull and accentuate the deformity include palmar subluxation of the metacarpophalangeal or wrist joint and contracture of the intrinsic muscles secondary to chronic flexion deformity of the metacarpophalangeal joint. In osteoarthritis, deformity typically starts with a stiff flexion deformity of the distal interphalangeal joint.

DEFORMITIES OF DISTAL INTERPHALANGEAL JOINT

In osteoarthritis and rheumatoid arthritis, deformities of the distal interphalangeal joint are usually secondary to collapse deformities. Specific deformities resulting from synovial invasion are uncommon; however, loosening of the distal attachment of the extensor tendon may cause a mallet or drop finger. Loosening of the collateral ligaments, erosive changes in the subchondral bone, and cartilage destruction in combination with external forces applied during daily activities may lead to joint instability. Complete joint destruction may also occur secondary to the severe resorptive changes seen in arthritis mutilans.

SURGERY FOR PROXIMAL INTERPHALANGEAL JOINT

In swan neck deformity, flexor synovitis is treated first. If the articular surfaces are preserved, hemitenodesis of the flexor digitorum superficialis tendon to the base of

the middle phalanx can be done at the same time to check the hyperextension deformity of the proximal interphalangeal joint. Usually, it is not necessary to lengthen the central slip in release of the swan neck deformity. It is important to obtain adequate release of the dorsal capsule, collateral ligaments, and palmar plate. A 10-degree flexion contracture (or greater) of

the proximal interphalangeal joint should be obtained and associated deformities of the contiguous joints corrected.

In a mild flexible deformity in weak hands, dermadesis is indicated, in which an elliptic wedge of skin (sufficient to create a 20-degree flexion contracture) is removed from the flexor aspect of the proximal interphalangeal

Plate 4.32

Hand and Finger

IMPLANT RESECTION ARTHROPLASTY FOR PROXIMAL INTERPHALANGEAL JOINT

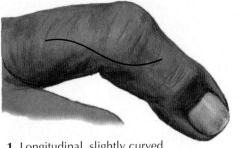

1. Longitudinal, slightly curved incision is made over proximal interphalangeal joint.

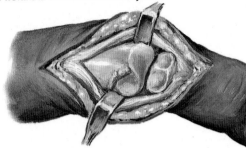

2. Central tendon incised, preserving insertion of middle phalanx, and each half retracted palmarly. Collateral ligament insertions on proximal phalanx preserved, if possible.

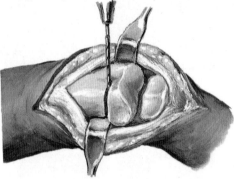

3. Head of proximal phalanx is resected using air drill with side-cutting burr or saw.

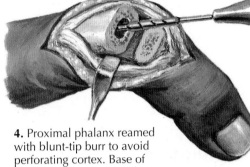

4. Proximal phalanx reamed with blunt-tip burr to avoid perforating cortex. Base of middle phalanx resected.

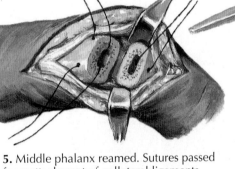

5. Middle phalanx reamed. Sutures passed for reattachment of collateral ligaments and central slip.

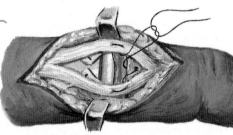

6. Largest implant that can be well seated is inserted first into proximal and then into middle phalanx.

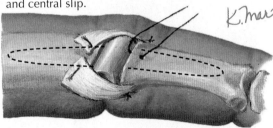

7. With joint extended, bone ends should not impinge on implant midsection. Collateral ligaments reattached, if possible.

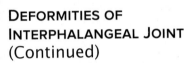

8. Halves of central tendon are drawn together and sutured through drill hole in base of middle phalanx.

DEFORMITIES OF INTERPHALANGEAL JOINT (Continued)

joint, preserving the underlying vessels and nerves. If the articular surfaces are inadequate, however, fusion of the proximal interphalangeal joint is preferred. Implant arthroplasty is rarely indicated.

Treatment of arthritic deformities of this joint includes realignment of the longitudinal arch of the digit. The joint can be treated by arthrodesis, resurfacing arthroplasty, or resection implant arthroplasty. Resurfacing of the proximal interphalangeal joint is indicated for painful, degenerative, or posttraumatic deformities with destruction. When subluxation of the joint cannot be corrected with soft tissue reconstruction alone or significant bone loss exists, implant resection arthroplasty is indicated. For deformities of the proximal interphalangeal joints of both the index and long fingers with osteoarthritis or early rheumatoid arthritis in a young person who performs heavy labor, the proximal interphalangeal joint of the index finger is fused in 20 to 40 degrees of flexion, and resurfacing or resection implant arthroplasty is performed for the proximal interphalangeal joint of the middle finger. The more stable index finger can be used in pinch, and the more flexible long finger can be used in grasp. Flexion of the proximal interphalangeal joints in the ring and little fingers is very important for grasping small objects, and function should be restored if possible.

Good results require adequate release of joint contractures. The collateral ligaments are left intact whenever possible and, if released, they should be released on both sides to prevent pivoting instability on the intact side. Rebalancing and postoperative capsuloligamentous healing will stabilize the joint when the postoperative protocol below is used. If the joint is severely contracted, more bone is removed, or if too great and the joint cannot reduced, an implant resection arthroplasty is used, allowing for even more bone resection. If the contracture persists, the palmar plate and collateral ligaments may be incised proximally or distally, as needed. The collateral ligaments are not required to be repaired. Resurfacing arthroplasty may be placed either press-fit because they have a bone ingrowth surface or cemented if a tight fit cannot be achieved. Importantly, the central tendon is advanced slightly distal on the middle phalanx, which ensures full extension postoperatively. A coexisting mallet deformity of the distal interproximal joint must be corrected at the time of surgery to rebalance the tendons and prevent a swan neck deformity.

The hand is dressed as in metacarpophalangeal joint surgery, and 2 or 3 days after surgery, hand-based thermoplastic splints are applied with the finger in 0 degrees of flexion for 3 to 4 weeks. Motion is initiated under supervision, and flexion is gradually increased after 3 weeks as long as full extension can be obtained. The

Plate 4.33

Upper Limb: PART I

MODULAR VERSUS IMPLANT RESECTION ARTHROPLASTY

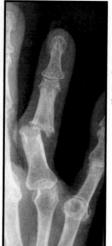

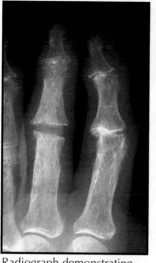

Radiograph demonstrating index finger PIP joint arthritis and long finger PIP joint Silastic arthroplasty

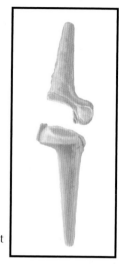

Radiograph of failed ring finger proximal interphalangeal (PIP) joint Silastic arthroplasty that has fractured, resulting in joint subluxation

Worn and fractured Silastic implant retrieved from patient in radiograph at left

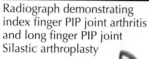

This type of modular PIP joint arthroplasty has a metal proximal stem/articular surface and a polyethylene surface on a metal distal articular stem design that mimics the natural joint surface. Stable aligned joints are required for a modular implant.

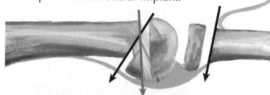

Modular PIP joint arthroplasties resect minimal bone.

Secure repair of the extensor mechanism by passage of suture through bone is critical to regaining normal finger extension.

DEFORMITIES OF INTERPHALANGEAL JOINT (Continued)

resting splint can be applied slightly to the radial or ulnar side of the digit to correct any residual tendency to deviate; it is worn at night and between exercise periods until adequate healing occurs.

In an alternative approach, the central tendon is preserved and the exposure is volar, releasing the cruciate pulley, displacing the flexor tendons, releasing the volar plate, and preserving the extensor tendon insertion. Postoperative motion is immediate and preferred for resection implant arthroplasty. However, visualization and correction of soft tissue and bony deformity for resurfacing arthroplasty is more difficult to achieve and may be incomplete.

Implant resection arthroplasty for proximal interphalangeal joints with collapse deformity requires adjustment of the tension of the central tendon and lateral bands as mentioned earlier. Compared with the lateral bands, the central tendon is relatively tight in the swan neck deformity and must be released, whereas in the boutonnière deformity, the central tendon is relatively loose and must be tightened.

Implant resection arthroplasty for boutonnière deformity is accompanied by reconstruction of the extensor tendon mechanism. The collateral ligaments are reefed or reattached to bone as needed. After surgery, extension of the proximal interphalangeal joint and flexion of the distal interphalangeal joint must be maintained. The proximal interphalangeal joint is immobilized in extension with a padded aluminum splint for 3 to 6 weeks; the distal joint is allowed to flex freely. Active flexion and extension exercises are started 3 to 4 weeks after surgery, and a splint should be worn at night for about 10 weeks.

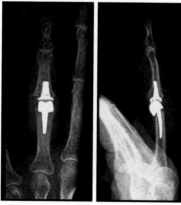

Radiographs of modular PIP joint arthroplasty

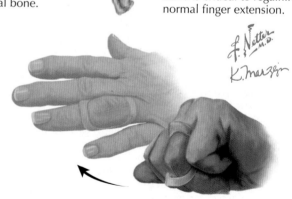

Early 6-week postoperative result of patient demonstrating near full range of motion restored. A ring splint is worn to prevent hyperextension during the first 3 months.

SURGERY FOR DISTAL INTERPHALANGEAL JOINT

If the distal interphalangeal joint is unstable, subluxated, or deviated or if there is articular damage, arthrodesis is the treatment of choice. Contractures of the joint may be treated with soft tissue release and temporary fixation with a Kirschner wire to allow some useful residual movement. Slight flexion movement of the distal interphalangeal joint is very important in finely coordinated activities, but if movement at the proximal interphalangeal joint is good, fixation in a functional position is acceptable.

Plate 4.34   Hand and Finger

PRESENTATION AND TREATMENT OF DUPUYTREN CONTRACTURE

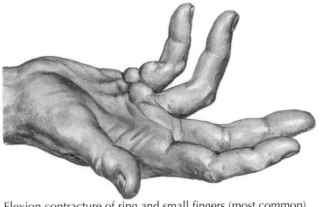

Flexion contracture of ring and small fingers (most common), dimpling and puckering of skin, and palpable fascial nodules near flexion crease of palm at base of involved fingers with cord-like formations extending to proximal palm.

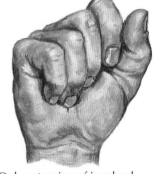

Only extension of involved fingers is limited. Flexion is not impaired because tendons are not involved.

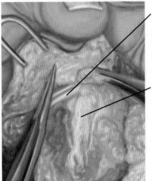

Ulnar digital nerve is pulled across the midline to the radial side by the Dupuytren cord.

Dupuytren cord

Digital nerve deviates from straight path shown by scissors due to Dupuytren cord pulling it across over years of growth.

DUPUYTREN CONTRACTURE

Dupuytren contracture is a progressive thickening and contracture of the palmar aponeurosis (fascia) that results in flexion deformities of the finger joints. Although its cause is unknown, trauma is not a factor in its origin (but can accelerate progression) and an increased familial incidence suggests a genetic component. Dupuytren contracture chiefly affects middle-aged White males, particularly those of Northern European descent. It most commonly affects the ring and small fingers, followed infrequently by long finger involvement. It rarely affects the index finger or the thumb.

CLINICAL MANIFESTATIONS

The first sign of the condition is a slowly enlarging, firm, and slightly painful nodule that appears under the skin near the distal palmar crease opposite the ring finger; other nodules may form at the bases of the ring and small fingers. Subcutaneous contracting cords develop later; they extend proximally from the nodule toward the base of the palm and distally into the proximal segment of a finger.

Flexion contractures gradually develop in the metacarpophalangeal joint and later in the proximal interphalangeal joint of the involved finger. The degree of the flexion deformities and their development rate vary, depending on the extent of thickening and contracture in the palmar fascia. Some contractures develop quickly over a few weeks or months; others take several years. Long remissions may occur, only to be followed by exacerbations and increasing deformity. As the flexion deformity progresses, secondary contractures occur in

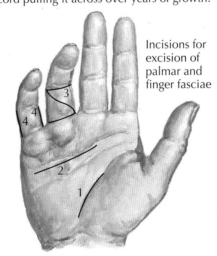

Incisions for excision of palmar and finger fasciae

1 and 2, incisions just distal to thenar and distal palmar creases; 3 and 4, alternative Z and midlateral finger incisions

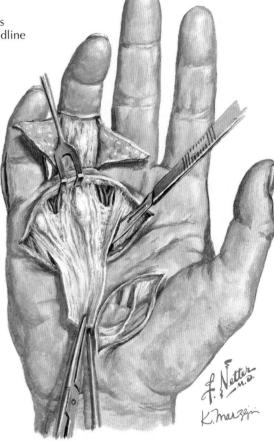

Partial excision of palmar fascia. Proximal portion of fascia divided and freed via thenar incision, then drawn up into palmar incision where it is further dissected with care to avoid neurovascular bundles. Dissection then continued into fingers. Nodules and cord-like fascial thickening are apparent.

the skin, nerves, blood vessels, and joint capsules. Because there is no tendon involvement, active flexion of the fingers remains complete. Involvement is usually bilateral, and in 5% of patients similar contractures occur in the feet.

Serious changes occur in the skin overlying the involved fascia. The short fascial fibers that extend from the palmar aponeurosis to the skin contract and draw folds of skin inward, producing dimpling, pitting,

fissuring, and puckering. The subcutaneous fat atrophies, and the skin becomes thickened, less mobile, and attached firmly to the underlying involved fascia. These changes occur particularly in the region of the distal palmar crease on the ulnar side of the palm. Except for the nodules, cords, and finger contractures, the patient has few complaints. Developing nodules may be slightly painful and tender. Finger deformities interfere with use of the hand, leading to disability in patients with

Plate 4.35

Upper Limb: PART I

SURGICAL APPROACH TO FINGER

Volar approach to finger

Incision site

Incision may be extended.

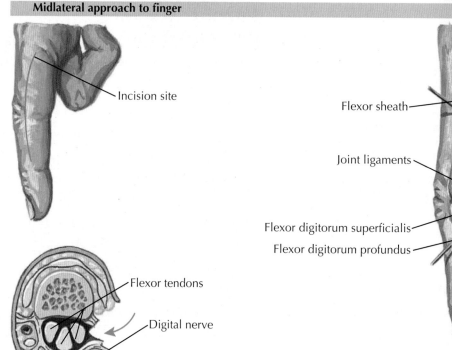

A1
C1
A2
C2

Digital nerve

Digital artery

A3
C3
A4

Flexor tendons

Flexor sheath

Grayson ligament

Digital nerve

Cleland ligament

Digital artery

Midlateral approach to finger

Incision site

Flexor sheath

Joint ligaments

Flexor digitorum superficialis

Flexor digitorum profundus

Flexor tendons

Digital nerve

Digital artery

JOHN A. CRAIG—AD

DUPUYTREN CONTRACTURE
(Continued)

certain occupations. The stages are not distinct and description of them is not essential.

TREATMENT

Surgery is the only effective treatment and should be done before the skin has deteriorated and the skin, nerves, and joint capsules have become too contracted. A typical timing for surgery is when the patient can no longer lay the hand flat on the table and definitely when contracture occurs at the proximal interphalangeal joint. Surgical repair should not be performed before contractures develop.

Partial fasciectomy, the most common treatment, removes all of the thickened and contracted aponeurosis without excision of the uninvolved portion. During fasciectomy, tourniquet hemostasis is essential because hematoma is the most common complication. Skin flaps must be reflected very carefully to avoid buttonholing of the skin and necrosis and the subsequent need for skin grafts. However, an open palm technique has been successfully used by making a distal palmar transverse crease; after full extension is obtained, the wound edges gap open often more than 2 cm. This can be treated with dressing changes, and it typically heals over time by wound contracture and epithelialization. In addition, great care must be taken to avoid any damage to the nerves and blood vessels that may be surrounded and distorted by the hypertrophic fibrous tissue. Neurovascular bundles are at times drawn across the midline of the finger, making them difficult to identify and easy to injure. Resection of Dupuytren contractures requires a keen knowledge of anatomy and surgical exposures to avoid neurovascular injury.

After surgery, the fingers are not initially splinted as was done in the past because this avoids overstretching the neurovascular bundles, which can lead to neurapraxia, followed by a dystrophic response and complex regional pain syndrome. After 5 to 7 days, splinting is initiated, and splints are adjusted weekly to bring the fingers gradually into the corrected extended position. Prolonged postoperative care, which may require several months, is necessary to obtain optimal results and includes splinting the hand in the flat position between exercise sessions.

Percutaneous fasciotomy or chemolysis of contractures with injectable collagenase *Clostridium histolyticum* is an office-based procedure that has very good success for single cord palmar disease. It is less successful for proximal interphalangeal joint contractures, and recurrence is higher than open operative resection. However, recovery is faster, and it has a definite place in the treatment algorithm.

Plate 4.36

Hand and Finger

INFECTIONS OF THE HAND

Before the introduction of antibiotics, infections of the hand often led to prolonged morbidity, severe deformity, amputation, and even death. Kanavel's classic article in 1939 on the pathways of purulent infection within the anatomic compartments of the hand opened the modern era of treatment for these problems. Although injuries in the industrial workplace are less prevalent than in Kanavel's time, wounds of the hand still account for a large percentage of hand infections. A high incidence of hand infections is also associated with societal problems, such as intravenous injection of drugs with contaminated needles, wounds inflicted with various weapons in gang-related incidents, and complications of treatment with immunosuppressive agents. Human and animal bites may also have severe consequences.

The evaluation of a hand wound must include the duration of time since the injury, the contamination likely at the site of injury, and the severity of the wound. After the initial evaluation of the patient's neurovascular and musculoskeletal status, the examiner must make a decision about further evaluation and treatment. It is generally better to err on the side of caution and thoroughly inspect the wound under surgical control in the operating room. Regional, intravenous, or general anesthesia is induced. In a fresh wound, exsanguination is performed with an elastic bandage; if the wound is already infected, elevating the limb for 2 minutes reduces the risk of forcing the inflammation deeper into normal tissue. Hemostasis is obtained with an upper arm pneumatic or an Esmarch forearm tourniquet.

Foreign material and devitalized tissue are debrided, and the wound is thoroughly irrigated. Pulsed lavage with 3 L or more of saline solution significantly reduces bacterial contamination. Reducing the bacterial population below 1 million organisms/mm^3 allows the normal immune defenses to control contaminants. After debridement, exposed tendons, vessels, nerves, and joints should be protected, but wound closure should be delayed. Fine-meshed gauze impregnated with petroleum and 3% bismuth tribromophenate and then gauze dampened with saline solution provides a nonstick, antibacterial, and moist dressing to protect the exposed tissues. The hand is overwrapped in gauze and immobilized with a splint and elevated, which is extremely effective in halting infection. This open treatment followed by repeat debridement at 3 to 5 days and with delayed primary closure produces excellent results. Some smaller wounds are left open and treated by whirlpool baths daily with damp to dry dressings changed twice daily until granulation and epithelialization gradually close the wound from the inside out, preventing anaerobic bacteria from being trapped in a prematurely closed, subsequently anoxic wound.

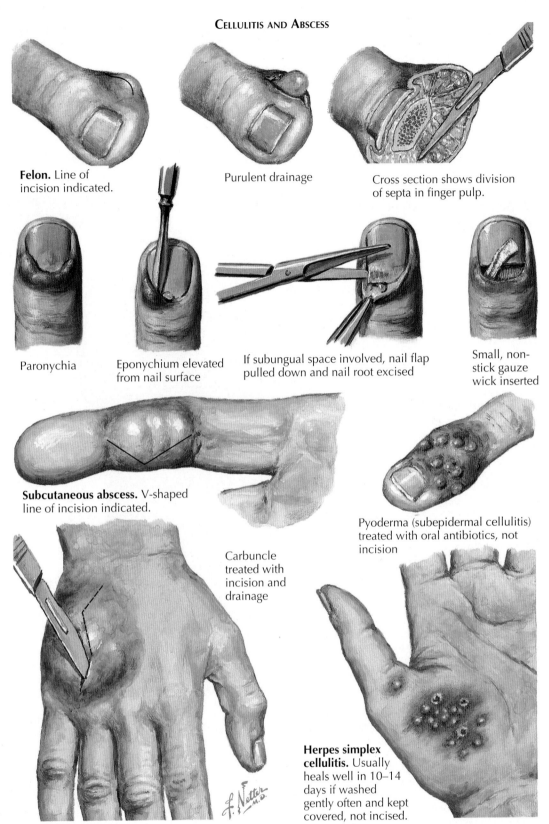

CELLULITIS AND ABSCESS

Felon. Line of incision indicated.

Purulent drainage

Cross section shows division of septa in finger pulp.

Paronychia

Eponychium elevated from nail surface

If subungual space involved, nail flap pulled down and nail root excised

Small, non-stick gauze wick inserted

Subcutaneous abscess. V-shaped line of incision indicated.

Carbuncle treated with incision and drainage

Pyoderma (subepidermal cellulitis) treated with oral antibiotics, not incision

Herpes simplex cellulitis. Usually heals well in 10–14 days if washed gently often and kept covered, not incised.

The same approach to postoperative care is appropriate after incision and drainage of abscesses. In the immediate postoperative period, the wrist is generally immobilized in dorsiflexion, the metacarpophalangeal joints in 30 to 40 degrees of flexion, and the proximal interphalangeal joints in relative extension. A bulky dressing provides pressure to reduce edema and capillary drainage to extract exudate. These measures minimize the likelihood of joint contractures due to immobility.

CELLULITIS AND EPIDERMAL ABSCESS

If possible, cultures should be obtained before beginning antibiotic therapy for any hand infection. Gram-positive cocci are responsible for most abscesses, particularly those resulting from infections incurred around the home or in the industrial workplace. Wounds due to agricultural or garden accidents are more likely to be contaminated with gram-negative or mixed organisms.

Plate 4.37

Upper Limb: PART I

TENOSYNOVITIS AND INFECTION OF FASCIAL SPACE

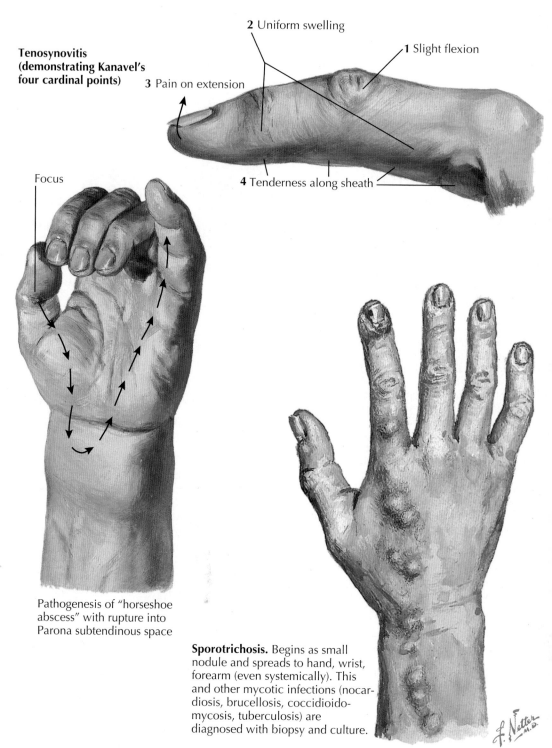

Tenosynovitis (demonstrating Kanavel's four cardinal points)

2 Uniform swelling

1 Slight flexion

3 Pain on extension

4 Tenderness along sheath

Focus

Pathogenesis of "horseshoe abscess" with rupture into Parona subtendinous space

Sporotrichosis. Begins as small nodule and spreads to hand, wrist, forearm (even systemically). This and other mycotic infections (nocardiosis, brucellosis, coccidioidomycosis, tuberculosis) are diagnosed with biopsy and culture.

INFECTIONS OF THE HAND (Continued)

FELON

A felon, or whitlow, may begin as a subepidermal abscess that penetrates a pulp space of the finger. Further extension into adjacent fibrofatty spaces causes distention with severe pain and throbbing. If the spread continues, osteomyelitis of the distal phalanx may result in loss of the tuft, septic arthritis of the distal interphalangeal joint, or infective tenosynovitis of the flexor tendon sheath.

In the earliest phase, release of the subepidermal abscess and antibiotic treatment may abort the infection. However, when the felon is well established, incision and drainage are imperative. A longitudinal incision is made directly over the site of drainage or necrosis to minimize the chance of injuring a digital nerve. Blunt breakdown of septa with a hemostat allows for thorough drainage. A fishmouth incision or through-and-through incision is seldom necessary. A wick of gauze is left in the wound for 1 or 2 days, after which irrigation or soaks may be started.

PARONYCHIA

Paronychia usually originates with an undetected break in the eponychium (cuticle) or with a hangnail. Dryness of the skin may be a factor, and the infectious organisms are often supplied from the patient's nasopharynx. The early signs are redness and burning that spread along the nail fold. Pain is often inordinate for the apparent degree of inflammation. At this early stage, gently lifting the eponychium with a No. 11 blade evacuates the pus, allowing the inflammation to resolve without further treatment. A partial finger block suffices for anesthesia.

If untreated, the infection may progress beneath the nail, causing it to loosen. At this stage, excision of the proximal nail produces satisfactory decompression. A radial incision in the nail fold should be avoided. Sometimes an incision halfway between the eponychium and the distal interphalangeal skin crease allows for direct drainage, accompanied by nail plate removal. Rarely, a mucous cyst simulates a paronychia or actually becomes infected. The infection may progress up the stalk of the cyst to the joint cavity, resulting in a septic distal interphalangeal joint.

SUBCUTANEOUS ABSCESS

Subcutaneous abscesses may occur anywhere in the fingers or hand and usually result from minute breaks in the skin that becomes infected. These infections present as pain, swelling, redness, and turgor. On the dorsum of the hand, abscesses are likely to originate in a hair follicle, or there may be several drainage sinuses that coalesce into a carbuncle.

Subcutaneous abscesses often have a purulent center, which aids identification. Incision and drainage are performed, with suitable regional anesthesia induced proximal to any obvious inflammation and avoiding areas of lymphangitis. The incision is centered over the fluctuant area, placed in skin creases, or angled at them obliquely. The incision should avoid underlying structures, particularly cutaneous nerves.

Pyoderma

Also called subepidermal or vesicular cellulitis, pyoderma is most often seen in children and usually involves the dorsal aspect of the two distal segments of a finger. This infection is often due to *Streptococcus* from the nasopharynx, although both *Staphylococcus* and *Pseudomonas* species may also be present. The blebs may be aspirated and the fluid cultured to obtain

Plate 4.38

Hand and Finger

TENOSYNOVITIS AND INFECTION OF FASCIAL SPACE (CONTINUED)

Common variation

Usual arrangement

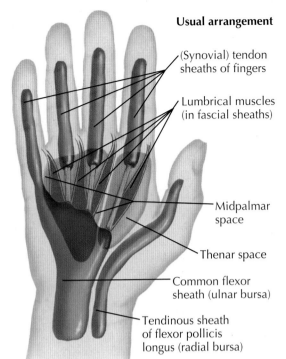

(Synovial) tendon sheaths of fingers

Lumbrical muscles (in fascial sheaths)

Midpalmar space

Thenar space

Common flexor sheath (ulnar bursa)

Tendinous sheath of flexor pollicis longus (radial bursa)

Intermediate bursa (communication between common flexor sheath [ulnar bursa] and tendinous sheath of flexor pollicis longus [radial bursa])

INFECTIONS OF THE HAND (Continued)

definitive diagnosis, but the lesions invariably respond to antibiotics and protection from contact with the mouth. Pyoderma is highly contagious, and precautions should be taken to avoid spreading it to family members or schoolmates.

Herpes Simplex Cellulitis

A vesicular cellulitis of the hand or fingers due to infection with herpes simplex virus occurs most often in dentists and healthcare workers. Although the infection is contagious and often quite uncomfortable, it tends to run a benign course: several crops of vesicles develop slowly and heal over 2 to 3 weeks. The vesicles may be punctured under sterile conditions. Involved hands must be kept clean and dry, and the patient must be very careful to avoid further self-contamination or cross-contamination.

TENOSYNOVITIS AND INFECTION OF FASCIAL SPACE

Tenosynovitis

Purulent tenosynovitis can be a devastating infection because it produces adhesions within the tenosynovial canal that markedly limit finger motion. If the infection affects one of the ulnar three fingers, the quadrigia effect may limit motion of the adjacent fingers as well. Once a granulation response has begun, the ability to restore full function is compromised. If treatment is delayed or the antibiotics used are insufficient or ineffective, the infection may convert to a subacute state that produces progressive destruction.

The infection is usually secondary to a puncture wound, and initial onset is insidious. Infection with a virulent organism such as *Staphylococcus*, however, can produce severe pain within a few hours. The four cardinal signs of tendon sheath infection (described by Kanavel) are uniform swelling, fixed flexion, pain on attempted passive extension of the finger, and tenderness along the course of the tendon sheath into the distal palm.

In the thumb and little finger, the tendon sheath usually extends into the radial and ulnar bursae, respectively, allowing infection to spread well into the distal forearm (see Plates 4.37 and 4.38). A communication between the two bursae allows the establishment of a horseshoe abscess that affects both the thumb and the little finger, although effective treatment with antibiotics has made this complication rare. By the time the horseshoe abscess occurs, irrevocable damage to the delicate gliding tissues of the tenosynovial sheath may have occurred. Avascular necrosis of the tendons follows quickly from vascular occlusion and intracompartmental pressure. Less virulent

For severe subacute purulent flexor tenosynovitis, open drainage and debridement is done by zigzag volar incision. Tendon sheath is opened by reflecting cruciate pulleys and preserving annular pulleys. With more prompt diagnosis, closed tendon sheath irrigation provides drainage while promoting healing and return of finger motion. An incision is made in the palm, releasing the A1 pulley. A second midlateral incision is made distally in the finger and the tendon sheath incised distal to the A4 pulley. A catheter is inserted into the proximal end of the tendon sheath and a drain in the distal end. The tendon sheath is irrigated until all purulent material is removed. Post-operatively, the catheter is kept in place for approximately 48 hours to allow intermittent saline irrigation of the tendon sheath.

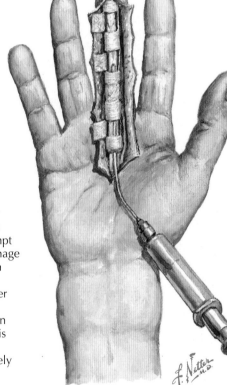

organisms cause a less acute infection, but if they are unrecognized and untreated, the residual effect may be no less detrimental.

A subcutaneous abscess directly over the tendon sheath may be confused with true purulent tenosynovitis. Therefore, if the diagnosis is not clear, incision and drainage should be performed. The initial incision is made over the site of maximum tenderness. If a

subcutaneous abscess is found and the underlying sheath appears transparent and free of effusion, further dissection is not necessary. However, if there is effusion, purulence, distention, or thickening and opacity of the sheath, the incision should be extended as a Brunner zigzag incision.

To ensure adequate drainage and perfusion of the sheath, one or more flaps are raised at the sites of the

Plate 4.39

Upper Limb: PART I

INFECTED WOUNDS OF HAND AND FINGERS

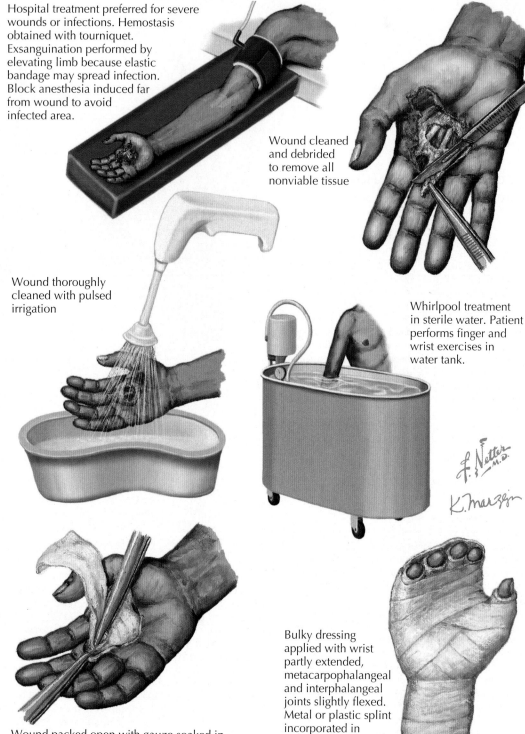

Hospital treatment preferred for severe wounds or infections. Hemostasis obtained with tourniquet. Exsanguination performed by elevating limb because elastic bandage may spread infection. Block anesthesia induced far from wound to avoid infected area.

Wound cleaned and debrided to remove all nonviable tissue

Wound thoroughly cleaned with pulsed irrigation

Whirlpool treatment in sterile water. Patient performs finger and wrist exercises in water tank.

Wound packed open with gauze soaked in dilute povidone-iodine solution, then covered with fluffed gauze

Bulky dressing applied with wrist partly extended, metacarpophalangeal and interphalangeal joints slightly flexed. Metal or plastic splint incorporated in outer layers of dressing.

INFECTIONS OF THE HAND (Continued)

cruciate pulleys. Any fluid should be aspirated and cultured immediately. If the tenosynovial sheath is inflamed, tissue samples should be sent for culture, Gram stain, and histologic examination. Determining the causative organism is essential because a number of unusual organisms, including *Brucella, Pasteurella multocida,* and various *Mycobacterium* species, may also induce tenosynovitis.

The tendon sheath can be milked by passive movements of the fingers. The sheath may also be irrigated through a small catheter, which is left in place for 1 or 2 days, and the effusion allowed to drain. The skin may be closed loosely to protect the underlying tendon. Active movement of the finger should be started once daily after surgery and continued under supervision but splinted and elevated between treatments. If the ulnar or radial bursa is involved, separate incisions are made at the wrist or the digital incisions extended, with care to preserve the transverse carpal ligament.

Sporotrichosis

Sporothrix schenckii, a fungus frequently found in soil or on garden plants, produces cutaneous and subcutaneous lesions and inflammation of the lymph vessels (lymphangitis). This indolent infection is characterized by a pilot lesion at the site of inoculation, followed by the appearance of a succession of satellite lesions, which progress proximally along a lymphatic chain. The lesions are raised, red, swollen, and usually about 1 cm in diameter; the center may ulcerate and drain. Pain is minimal. Diagnosis requires isolating the organism from the ulcerations.

The treatment of choice is topical application of potassium iodide, which is effective in the benign form of the disease. Lesions heal in 2 to 3 weeks. Sporotrichosis may remain localized or spread systemically to involve other organ systems.

INFECTION OF DEEP COMPARTMENTS

The deep compartments of the hand may become infected by direct inoculation via penetrating wounds or by extension of infection in adjacent areas. Such infections are relatively infrequent but, when present, they cause rapid deleterious changes and are prone to spreading. Unless treated with incision and drainage, deep infection may cause permanent deformity.

Infection of Midpalmar Space

The midpalmar space lies under the flexor tendons of the ulnar three fingers and over the deep fascia covering the intrinsic muscles. Ulnarly, the hypothenar muscles

and, radially, the adductor pollicis muscle define the space, which is partially separated by fibrous septa that attach the palmar floor to the central ridges of the metacarpal shafts. Purulence may enter or extend through the lumbrical canals or break through into the carpal canal or thenar space.

Symptoms such as pain on movement, swelling, and marked tenderness may rapidly increase in severity. The dorsum of the hand swells as the lymphatic drainage becomes involved. Tenosynovitis may also develop. The diagnosis is suggested by exquisite tenderness over the palm.

Plate 4.40   Hand and Finger

INFECTION OF DEEP COMPARTMENTS OF HAND

Infection of midpalmar space secondary to tenosynovitis of middle finger. Focus is infected puncture wound at distal crease. Line of incision indicated.

INFECTIONS OF THE HAND
(Continued)

Treatment is by incision, which follows skin creases and is centered to allow access to the midpalmar space and retraction of the flexor tendons. The neurovascular bundles must be carefully identified and retracted. Usually, the purulence is under pressure when the midpalmar space is opened and can be aspirated and the space irrigated. Extensions into adjacent spaces can be identified by massaging the palm, starting at the perimeter. Drains are inserted and kept in place for 1 or 2 days.

Infection of Thenar Space

The thenar space lies under the flexor tendons of the index finger and over the adductor pollicis muscle. The septum to the third metacarpal defines the ulnar border, and the thenar muscles define the radial border. The infection may extend into the lumbrical canal of the index finger and over the distal aspect of the adductor pollicis muscle. A dorsal thenar space infection on the dorsal aspect of the adductor pollicis muscle may dissect under the first dorsal interosseous muscle. An incision along the thenar space must avoid the recurrent motor branch of the median nerve. The nerve is identified by surface anatomic landmarks, using Kaplan's cardinal line intersection with the thenar crease. The incision can be extended distally as a Z-plasty over the first web space.

Collar Button Abscess

These types of abscesses derive their name from the dumbbell-shaped contour of the abscess around the margin of the superficial transverse metacarpal ligament in one of the web spaces. Thus they may present on both dorsal and volar aspects of the hand. Drainage is through a zigzag incision over the distal web space.

Infection in the Space of Parona

The space of Parona lies deep to the flexor tendon sheaths in the distal forearm and volar to the pronator quadratus muscle. Infections are usually due to direct inoculation or extension from an infection of the tendon sheaths. An abscess may be drained through a direct palmar incision if the radial and ulnar bursae are involved. The median nerve must be identified and protected. If the tendon sheaths are not involved, an incision between the flexor tendons and ulnar neurovascular bundle allows access to the space of Parona, as does a direct ulnar incision sliding along the pronator quadratus muscle.

Infections from Human and Animal Bites

Teeth carry a variety of virulent organisms, and a bite may inoculate these organisms deeply into tissues of

Dorsal edema characteristic of palmar infections. Should not be incised unless fluctuant or pointing.

Branch of median nerve to thenar muscles (in phantom)

Infection of thenar space from tenosynovitis of index finger due to puncture wound. Note: thenar space also extends dorsal to adductor pollicis muscle. Line of incision indicated.

Infection of thenar web space in infant. Incision line for Z-plasty indicated.

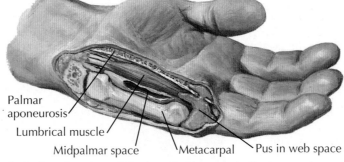

Palmar aponeurosis
Lumbrical muscle
Midpalmar space
Metacarpal
Pus in web space

Sagittal section shows infection of web space (collar button abscess).

Collar button abscess treated with incision and drainage

the hand. Most dogs and cats are carriers of *Pasteurella multocida,* an organism that produces a rapidly spreading inflammation that may penetrate subcutaneous and subfascial spaces as well as tendon sheaths and deep compartments. More aggressive and earlier treatment is required for cat bites because delayed surgical treatment leads to very slow resolution of infection. Human bites carry streptococcal, staphylococcal, spirochetal, and gram-negative organisms. *Eikenella corrodens* is an especially invasive organism that is difficult to eradicate. Penetration of the metacarpophalangeal joint by an incisor may lead to a destructive septic arthritis and dissemination of infection into the adjacent spaces. Treatment of this type of infection requires early recognition, adequate incision, and irrigation.

Plate 4.41

Upper Limb: PART I

LYMPHANGITIS

INFECTIONS OF THE HAND
(Continued)

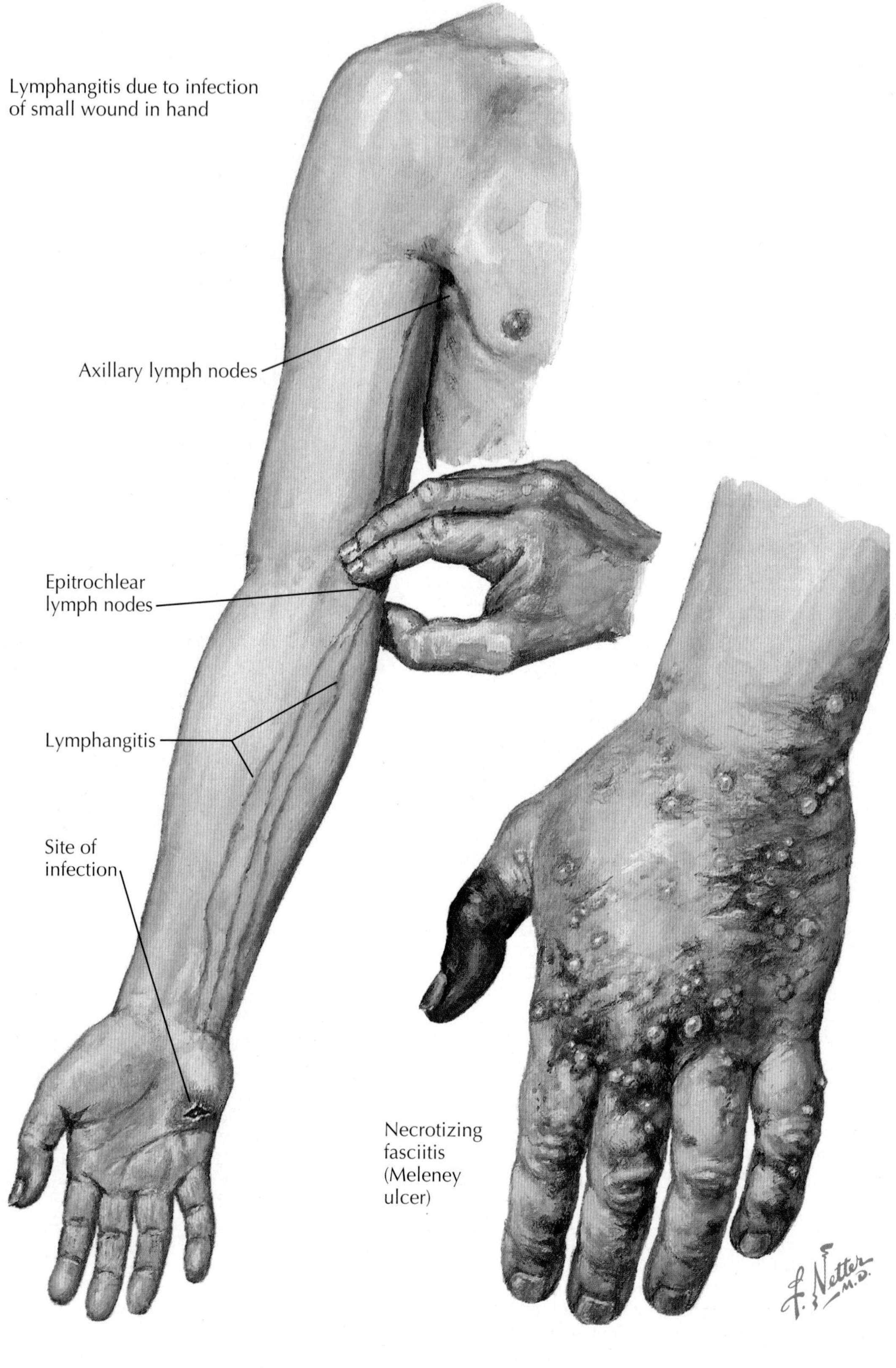

LYMPHANGITIS

Lymphangitis often originates from an insignificant break in the skin or a small wound in the hand. Pain and a burning erythema develop at the site of inoculation. Lymphangitic erythematous streaks begin to form over the dorsum of the hand, progressing in just a few hours into the forearm and then into the arm. Pain intensifies and fever and chills develop. The axilla and epitrochlear areas become tender and swollen.

On examination, the patient appears anxious, protects the involved arm, and may shiver with chills. The wound and the lymphangitic streaks are tender to the touch, as are the soft, swollen epitrochlear and axillary nodes. There may be a small serous drainage at the wound site, which should be cultured and Gram stained. Because streptococci are the usual causative organisms, treatment with penicillin or cephalosporin is started immediately. The perimeter of the erythema at the wound site and the lymphangitic streaks can be marked with a pen for later reference, and the size of the nodes is noted. If the infection does not respond to treatment with antibiotics or if the signs worsen in 12 to 24 hours, a culture sample should be obtained by aspiration or incision or the antibiotic regimen should be changed.

Necrotizing Fasciitis

Also called a Meleney ulcer, necrotizing fasciitis is a severe manifestation of lymphangitis that progresses in a frightening manner within a few hours. Anaerobic or microaerophilic streptococci are believed to be the usual cause, but these microorganisms are difficult to culture. Tissue necrosis develops rapidly behind an advancing wall of inflammation that limits penetration by antibiotics. Desquamation followed by gangrene may be relentless. The clinical signs of pain, hyperpyrexia, and chills are severe.

The skin lesions are incised and drained or aspirated to obtain fluid for culture. Intravenous infusion of aqueous penicillin must be instituted immediately; additional antibiotics may be recommended by an infectious disease specialist. The progress of the inflammation and necrosis must be carefully monitored. Surgical intervention within hours is often required to save life and limb. Even when the necrotizing lymphangitis is controlled early, however, autoamputation may be a sequela and death is an occasional outcome.

Other Hand Infections

The preceding discussion is merely an introduction to the greater scope of infections of the hand. Mycobacterial tenosynovitis and arthritis still occur. *Mycobacterium*

Lymphangitis due to infection of small wound in hand

Axillary lymph nodes

Epitrochlear lymph nodes

Lymphangitis

Site of infection

Necrotizing fasciitis (Meleney ulcer)

marinum is an organism frequently associated with injuries due to marine activities. Gonococcal septic arthritis rapidly destroys involved joints. Rare invaders of the musculoskeletal system are fungal infections, including coccidioidomycosis and blastomycosis. *Clostridium perfringens* may colonize crushed muscle in the hand, producing gas gangrene. Rare viral infections transmitted from domestic animals occasionally produce lesions on the hand, and inflammation that mimics

infection (e.g., calcium pyrophosphate dihydrate disease) should also be considered in the differential diagnosis.

The introduction of antibiotics has dramatically improved the prognosis for infections of the hand. For optimal treatment, however, the correct diagnosis must be established, the organism identified, the purulence drained, and an appropriate rehabilitation program instituted.

Plate 4.42

Hand and Finger

BIER BLOCK ANESTHESIA

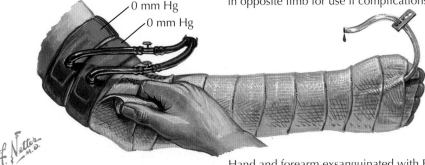

0 mm Hg
0 mm Hg

Double pneumatic tourniquet placed on arm but not yet inflated. Butterfly needle introduced into dorsal vein of hand and taped in place. Intravenous line also established in opposite limb for use if complications develop.

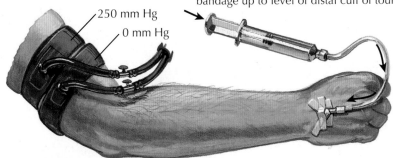

0 mm Hg
0 mm Hg

Hand and forearm exsanguinated with Esmarch or elastic bandage up to level of distal cuff of tourniquet

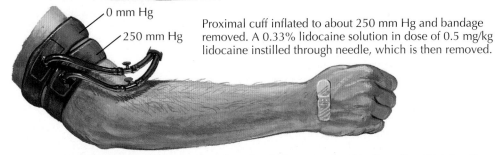

250 mm Hg
0 mm Hg

Proximal cuff inflated to about 250 mm Hg and bandage removed. A 0.33% lidocaine solution in dose of 0.5 mg/kg lidocaine instilled through needle, which is then removed.

0 mm Hg
250 mm Hg

In about 10 minutes, adequate anesthesia develops from level of proximal cuff to fingertips. Distal cuff then inflated to 250 mm Hg and proximal cuff deflated, transferring level of compression into anesthetized area, where it is well tolerated. Cuff remains inflated throughout surgical or manipulative procedure, after which it is slowly deflated, then inflated again, and again slowly deflated, to avoid sudden flush of anesthetic into systemic circulation. For same reason, constriction must be maintained for at least 20 minutes to allow adequate tissue binding of lidocaine. Anesthesia dissipates in about 10 minutes.

ANESTHESIA FOR HAND SURGERY

REGIONAL ANESTHESIA

For procedures lasting more than 45 minutes and/or bony procedures with significant pain expected, surgeons often prefer to use regional anesthesia. This allows for longer tourniquet times without discomfort and continuous pain relief for 12 to 24 hours postoperatively. The choice of supraclavicular versus axillary block and the mixture of short- versus long-acting anesthetic is chosen by the anesthesiologist in consultation with the surgeon, directing the anesthesia to the nerves affecting the region of the hand being operated upon.

BIER BLOCK ANESTHESIA

The usual risks of general anesthesia can also be avoided with the use of Bier block regional anesthesia. Axillary and supraclavicular blocks are often time consuming, especially in patients who are in significant pain and unable to fully cooperate with the examiner. Intravenous regional, or Bier block, anesthesia is a good choice for reductions of the forearm fractures and for elective procedures in the hand. The method is safe and reliable, producing adequate muscle relaxation and pain relief for up to 45 minutes without tourniquet discomfort.

First, an intravenous line is established in the normal, uninjured forearm to provide immediate access for the administration of sedative medications. In the injured limb, a butterfly needle is placed in a dorsal vein

in the hand, distal to the fracture site. A 0.33% lidocaine solution is given in a dose of 0.5 mg/kg. (A 1% lidocaine solution is diluted threefold with normal saline to produce a 0.33% lidocaine solution.) The syringe containing the dilute anesthetic solution is then attached to the butterfly needle. The arm is exsanguinated either by elevating it for 3 to 4 minutes or by wrapping it carefully with an elastic bandage. A double pneumatic

tourniquet is placed on the arm proximal to the fracture site. The more proximal of the two cuffs is inflated to 250 to 300 mm Hg. Within 1 minute after the injection, the patient usually experiences significant relief of pain. Mottling of the skin is another indication that the block is effective.

If tourniquet pain develops before the procedure is completed, the distal cuff of the tourniquet can be

Plate 4.43

Upper Limb: PART I

THUMB CARPOMETACARPAL INJECTION, DIGITAL BLOCK, AND FLEXOR SHEATH INJECTION

Thumb carpometacarpal injection

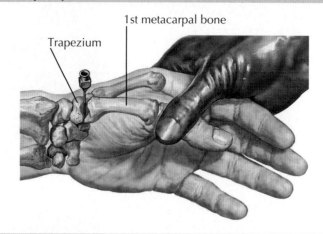

Trapezium

1st metacarpal bone

Digital block

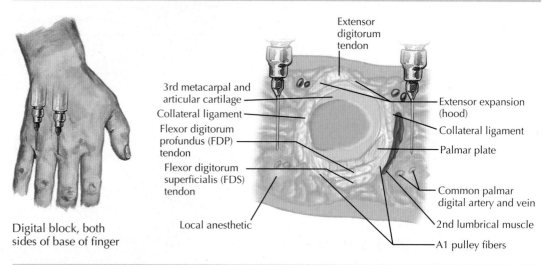

Extensor digitorum tendon

3rd metacarpal and articular cartilage

Collateral ligament

Flexor digitorum profundus (FDP) tendon

Flexor digitorum superficialis (FDS) tendon

Extensor expansion (hood)

Collateral ligament

Palmar plate

Common palmar digital artery and vein

2nd lumbrical muscle

A1 pulley fibers

Local anesthetic

Digital block, both sides of base of finger

ANESTHESIA FOR HAND SURGERY (Continued)

inflated and the proximal cuff released; because the area under the now inflated distal cuff is anesthetized by the block, the tourniquet can remain inflated longer without causing discomfort. After 30 to 45 minutes, most of the lidocaine has been bound to tissues in the forearm; therefore removing the tourniquet at this time does not release a large dose of lidocaine into the general circulation. When the tourniquet is released, however, the patient's pulse and respirations must be monitored because cardiac arrhythmias and seizures have occurred in some patients. A conservative practice is to maintain the tourniquet for 45 minutes (20 minutes has been used routinely as a minimum time), then release it slowly while monitoring vital signs. Moderately long-acting local anesthesia is required for postprocedural pain relief and is given locally around the site of fracture or surgery before discontinuing the Bier block.

In practice, use of forearm single-cuff tourniquets with less anesthetic volume is very effective for short procedures, and compression of the forearm is better tolerated than the upper arm.

DIGITAL BLOCK AND LOCAL ANESTHESIA

For smaller procedures in the fingers distal to the metacarpophalangeal joints, a digital block gives excellent anesthesia and is easily administered. A dorsal approach to the web space is made with the needle, and

Flexor sheath injection

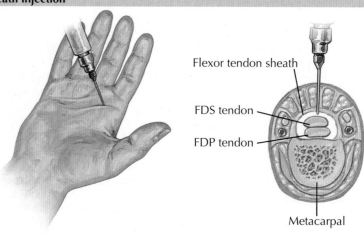

Flexor tendon sheath

FDS tendon

FDP tendon

Metacarpal

a bolus of 1 to 2 mL of 1% to 2% lidocaine is placed under the skin as the needle is placed more volar, down to the subcutaneous layers bathing the neurovascular bundle. Through the same insertion site, the needle is passed across dorsally, subcutaneously infiltrating another 1 to 2 mL until the next web space. A new insertion site is then made in the already anesthetized web space on the other side of the finger, dispensing another 1 to 2 mL of lidocaine down to the volar neurovascular bundle. Local anesthesia placed subcutaneously can

be used for small procedures directly over the site of incision.

JOINT AND TENDON SHEATH INJECTIONS

It is very common for patients with arthritis or tendonitis to require an injection of corticosteroid as an antiinflammatory agent. These injections are typically given in a mixture with local anesthetic to ease the discomfort during the postinjection phase.

Plate 4.44

Hand and Finger

TRIGGER FINGER AND JERSEY FINGER

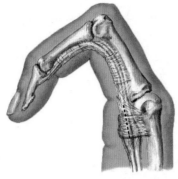

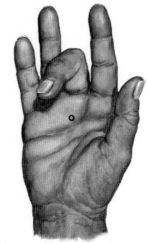

Inflammatory thickening of fibrous sheath (pulley) of flexor tendons with fusiform nodular enlargement of both tendons. Broken line indicates line for incision of lateral aspect of pulley.

Patient unable to extend affected finger. It can be extended passively, and extension occurs with distinct and painful snapping action. Circle indicates point of tenderness where nodular enlargement of tendons and sheath is usually palpable.

Incision of thickened pulley via small transverse skin incision just distal to distal flexion crease releases constriction, permitting flexor tendons to glide freely and inflammation to subside.

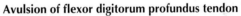

Avulsion of flexor digitorum profundus tendon

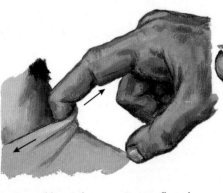

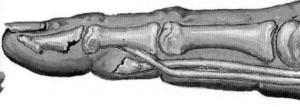

Caused by violent traction on flexed distal phalanx, as in catching on jersey of running football player

Flexor digitorum profundus tendon may be torn directly from distal phalanx or may avulse a small or large bone fragment. Tendon usually retracts to about level of proximal interphalangeal joint, where it is stopped at its passage through flexor digitorum superficialis tendon; occasionally, it retracts into palm. Early open repair of tendon and its torn fibrous sheath is indicated.

TENDON DISORDERS IN THE HAND

TRIGGER FINGER

Trigger finger is the result of localized tenosynovitis of the superficial and deep flexor tendons in the region of the fibrous sheath (annular ligament, or pulley) at a metacarpal head (A1). It occurs most often in the long or ring fingers (occasionally in the thumb) of middle-aged women, but its exact cause has not been determined. Trigger finger may also be associated with rheumatoid arthritis and diabetes involving several fingers.

The localized inflammation causes a thickening and narrowing of the sheath, and a nodular or fusiform enlargement develops in the tendons distal to the pulley. These changes interfere with—and may actually prevent—the smooth gliding of the tendons through the fibrous sheath.

Clinical Manifestations

In the early stage, the nodule produces a slightly painful clicking or grating as it passes through the constricted sheath when the finger is flexed and extended. As the pathologic changes in tendon and sheath advance, flexion of the finger is arrested in the middle range; as more force is required to pull the nodule through the constricted pulley, the finger snaps painfully into full flexion or extension. Later, the tendon nodule may not pass through the stricture, and the finger is partially fixed in extension or flexion, usually the latter. Passive manipulation of the flexed finger may force the nodule through the sheath, producing a painful snap into extension.

On examination, the patient can usually demonstrate the trigger finger and may be able to demonstrate the finger locking in flexion; flexion and extension produce crepitation. Palpation over the metacarpal head reveals a tender nodule that moves with the tendon.

Treatment

Although trigger finger often subsides spontaneously, a cortisone injection into the tendon sheath may alleviate the triggering in up to 80% of patients. If painful triggering continues, a minor operation can provide permanent relief. A 0.25-inch transverse or longitudinal incision is made just distal to the distal flexion crease over the metacarpal head, exposing the flexor tendons and sheath. The constriction is relieved by completely incising the thickened A1 pulley longitudinally along its radial or ulnar aspect, taking care to avoid the digital nerves. Thick inflamed tenosynovium is removed, freeing the movement of the superficialis (sublimis) and profundus tendons. The patient can now actively flex and extend the finger freely and comfortably, and the pulley heals again but has a larger diameter.

FLEXOR TENDON REPAIR

Flexor tendon injuries can occur by various mechanisms, but the most common injury is a laceration. "Jersey finger" is an avulsion of the flexor digitorum

Plate 4.45

Upper Limb: PART I

REPAIR OF TENDON

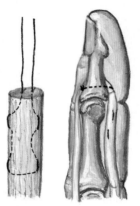

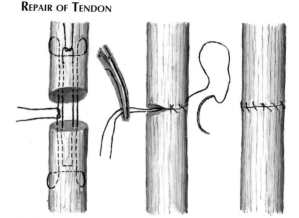

For tears of flexor digitorum profundus tendon at distal phalanx, tendon is repaired to the native footprint.

Traditionally, tendons are repaired with 4-0 polyester Kessler core suture with knot in gap, followed by circumferential repair with running epitenon suture of 6-0 or 7-0 nylon.

More recent suture configurations achieve four core sutures but put the knots away from the repair site. A similar running epitenon suture is used.

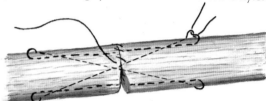

Flexor digitorum superficialis tendon

Flexor digitorum profundus tendon

Camper chiasm

Flexor digitorum superficialis tendon runs volar to flexor digitorum profundus tendon but splits over proximal phalanx to allow passage of flexor digitorum profundus tendon. Two slips of flexor digitorum superficialis tendon insert on the middle phalanx dorsal to flexor digitorum profundus tendon. In injury involving zone of divided flexor digitorum superficialis tendon (Camper chiasm), one, two, or three tendon slips may be divided and require careful suturing.

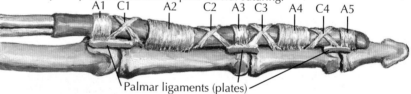

A1   C1   A2   C2   A3   C3   A4   C4   A5

Palmar ligaments (plates)

Flexor digitorum superficialis and profundus tendons are encased in synovial sheaths bound to bones of digits by fibrous sheaths made up of alternating strong annular (A) and weaker cruciate (C) pulleys. When sheath must be opened to repair severed tendon, opening should be made in zones of cruciate pulleys because anatomic annular pulleys are critical to function.

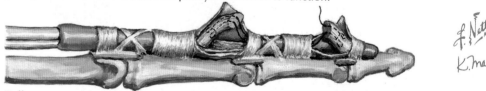

Pulley system must be preserved. If synovial sheath must be incised to repair flexor tendons, small funnel-shaped openings made in cruciate pulley area are subsequently meticulously repaired to prevent catching during gliding of tendons.

TENDON DISORDERS IN THE HAND (Continued)

profundus tendon that occurs typically in the ring finger as a result of a forced gripping versus resistance, as seen when the finger gets tied up in an opponent's jersey during a football tackle. Flexor tendon laceration often occurs in the household on broken glass, from tin can lids, or inadvertently with a kitchen knife. Laceration can occur anywhere along the length of the finger, with the most complex occurring in zone 2 over the proximal phalanx where the profundus and sublimis tendons travel together in a fibro-osseous sheath. Typically, the hand is clenched and therefore the skin injury is more proximal than the tendon injury, requiring careful attention to the physical examination.

Primary repair in the first 6 weeks produces acceptable functional results; after 6 weeks, tendon grafting or arthrodesis of the distal interphalangeal joint is the treatment of choice. Repair of a lacerated or avulsed flexor digitorum profundus tendon to the distal phalanx is typically performed by using a bone suture anchor placed in the distal phalanx or passage of the locking suture weave placed in the tendon through the bone from palmar to dorsal and tying the sutures over the dorsal cortex. Postoperatively, a dorsal splinting protocol prevents maximal extension during the early phases of healing, with early passive motion and active flexion initiated by 3 weeks. Strengthening is begun at the 6-week mark.

Tendon repair is most successful after a sharp laceration of the tendons as opposed to tearing seen with saw injuries. The goal is to obtain a strong repair with the least amount of bulk in the tendon so the tendons will pass smoothly through the pulleys in the fibro-osseous sheath. The flexor tendon repair consists of two layers of sutures. The first layer is a core stitch, most commonly performed to obtain at least four passes across the tendon repair. This provides significant strength to allow early active range of motion. The second layer is a circumferential epitendinous stitch with a fine nonabsorbable suture that adds strength but

also helps reduce the volume and friction of the repair. Owing to the site of laceration, at times a four-strand repair is not possible and separate two-strand core stitches are placed in each stump and then tied to work around the pulleys. A second core stitch can then be placed in a horizontal mattress fashion, providing a total of four core stitches.

Therapy after flexor tendon repair requires highly skilled hand therapists to work closely with patients to

reduce edema and guide the patient through the different stages of recovery. The initial stage is typically passive motion to initiate tendon gliding in a safe manner, followed by active range of motion and later strengthening. Full recovery can take up to 6 months, and it is not uncommon that a secondary operative procedure is required to perform a tenolysis to break down the adhesions that occur after wound and tendon healing.

Plate 4.46

Hand and Finger

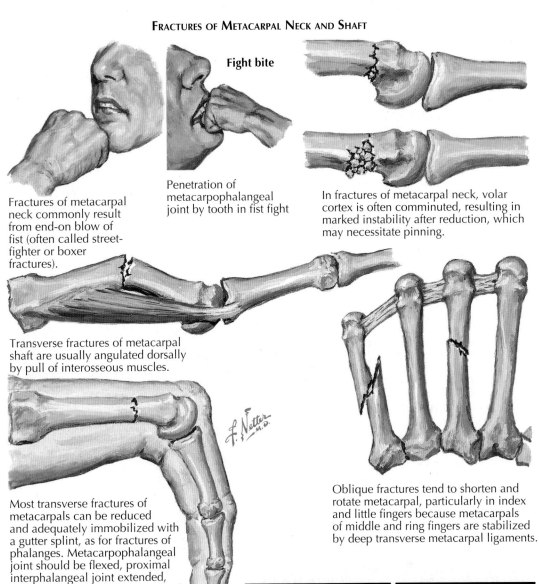

Fight bite

Fractures of metacarpal neck commonly result from end-on blow of fist (often called street-fighter or boxer fractures).

Penetration of metacarpophalangeal joint by tooth in fist fight

In fractures of metacarpal neck, volar cortex is often comminuted, resulting in marked instability after reduction, which may necessitate pinning.

Transverse fractures of metacarpal shaft are usually angulated dorsally by pull of interosseous muscles.

Most transverse fractures of metacarpals can be reduced and adequately immobilized with a gutter splint, as for fractures of phalanges. Metacarpophalangeal joint should be flexed, proximal interphalangeal joint extended, and active movement encouraged to avoid flexion deformity. Frequent radiographic follow-up is important.

Oblique fractures tend to shorten and rotate metacarpal, particularly in index and little fingers because metacarpals of middle and ring fingers are stabilized by deep transverse metacarpal ligaments.

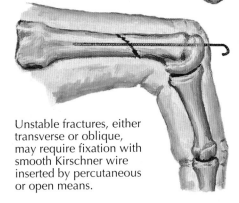

Unstable fractures, either transverse or oblique, may require fixation with smooth Kirschner wire inserted by percutaneous or open means.

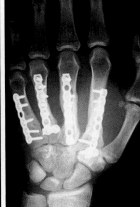

Plate fixation of multiple metacarpal fractures

FRACTURE OF METACARPALS

The carpal and metacarpal bones form a longitudinal arch within the osseous framework of the hand, with transverse arches formed by the metacarpals. The treatment of metacarpal fractures must restore the architecture of the hand so that the metacarpals of the mobile groups—the thumb on the radial side and the ring and small fingers on the ulnar side—maintain their important relationship with the stable central ray, which includes the metacarpals of the index and long fingers.

FRACTURE OF METACARPAL NECK

The most common metacarpal fracture occurs at the neck of the fifth metacarpal. Although often called the boxer fracture, it is more aptly named the "street-fighter (brawler)" fracture because trained boxers attempt to strike their opponent with the radial side of the hand, which is more stable than the ulnar side. Most fractures of the neck of the fifth metacarpal are significantly comminuted on the volar side, resulting in apex dorsal angulation at the fracture site. These fractures are usually treated with closed reduction and immobilization in an ulnar gutter splint, which holds the metacarpophalangeal joint in 70 to 90 degrees of flexion.

Most fractures heal satisfactorily. Maintaining adequate rotational alignment is important, but some residual dorsal angulation is acceptable because the flexible ulnar side of the hand can adapt to slight deformity. Some extensor lag commonly persists after fracture healing. Open reduction is indicated only if rotational alignment cannot be maintained or the fracture angulates greater than 60 degrees. In any fracture of this type, the physician must carefully search for a laceration of the adjacent metacarpophalangeal joint caused by impact with a tooth; lacerations could lead to significant infection and marked disability if left untreated. Careful examination of a fight wound over the metacarpophalangeal joint requires a high index of suspicion because the extensor tendon laceration from a tooth is more proximal than the skin laceration when the hand is examined in the extended position; during making of a fist the tendon and skin laceration line up, as does the cartilage injury to the metacarpal head.

FRACTURE OF METACARPAL SHAFT

Most transverse fractures of the metacarpal shaft are angulated dorsally by the pull of the intrinsic muscles of the hand. The metacarpals of the long and ring fingers, however, are stabilized by the adjacent border metacarpals and their deep transverse metacarpal ligaments; therefore they do not generally shorten even if the

fracture is comminuted. Oblique or spiral fractures of the metacarpals of the small and index fingers do tend to shorten because they are not adequately splinted by stable metacarpals on either side.

Fractures of the metacarpal shaft can be treated adequately with immobilization in a plaster cast, with the metacarpophalangeal joint flexed 70 degrees and the proximal interphalangeal joint in full extension. This "position of function" relaxes the pull of the intrinsic muscles and allows the physician to monitor

apposition, length, and rotational alignment of the metacarpals. Early motion can be achieved by the use of a single retrograde intramedullary screw started intraarticularly in the upper third of the metacarpal head and advanced and buried under the articular surface. Massive crush injuries of the hand, with multiple fractures and considerable soft tissue damage, require open reduction and internal fixation. Surgical repair allows early active motion and produces a good functional result.

Plate 4.47

Upper Limb: PART I

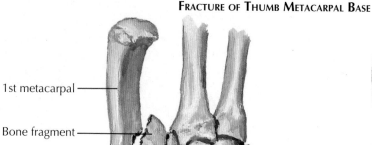

FRACTURE OF THUMB METACARPAL BASE

1st metacarpal

Bone fragment

Trapezium

Abductor pollicis
longus tendon

FRACTURE OF METACARPALS
(Continued)

FRACTURE OF BASE OF METACARPAL OF THUMB

Mobility of the carpometacarpal joint of the thumb is essential for adequate hand function. Therefore treatment of all fractures of the thumb must achieve and maintain good reduction and alignment. Two particularly troublesome fractures are intraarticular fractures of the base of the first metacarpal.

Type I Intraarticular Fracture (Bennett Fracture)

This fracture within the joint is often associated with proximal dislocation of the metacarpal shaft. The abductor pollicis longus tendon inserts on the base of the metacarpal of the thumb and tends to abduct and pull the metacarpal shaft proximally. The very strong volar ligament, which is attached to the base of the articular facet of the metacarpal, maintains the alignment of the proximal fragment with the trapezium.

Bennett fractures usually require surgical fixation because reduction is difficult to maintain in a plaster cast. If a very small fragment of the metacarpal base remains on the ulnar side, the dislocated metacarpal can be reduced easily by applying traction and holding the thumb in abduction. The reduction is maintained with Kirschner wires inserted percutaneously. If the intraarticular fragment is very large, open reduction should be considered to restore the anatomy of the joint to as normal as possible. The reduction can be stabilized with screws, Kirschner wires, or a small buttress plate.

Often, a small displaced fragment appears innocuous on the radiograph, and the dislocation is missed. The most important aspects of the treatment of Bennett fractures are recognizing that the injury is a fracture dislocation rather than just an intraarticular fracture and achieving and maintaining an adequate reduction.

Type II Intraarticular Fracture (Rolando Fracture)

This comminuted fracture involves the articular surface of the metacarpal. Unlike the type I fracture, there is no significant proximal displacement of the metacarpal shaft. The comminution extends radially along the base of the metacarpal of the thumb and distally to the insertion of the abductor pollicis longus tendon.

In a Rolando fracture, the amount of comminution determines the method of treatment. If there are two or three large fragments that can be adequately reduced, open reduction and internal fixation can be attempted. Usually, however, good reduction is achieved only with great difficulty. Extensive

Type I (Bennett fracture). Intraarticular fracture with proximal and radial dislocation of first metacarpal. Triangular bone fragment sheared off.

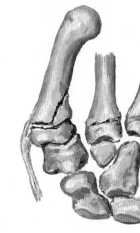

Type II (Rolando fracture). Intraarticular fracture with Y-shaped configuration.

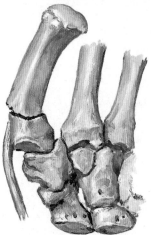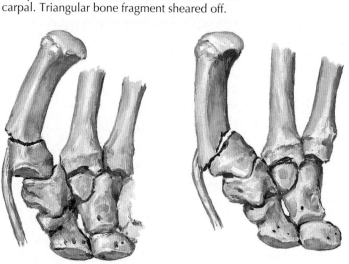

Type IIIA. Extraarticular transverse fracture.

Type IIIB. Extraarticular oblique fracture.

Type IV. Epiphyseal fracture with separation in child.

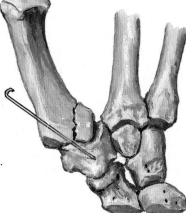

Percutaneous pinning of Bennett fracture. Note: First metacarpal pinned to trapezium; pin must not pass through bone fragment.

comminution of the base of the metacarpal indicates the need for skeletal or skin traction to maintain the reduction.

Intraarticular fractures of the base of the thumb often lead to osteoarthritis of the carpometacarpal joint. Arthrodesis of the carpometacarpal joint of the thumb may be required later to relieve pain and instability.

Types III and IV Fractures

Type III fractures of the first metacarpal are extraarticular; that is, they do not involve the joint. Type IV (epiphyseal) fractures commonly occur in children and involve the growth plate; they should be recognized as extraarticular, not intraarticular, fractures. Extraarticular fractures are treated with closed reduction and immobilization; they rarely require surgery.

Plate 4.48

Hand and Finger

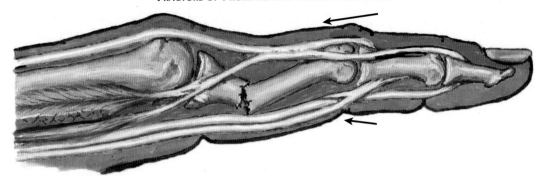

FRACTURE OF PROXIMAL AND MIDDLE PHALANGES

Transverse fractures of proximal phalanx tend to angulate volarly because of pull of interosseous muscles on base of proximal phalanx and collapsing action of long extensor and flexor tendons.

INJURY TO FINGERS

The hand has both mechanical and sensory functions. Therefore injuries to the hand not only disrupt mechanical ability but also compromise the sensory function of the upper limb. Most hand injuries cause pain, swelling, and often discoloration. Because the flexor and extensor tendons and the bones lie close to the skin, each major anatomic structure can be examined easily and its functional status determined. Radiographs of the whole hand itself are not needed if only the wrist or finger is injured, but anteroposterior, lateral, and oblique views of the specific site of injury are essential for a complete evaluation.

FRACTURE OF PROXIMAL AND MIDDLE PHALANGES

Diagnosis of fractures of the phalanges requires anteroposterior, lateral, and oblique radiographs and careful clinical examination of the soft tissues—specifically the flexor and extensor tendons—to verify the extent of the injury. Because finger injuries are often caused by crushing forces, open fractures of the fingers are common.

Several muscle forces contribute to deformity in fractures of the proximal or middle phalanx. The insertion of the flexor digitorum superficialis (sublimis) tendon along the middle phalanx affects the angulation of a fracture, depending on the location of the break. If the fracture of the middle phalanx is distal to the insertion of the flexor digitorum superficialis tendon, the fractured bone angulates volarly. Fractures proximal to the insertion of the flexor digitorum superficialis tendon angulate dorsally. In fractures of the proximal phalanx, the insertions of the interosseous muscle at the base of the proximal phalanx tend to flex the proximal fragment and the flexor and extensor tendons angulate the fracture volarly.

For reduction of a fracture of the phalanx, correct rotational alignment is just as essential as alignment in the anteroposterior and lateral planes. In the normal hand, the tips of all the flexed fingers point toward the tuberosity of the scaphoid. Inadequate reduction and persistent rotational malalignment adversely affect the patient's ability to grasp. Often, the rotational malalignment is not noticeable when the fingers are extended, but it is always obvious when the fingers are flexed. Although judging the reduction of any phalanx fracture in both flexion and extension may be difficult, this step is most important.

The high-energy forces that cause transverse and comminuted fractures of the phalanx often produce significant injury to the soft tissues of the finger as well. Successful treatment of phalanx fractures demands careful attention to the potential consequences of the

Fractures of neck of middle phalanx usually angulate volarly because of pull of flexor digitorum superficialis tendon, which inserts into proximal fragment.

Fractures of base of middle phalanx are often dorsally angulated by traction of central band of long extensor tendon on proximal fragment plus tension of both long flexor tendons.

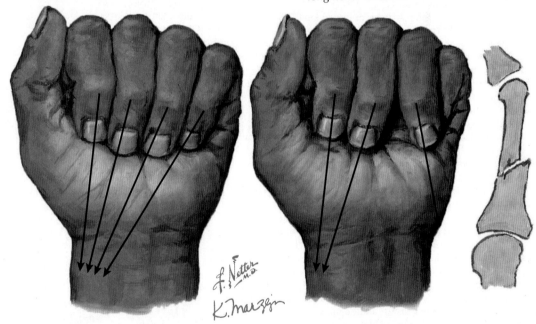

Reduction of fractures of phalanges or metacarpals requires correct rotational as well as longitudinal alignment. In the normal hand, tips of flexed fingers point toward tuberosity of scaphoid, as in hand at left. Hand at right shows result of healing of ring finger in rotational malalignment. Rotational malalignment, usually discernible clinically, may also be evidenced on radiographs by discrepancy in cross-sectional diameter of fragments, as shown at extreme right. Discrepancy in diameter is most apparent in a true lateral radiograph but is visible to some extent in the anteroposterior view.

soft tissue injuries. Even though the fracture may heal in adequate alignment, injuries to the flexor and extensor mechanisms can lead to significant long-term dysfunction.

MANAGEMENT OF FRACTURE

Correction of deformity, preservation of motion, and care of the soft tissues are all important in the treatment

of hand injuries. Adherence to the basic principles of fracture care is essential for good functional results. These principles are (1) alignment of the distal fragment with the proximal fragment, (2) adequate immobilization to allow healing, and (3) preservation of motion and soft tissue function. The primary goal in treating any hand injury is to maintain function, particularly full active motion of all joints. Persistent stiffness in the interphalangeal and metacarpophalangeal

Plate 4.49

Upper Limb: PART I

MANAGEMENT OF FRACTURE OF PROXIMAL AND MIDDLE PHALANGES

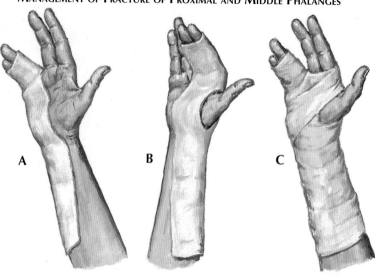

Most fractures of proximal or middle phalanx can be treated with closed reduction and, if stable, satisfactorily immobilized in a plaster gutter splint. **A**. Ulnar splint used for ring and little finger. **B**. Radial splint for index and middle fingers. **C**. Splints held in place with elastic bandage. Metacarpophalangeal joints flexed 70 to 90 degrees, proximal interphalangeal joints extended.

INJURY TO FINGERS (Continued)

joints and adduction contracture of the thumb produce a functional loss that can be debilitating.

Immobilization should maintain the hand in a "position of function": 45 degrees of extension of wrist, 70 degrees of flexion of the metacarpophalangeal joint, 20 degrees of flexion of the proximal interphalangeal joints, and maximal abduction of the thumb. If scarring occurs, this position will preserve as much soft tissue length and joint flexibility as possible. In any significant hand injury, only fingers requiring immobilization should be placed in a cast or splinted; the other fingers should remain free to move.

Some fractures of the phalanges are considered stable; these include most nondisplaced fractures, long spiral fractures, and minimally displaced intraarticular fractures that do not displace with gentle early motion. Stable fractures can be treated by taping the injured finger to the normal adjacent finger (buddy taping) and initiating early active motion. Frequent and careful follow-up during the healing phase ensures that early motion does not displace the fracture fragment.

Most displaced fractures of the proximal and middle phalanges can be treated with closed reduction and cast immobilization using an ulnar or radial gutter splint. The plaster must be applied with great care to avoid excessive pressure on the soft tissues, which can cause ulceration of the skin. The fracture is checked at weekly intervals for 4 to 6 weeks. In fractures of the phalanges, radiographic evidence of healing appears slowly, and radiographs do not show union for many weeks. However, most uncomplicated fractures are clinically stable in 4 to 6 weeks. If examination at that time detects minimal swelling, no tenderness, and no instability, the patient can begin gentle protected motion, but the fracture should be protected for an additional few weeks with intermittent splinting or buddy taping.

Fractures that require open reduction and internal fixation or closed reduction and pin fixation include unstable fractures, fractures that cannot be adequately reduced and maintained with closed means, displaced intraarticular fractures, multiple fractures with soft tissue injuries, and fractures in patients who repeatedly remove their casts.

Oblique fractures are often unstable and tend to shorten the finger. Closed reduction under radiographic control followed by percutaneous pinning restores stability, maintains the reduction, and allows early motion. Transverse fractures of the proximal or middle phalanx are very unstable, often requiring internal fixation. Inserted through a dorsal or midaxial incision, crossed Kirschner wires stabilize the fracture with only minimal disruption of the soft tissues; the wires are removed under local anesthesia without significant soft tissue dissection. Small compression plates may be

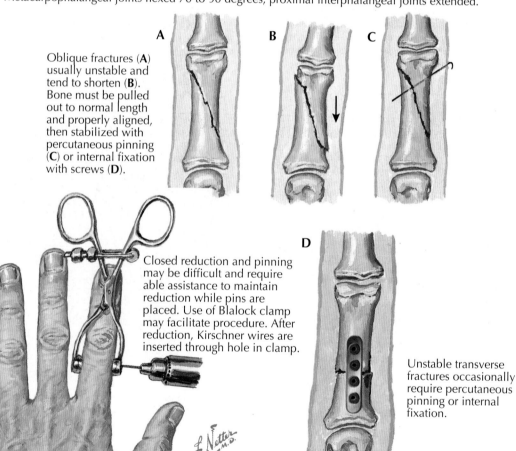

Oblique fractures (**A**) usually unstable and tend to shorten (**B**). Bone must be pulled out to normal length and properly aligned, then stabilized with percutaneous pinning (**C**) or internal fixation with screws (**D**).

Closed reduction and pinning may be difficult and require able assistance to maintain reduction while pins are placed. Use of Blalock clamp may facilitate procedure. After reduction, Kirschner wires are inserted through hole in clamp.

Unstable transverse fractures occasionally require percutaneous pinning or internal fixation.

used. Early motion can be achieved by the use of a single or double anterograde intramedullary screw started at the proximal ulnar and/or radial corner and advanced and buried under the bony surface.

When a fracture is stabilized with either closed reduction and pin fixation or open reduction and internal fixation, the finger is left undisturbed for 8 to 10 days for

the initial phase of soft tissue healing; then active supervised motion is begun to preserve soft tissue function.

Massive crushing injuries with multiple fractures of the phalanges and significant destruction of soft tissue require open reduction and stabilization. Fortunately, the incidence of postoperative infection in open hand fractures is quite low.

Plate 4.50

Hand and Finger

SPECIAL PROBLEMS IN FRACTURE OF MIDDLE AND PROXIMAL PHALANGES

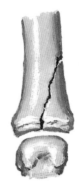

Intraarticular fractures of phalanx that are nondisplaced and stable may be treated with buddy taping, careful observation, and early active exercise.

INJURY TO FINGERS (Continued)

SPECIAL PROBLEMS IN FRACTURE OF PHALANGES

Management of fractures of the phalanges is complicated by numerous problems. Because of the intricate relationship between the flexor and extensor tendons, the joints, and the architecture of the phalanges, neglect or inadequate treatment can lead to significant disability.

Treatment of Oblique Fractures

The pull of the flexor muscles tends to shorten oblique fractures of the proximal and middle phalanges. Resulting soft tissue adhesions contribute to stiffness of the proximal interphalangeal joint. In addition, a bone spike protrudes volarly, creating a mechanical block to full flexion of the proximal interphalangeal joint. Such problems can be managed in a number of ways. If the alignment of the proximal phalanx is adequate but joint motion is limited, the volar spike can be removed surgically and the tendon adhesions freed. These procedures increase flexion and extension of the proximal interphalangeal joint. Inadequate bone alignment necessitates osteotomy of the proximal phalanx and internal fixation with Kirschner wires or intramedullary screws.

Treatment of Stable Intraarticular Fractures

Most intraarticular fractures of the metacarpophalangeal joint that have large nondisplaced fragments can be treated with buddy taping. However, close follow-up is essential to ensure that the fragment does not subsequently displace.

Treatment of Fracture of Condyles

Intraarticular fractures of the interphalangeal joints that involve the condyles of the proximal or middle phalanx are usually unstable. To avoid missing the fractured condyle and to assess the degree of displacement, radiographic examination must include anteroposterior, lateral, and oblique views. However, even after adequate open reduction, stable internal fixation, and fracture healing, stiffness usually persists in the distal or proximal interphalangeal joint.

Treatment of Malunion and Nonunion

Even with proper treatment and adequate follow-up, fracture malunion may occur. In most cases, a malunion does not require any further care, but if it causes pain, limits hand function, or is cosmetically displeasing, surgical intervention should be considered. Osteotomy at the fracture site or at an adjacent area of metaphyseal bone is the usual procedure for realigning the phalanx. The osteotomy is stabilized with an internal fixation device.

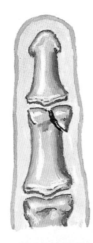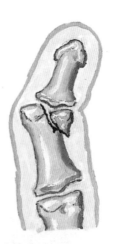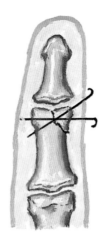

Condylar fractures tend to angulate and require open reduction and pinning, even if fragment is small.

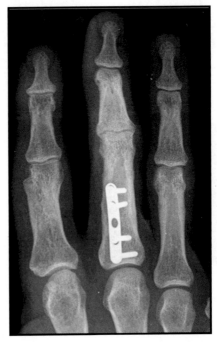

Long finger fracture fixation by plating. Malunion of index proximal phalanx fracture treated nonoperatively.

Nonunion is rare in phalanx fractures and often remains asymptomatic. For symptomatic nonunion, treatment with open reduction and internal fixation combined with bone grafting usually results in healing.

Treatment of Tendon Adhesions

Because injuries to the phalanges damage soft tissue as well as bone, adhesions may develop between the flexor and extensor tendons and the fracture site. The primary clinical sign of this complication is a limitation of active flexion. The need for assistance to achieve full flexion usually indicates the presence of adhesions within the sheath of the flexor tendon. Vigorous physical therapy can help restore motion, but surgical tenolysis of the flexor sheath at the level of the healed fracture is occasionally required. Extensor tendon adhesions also limit active finger flexion and require the same treatment.

Plate 4.51

Upper Limb: PART I

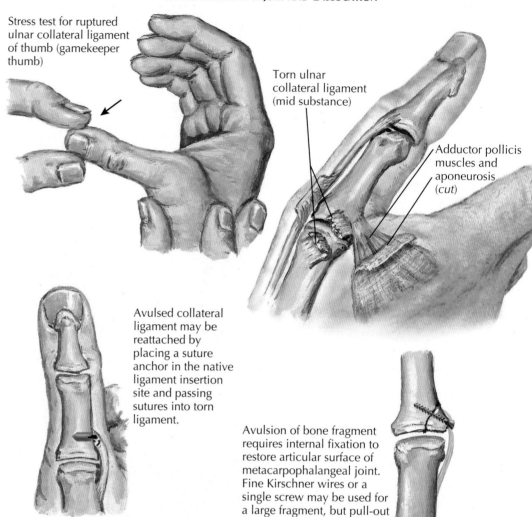

Stress test for ruptured ulnar collateral ligament of thumb (gamekeeper thumb)

Torn ulnar collateral ligament (mid substance)

Adductor pollicis muscles and aponeurosis (*cut*)

Avulsed collateral ligament may be reattached by placing a suture anchor in the native ligament insertion site and passing sutures into torn ligament.

Avulsion of bone fragment requires internal fixation to restore articular surface of metacarpophalangeal joint. Fine Kirschner wires or a single screw may be used for a large fragment, but pull-out sutures or a suture anchor may be advantageous for a small fragment.

Pure dislocation of carpometacarpal joint of thumb without fracture is reducible but unstable. It should be pinned to trapezium, as for Bennett fracture.

Position of hand on cassette for Robert view (true anteroposterior) radiograph. Robert view best visualizes carpometacarpal joint of thumb, and pathologic process may be missed if this view is not taken.

CARPOMETACARPAL AND METACARPOPHALANGEAL INJURIES OTHER THAN FRACTURE

The thumb acts as a very mobile post that opposes the actions of the index, middle, ring, and small fingers. The stability of the thumb is therefore very important in hand function.

INJURY TO ULNAR COLLATERAL LIGAMENT OF THE THUMB

In the metacarpophalangeal joint of the thumb, injury to the ulnar collateral ligament destroys joint stability and impairs the ability to pinch. Known as the gamekeeper thumb, this injury is a common consequence of skiing, motor vehicle, and occupational accidents.

Any injury to the ulnar side of the metacarpophalangeal joint of the thumb must be evaluated with a stress test to determine the integrity of the ulnar collateral ligament. The stress test should be performed using digital block anesthesia. If the test shows joint instability, the ulnar collateral ligament should be repaired surgically.

Surgical examination often reveals the adductor tendon aponeurosis interposed between the torn ends of the ulnar collateral ligament; this condition, called the Stener lesion, prevents healing. A tear in the substance of the ligament itself is repaired with interrupted sutures. If the ligament is avulsed from the bone, repair with a pull-out wire or bone suture anchor is needed. Primary repair can be augmented by incorporating a nonabsorbable suture tape into the repair and anchoring it proximally and distally. Avulsion of a bone fragment together with the ligament requires reduction of the fragment and fixation with a small screw, a pull-out wire, or Kirschner wires.

To ensure stability, a Kirschner wire is sometimes placed across the joint to relieve the tension on the repaired ligament. After ligament repair, the thumb is immobilized in a cast for at least 4 weeks. The patient can begin guarded activity at 4 weeks, after the cast and pin are removed. Early anatomic repair of gamekeeper thumb produces quite satisfactory results.

DISLOCATION OF CARPOMETACARPAL JOINT

This thumb injury can also be quite disabling. Because of the configuration of the carpometacarpal joint, dislocations are inherently unstable. Although reduction of the carpometacarpal dislocation is easy, maintaining the reduction in a plaster cast is very difficult.

Plate 4.52

Hand and Finger

CARPOMETACARPAL AND METACARPOPHALANGEAL JOINT INJURY

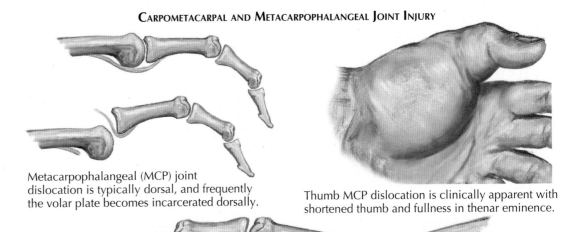

Metacarpophalangeal (MCP) joint dislocation is typically dorsal, and frequently the volar plate becomes incarcerated dorsally.

Thumb MCP dislocation is clinically apparent with shortened thumb and fullness in thenar eminence.

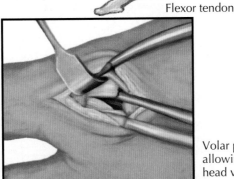

Flexor tendon

Lumbrical

Volar plate is flipped through joint and dorsal to metacarpal head. Closed reduction is often impossible due to noose created by lumbrical radially and flexor tendons ulnarly that tighten around metacarpal neck with traction on finger, preventing head from slipping through.

Volar plate is split via a dorsal approach, allowing it to be passed around metacarpal head volarly and relocating the joint.

CARPOMETACARPAL AND METACARPOPHALANGEAL INJURIES OTHER THAN FRACTURE (Continued)

Therefore, in most carpometacarpal dislocations, the reduction must be pinned to ensure stability. The pin is placed across the joint and maintained for 4 to 6 weeks to allow the joint capsule to heal. Chronic, undiagnosed, or recurrent dislocations of the carpometacarpal joint of the thumb can be treated either with ligament reconstruction, using the flexor carpi radialis tendon, or with arthrodesis of the carpometacarpal joint.

Dislocation of the carpometacarpal joint is also common in the small finger and lesser in the ring finger and is usually due to a punch against a wall in a fit of anger. Because there is significant mobility in the ring and small finger carpometacarpal joint, it remains unstable unless reduced and it often requires temporary pinning. There is also a high incidence of fracture of either the base of the metacarpal or the dorsal articular surface of the hamate that requires open reduction and internal fixation to restore the articular surface.

DISLOCATION OF METACARPOPHALANGEAL JOINT

Dorsal dislocation of the metacarpal phalangeal joint occurs more commonly in the thumb than in the lesser fingers, and the direction of dislocation is defined by the direction of the distal bone. These can be difficult to reduce owing to the interposition of the volar plate, which makes closed reduction difficult at times. Open reduction in the thumb is often easily achieved from a dorsal incision, and then the volar plate that is reduced to the palmar position scars back down in place after immobilization of the joint in 30 degrees of flexion. If

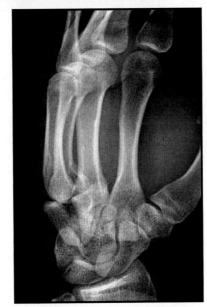

Small finger MCP joint fracture dislocation with coronal split of hamate and base of metacarpal dislocated into hamate

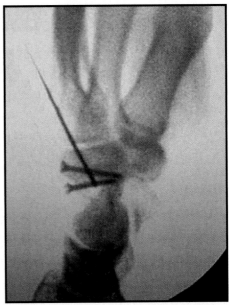

Postreduction and screw fixation of the hamate and pinning of metacarpal to hamate to maintain reduction

unstable, this joint can be held with a pin across the metacarpophalangeal joint for 4 weeks. A palmar approach to the metacarpophalangeal joint allows for direct repair of the volar plate to the volar neck of the metacarpal with a bone anchor.

In the lesser fingers, closed reduction becomes a challenge not only because the volar plate is trapped but also because the flexor tendons wrap around one side of the metacarpal neck and the lumbrical muscle around the opposite side and any kind of traction tightens this "noose," preventing reduction of the palmarly displaced metacarpal head. Both dorsal and volar approaches have been described to open reduce this dislocation. More uncommonly, palmar dislocations of the thumb and lesser fingers do occur and operative reduction is usually required.

Plate 4.53

Upper Limb: PART I

Dorsal and Palmar Interphalangeal Joint Dislocations

Dorsal dislocation (most common) is usually reducible by closed means, immobilized with dorsal splint for 1 week, then active range-of-motion exercises begun with dorsal blocking splint preventing full extension.

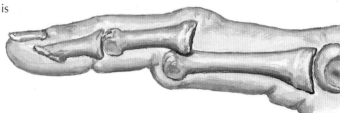

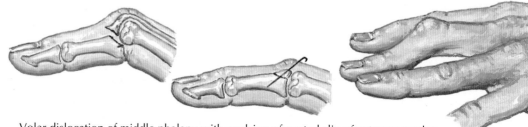

Volar dislocation of middle phalanx with avulsion of central slip of extensor tendon, with or without bone fragment. Failure to recognize and properly treat this condition results in boutonnière deformity and severely restricted function.

Palmar dislocation (uncommon) causes boutonnière deformity. Central slip of extensor tendon often torn, requiring open fixation, followed by palmar splinting to allow passive and active exercises of distal interphalangeal joint.

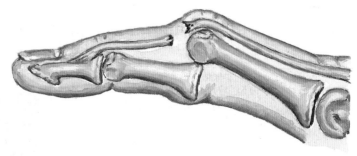

Dislocation of Proximal Interphalangeal Joint

The proximal interphalangeal joint is basically a hinge joint supported by the architecture of the bone and by strong collateral ligaments on either side, which are, in turn, reinforced by a strong volar ligament or plate. The dorsal capsule of the proximal interphalangeal joint is strengthened by the central slip of the extensor tendon and by the insertions of the lateral bands of the extensor tendon hood. Ligament injuries of the proximal interphalangeal joint, the most common injuries of the hand, include simple sprains of the collateral ligament or the volar plate (most common), complete dislocations, and the most severe injuries—fracture-dislocations.

Any injury to the proximal interphalangeal joint can significantly affect motion and function of the finger and hand because the lesser fingers typically work in concert together and dysfunction of one finger hinders the remaining fingers. During the diagnostic evaluation, the examiner must palpate specific areas for tenderness and assess the stability of the joint both actively, as the patient flexes the finger, and, passively, as the examiner moves the finger.

The most common dislocation of the proximal interphalangeal joint, the *dorsal* dislocation, is often called the coach's finger. Frequently occurring in athletic events, the dorsal dislocation is usually reduced by trainers or coaches shortly after injury. The uncommon *volar* dislocation of the proximal interphalangeal joint is a more serious injury because it disrupts the central slip of the extensor mechanism. Unless properly treated by splinting with the joint in extension, volar dislocation can result in a disabling boutonnière deformity. *Rotational* dislocations are rare. A unique aspect of this type of dislocation is the appearance of the phalanges

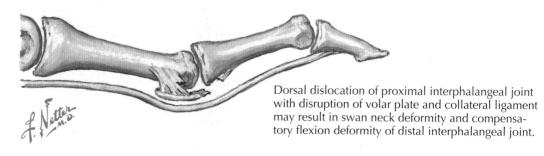

Dorsal dislocation of proximal interphalangeal joint with disruption of volar plate and collateral ligament may result in swan neck deformity and compensatory flexion deformity of distal interphalangeal joint.

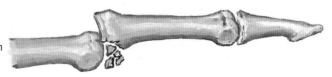

Fracture-dislocation of middle phalanx with fragmented volar lip. This disabling injury is often missed because of failure to take a true lateral radiograph.

on the lateral radiograph: the proximal phalanx is seen in an oblique plane and the middle phalanx in a true lateral plane.

TREATMENT OF DORSAL AND ROTATIONAL DISLOCATIONS

Although closed reduction usually produces a satisfactory result, open reduction is occasionally required to restore the phalanges to their anatomic positions. If there is evidence of instability after reduction, simple dorsal and rotational dislocations of the proximal interphalangeal joint can be treated with splinting for 3 weeks; if the joint is stable, early active motion with buddy taping is prescribed for 4 to 6 weeks.

Fracture-dislocations are the most severe and disabling injuries of the proximal interphalangeal joint. In addition to dislocation, a fracture disrupts the volar

Plate 4.54

Hand and Finger

TREATMENT OF PROXIMAL INTERPHALANGEAL JOINT DISLOCATION

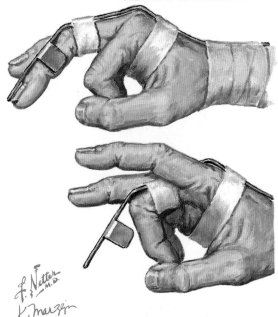

Extension block splint useful for dislocation of proximal interphalangeal (PIP) joint with small or comminuted fragment from base of middle phalanx. After reduction achieved and radiographically documented, amount of flexion necessary to maintain reduction determined, and splint adjusted to permit no extension beyond that. Proximal phalanx must be secured to splint with adhesive tape. Active flexion at PIP joint is encouraged. Extension block splint gradually and progressively adjusted so that functional range of motion achieved in 3–4 weeks.

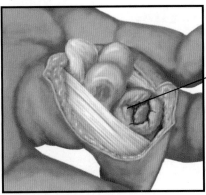

Depressed volar fragment

Depressed, arthritic volar half of middle phalangeal base

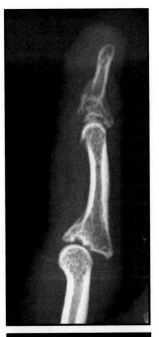

Healed and arthritic PIP joint after dorsal fracture dislocation with residual dorsal subluxation

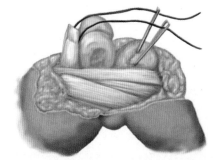

Volar plate arthroplasty is performed by attaching the volar plate to the middle of the base with sutures passed through bone and tied dorsally. This relocates the joint and creates a smooth articulating surface.

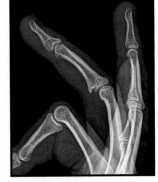

View after volar plate arthroplasty demonstrating joint relocated and joint space preserved

DISLOCATION OF PROXIMAL INTERPHALANGEAL JOINT (Continued)

surface of the middle phalanx, resulting in both dorsal and volar instability. These injuries are often missed because the dislocation reduces spontaneously and patients do not come to medical attention and/or the fracture of the volar lip of the middle phalanx appears quite insignificant on the radiograph to a non-hand specialist and restricted motion is not instituted, with subsequent resultant subluxation and joint degeneration.

Some fracture-dislocations can be treated with closed reduction of the dislocation and use of an extension block splint. The splint allows full flexion of the finger and a range of extension that maintains the reduction and stability of the proximal interphalangeal joint. This method of treatment requires close radiographic follow-up. As healing increases the stability on the volar side, the amount of extension can be gradually increased until the joint remains stable in full extension.

Fracture-dislocation with a large fragment from the volar lip requires open reduction with Kirschner wire or screw fixation. Late reconstruction of this injury involves either arthrodesis, volar plate interposition arthroplasty, or prosthetic arthroplasty.

In all injuries of the proximal interphalangeal joint, the patient should be informed that the joint will remain enlarged for a long time, possibly many years, and that some loss of motion is quite common.

TREATMENT OF VOLAR DISLOCATIONS

In the more severe volar dislocation, the proximal interphalangeal joint must be splinted in extension for

4 to 6 weeks to avoid creating a boutonnière deformity. A rare injury of the proximal interphalangeal joint, fracture of the dorsal lip of the middle phalanx results in an avulsion of the central slip of the extensor mechanism. This injury must be treated with open reduction and, if necessary, pin or screw fixation of the fracture

fragment. Failure to recognize this injury and restore the attachment of the central slip to the middle phalanx leads to a boutonnière deformity, with chronic pain and instability. If boutonnière deformity develops, arthrodesis of the proximal interphalangeal joint is often the only salvage procedure possible.

Plate 4.55

Upper Limb: PART I

Mallet finger

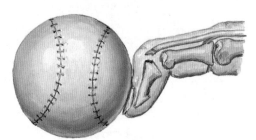

Usually caused by direct blow on extended distal phalanx, as in baseball, volleyball, or basketball

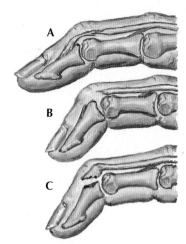

Degrees of mallet finger injury. A. Extensor tendon stretched but not completely severed; mild finger drop and weak extensor ability retained. **B**. Tendon torn from its insertion. **C**. Bone fragment avulsed with tendon. In **B** and **C** there is a 40- to 45-degree flexion deformity and loss of active extension.

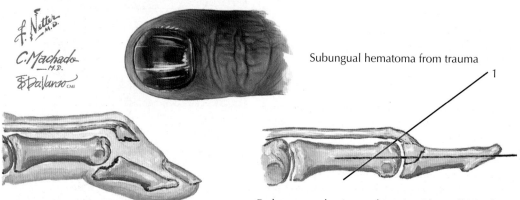

Treatment for mallet finger of tendon origin. A. Padded dorsal splint. **B**. Unpadded volar splint. **C**. Stack splint. Proximal interphalangeal joint left free for active exercise.

INJURIES TO THE FINGERTIP

As the sensory input to the upper extremities, the fingertips encounter their environment first and are often unfortunately injured. Whether it be on a sporting field or in the workplace, the fingertips are subject to cuts, burns, punctures, and sudden impact and crushing injuries. It is of paramount importance to try and restore the fingertips for optimal hand and upper extremity function.

FRACTURE OF THE DISTAL PHALANX AND SUBUNGUAL HEMATOMA

Impact injury to the fingertip often causes a hematoma due to bleeding from either the nail bed or an underlying fracture of the distal phalanx. This hematoma is often trapped under the nail plate, causing significant pressure to build up and resultant pain. When the pain is significant, this can be relieved by drainage of the hematoma. It is important to obtain a radiograph to rule out a fracture because, once drained, this hole in the nail plate becomes a portal to an infection in the distal phalangeal bone if not cared for appropriately. An old treatment of heating a paperclip under a flame does not properly sterilize the metal tip, and therefore only a sterile needle should be used. A 22-gauge needle can be used by hand to adequately drill a small perforation in the nail plate and provide evacuation of the hematoma. The patient should be given an antibiotic if the injury dictates, and the nail plate should be kept clean. A short splint blocking the distal interphalangeal joint will allow for pain relief and protection of the underlying injured fingertip.

MALLET FINGER

Hyperflexion that disrupts the extensor mechanism of the distal phalanx causes a mallet finger, an injury common in ball players. Three types of injury occur: stretching of the extensor tendon past its elastic limit, which causes multiple interstitial tears; complete disruption of the extensor tendon; and avulsion fracture of the base of the distal phalanx. The patient with mallet finger often does not appreciate the severity of the injury, and even the examining physician may not recognize the injury. The acute signs are tenderness over the dorsum of the distal interphalangeal joint and inability to actively extend the distal phalanx.

Treatment consists of splinting the distal interphalangeal joint in extension. The splint should be placed on the dorsal aspect during the day so the volar surface

Subungual hematoma from trauma

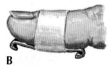 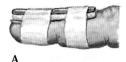 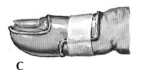

Mallet finger of bone origin. Avulsion of bone fragment and volar subluxation of distal phalanx.

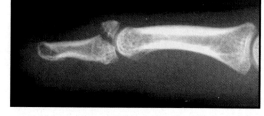

Early open reduction and repair with small Kirschner wire indicated, but difficulty of exposure and small size of fragment present problems. Displaced dorsal fragment prevented from retraction with wire 1 and subluxation with wire 2.

With subluxation and flexion at the DIP joint, a compensatory hyperextension occurs at the PIP joint, creating a swan neck deformity.

of the finger can still be used in opposition; it is worn continuously for 6 to 8 weeks, then only at night for an additional 3 to 4 weeks. A palmar splint is used at night to relieve the continuous pressure on the dorsal skin. The patient should be warned that splinting may cause some skin loss over the dorsum of the distal phalanx and that full extension may never be regained.

Mallet finger with avulsion of a large bone fragment may be associated with volar subluxation of the distal interphalangeal joint. Surgical repair, although indicated, is difficult because the blood supply to the skin is poor, the fragment is quite small, and a good reduction with Kirschner wires is often difficult to maintain. Therefore a dorsal blocking pin is more effective to prevent proximal retraction of the tendon-bone complex. A pin across the joint ensures concentric reduction and good soft tissue healing to avoid recurrent subluxation.

Plate 4.56

Hand and Finger

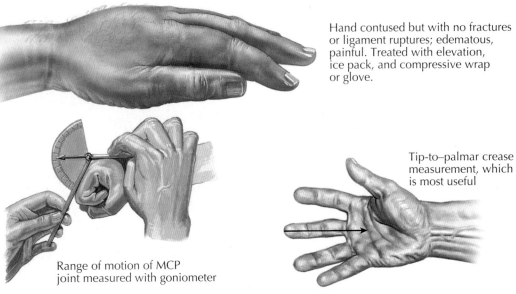

Hand contused but with no fractures or ligament ruptures; edematous, painful. Treated with elevation, ice pack, and compressive wrap or glove.

Range of motion of MCP joint measured with goniometer

Tip-to–palmar crease measurement, which is most useful

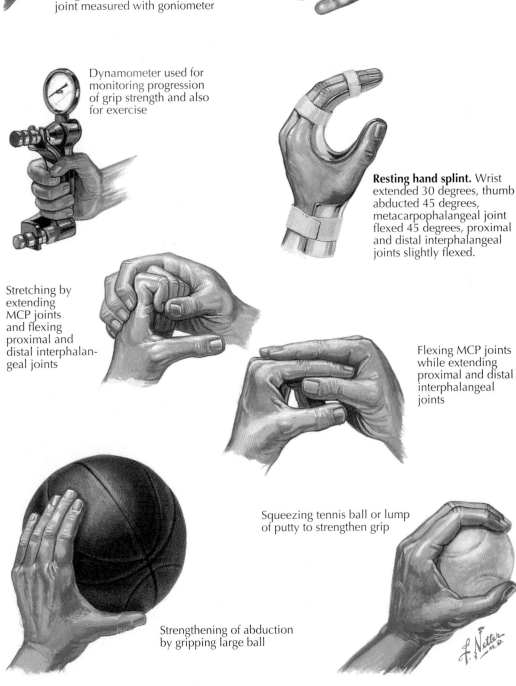

Dynamometer used for monitoring progression of grip strength and also for exercise

Resting hand splint. Wrist extended 30 degrees, thumb abducted 45 degrees, metacarpophalangeal joint flexed 45 degrees, proximal and distal interphalangeal joints slightly flexed.

Stretching by extending MCP joints and flexing proximal and distal interphalangeal joints

Flexing MCP joints while extending proximal and distal interphalangeal joints

Squeezing tennis ball or lump of putty to strengthen grip

Strengthening of abduction by gripping large ball

REHABILITATION AFTER INJURY TO HAND AND FINGERS

Failure to identify a significant hand injury may result in prolonged disability due to excessive scarring, which can significantly reduce hand and finger motion. Early diagnosis and treatment and proper rehabilitation are needed to establish full function. The goal of treatment of hand and finger injuries is to promote healing of the injured structures while maintaining a functional range of motion and preventing the formation of joint contractures. Because certain structures of the hand are fragile, the rehabilitation team must clearly understand the extent and severity of the injury and take appropriate precautions, as identified by the attending hand surgeon, before initiating rehabilitation therapy.

The first step in hand and finger rehabilitation consists of assessment of muscle strength and restriction of range of motion, with formal measurement of the motion of each involved joint on both hands. After the baseline factors are established, progress should be monitored at weekly or biweekly intervals. During passive range-of-motion exercises, the range of motion should be increased to the point of discomfort, but not beyond. As the injury heals, a more aggressive program can be adopted, including active and active-assisted range-of-motion exercises of the affected joints. Importantly, soft tissue swelling must resolve before full range of motion can be achieved, and all efforts should be placed on this goal.

If possible, the hand should be warmed in a paraffin bath or deep moist or dry heat before the range-of-motion activity. The hand should then be kept in the stretched position until it has cooled to normal temperatures. Exercises can be performed by the patient at home, with weekly monitoring by the physical therapist.

Plate 4.57

Upper Limb: PART I

AMPUTATION OF PHALANX

Amputation of distal phalanx

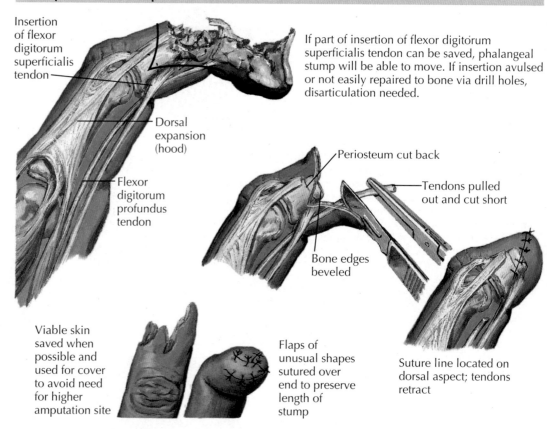

Formation of flap

Nail matrix completely removed

Sharp bone edges rounded

Periosteum cut back

Soft tissues mobilized from bone

Scar on dorsal aspect; end cover ample but not redundant

Amputation of middle phalanx

Insertion of flexor digitorum superficialis tendon

Dorsal expansion (hood)

Flexor digitorum profundus tendon

If part of insertion of flexor digitorum superficialis tendon can be saved, phalangeal stump will be able to move. If insertion avulsed or not easily repaired to bone via drill holes, disarticulation needed.

Periosteum cut back

Tendons pulled out and cut short

Bone edges beveled

Viable skin saved when possible and used for cover to avoid need for higher amputation site

Flaps of unusual shapes sutured over end to preserve length of stump

Suture line located on dorsal aspect; tendons retract

AMPUTATION IN THE HAND

Amputations in the hand are almost always traumatic in origin; only rarely is amputation required to treat gangrene, infection, or tumor. Traumatic injuries to the hand are quite common, particularly in persons who use power tools in the workplace or the home. The general principles of amputation apply to procedures in the hand, and preservation of length is especially critical. Every effort should be made to salvage as much of each digit as possible.

The most important digit is the thumb, and it is absolutely essential to try to preserve both its length and function after injury. Often, severe injury or amputation of one of the other four fingers is best treated with primary amputation, because the remaining fingers can readily assume most functions. If the other digits are healthy, then prolonged or repeated attempts to reimplant a single finger or restore function to a finger (as distinguished from the thumb) may be time consuming, costly, and frustrating for the patient. Immediate amputation, combined with an aggressive and immediate rehabilitation program, may often be best for the patient. When multiple fingers are injured, however, the decision to amputate any injured finger must be considered very carefully.

After injury to the hand, amputation should be considered only when three or more of the five tissue areas (skin, tendon, nerve, bone, and joint) require special procedures for salvage. Age is also a factor in the decision to amputate. Amputation is rarely indicated in a child, even after a severe injury. In patients older than 50 years, however, removal of a single finger, except the thumb, is often the preferred option, particularly when both the digital nerves and the flexor tendons have been transected.

AMPUTATION OF FINGERTIP

With fingertip amputations, it is also important to preserve as much length as possible. The primary factor influencing the ability to preserve length is the integrity of the volar skin. In fingertip injuries, the volar skin should be preserved, if possible, for use as a flap; this area comprises the best tissue for digital function. If the volar skin has been amputated or destroyed, the finger must be shortened to ensure that the volar surface of the residual digit is covered with full-thickness, sensate skin that will be durable and functional. The digital nerves should be assessed carefully. Each nerve should be transected under gentle traction and allowed to retract deep into the soft tissues to avoid painful neuromas at the end of the finger. The end of the bone should be contoured to eliminate bony prominences and a club-shaped stump. The flap should cover the end of the

Plate 4.58

Hand and Finger

AMPUTATION OF THUMB AND DEEPENING OF THENAR WEB CLEFT

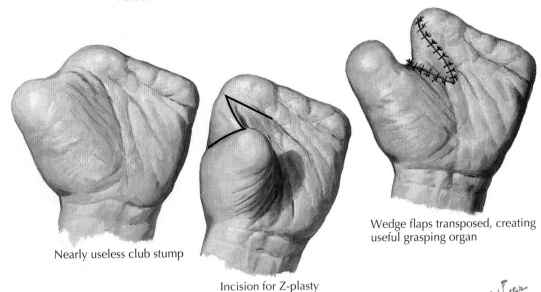

Nearly useless club stump

Incision for Z-plasty

Wedge flaps transposed, creating useful grasping organ

AMPUTATION IN THE HAND (Continued)

stump securely, but a redundant skin flap should be avoided. Excessive tension on the skin edges must also be avoided to prevent further necrosis of the skin flaps. It is not advisable to trim corners significantly because scar contraction and stump molding in therapy will provide adequate contouring.

When the very tip of the finger has been amputated, the roughened end of the distal phalanx should be smoothed and any protruding bony spikes removed. The volar skin can be mobilized distally by careful dissection along deep tissue planes just superficial to the flexor tendon sheath. The flap is brought up to and sutured to the fingernail, allowing wound closure and the resultant scar to be positioned on the dorsal aspect of the finger, away from the area that will be exposed to repetitive trauma.

When it is essential to preserve length, larger defects that cannot be closed primarily are treated with a *thick* split-thickness skin graft. The amputation bed is debrided of all necrotic and potentially infected tissue. A thick split-thickness skin graft can be harvested from the volar aspect of the forearm or the medial aspect of the arm just below the axilla. The donor site is closed primarily and the free graft sutured securely over the raw amputation stump. *Thin* split-thickness skin grafts should be avoided because they are not durable and will break down with repeated use, necessitating later revision of the amputation to a higher level.

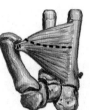
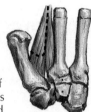
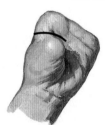

Distal portion of adductor pollicis muscle removed (*broken line*). Insertion reattached, if necessary.

Thenar half of first dorsal interosseous muscle removed

Insertion of flexor pollicis brevis muscle reattached, if necessary

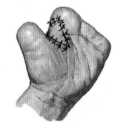

Use of skin graft

Transverse incision

Full-thickness skin graft in place

Skin graft can also be used to deepen cleft.

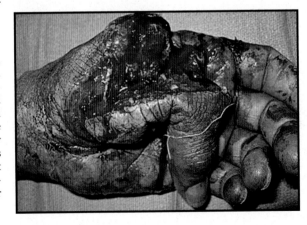

Traumatic saw injury to the thumb spared vascular structures, allowing for easier reconstruction compared with grinder injury.

AMPUTATION OF DISTAL PHALANX

If the injury damages the distal phalanx—particularly when the damage extends into the nail matrix—the nail will probably be irregular and painful when it grows back. Therefore, in traumatic amputations through the distal phalanx that involve most of the fingernail, the entire nail matrix should be removed. Because the nail matrix extends considerably proximal to the skin fold, extensive dissection may be necessary to remove it completely. The distal portion of the phalanx should be

removed as well, but the insertions of the extensor and flexor tendons on the most proximal portion of the distal phalanx should be left intact. The entire nail matrix is identified and sharply excised, and the periosteum overlying the distal phalanx is resected to avoid creating a bone spur. As in fingertip amputations, a volar skin flap is created and the wound closure positioned dorsally. Enough skin should be left to allow closure without tension but also without redundant tissue.

AMPUTATION THROUGH MIDDLE PHALANX

A crushing injury that destroys the distal phalanx and a portion of the middle phalanx necessitates amputation through the middle phalanx. If the insertion of the flexor digitorum superficialis into the base of the middle phalanx can be preserved, some function of the proximal interphalangeal joint may be preserved as well. If the insertion of the tendon has been

Plate 4.59

Upper Limb: PART I

THUMB LENGTHENING POST AMPUTATION

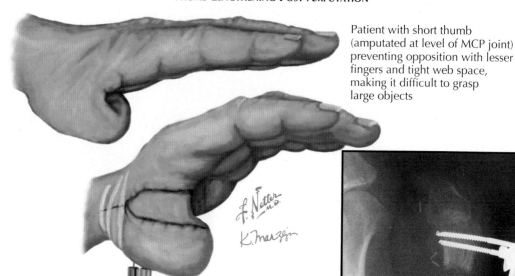

Patient with short thumb (amputated at level of MCP joint) preventing opposition with lesser fingers and tight web space, making it difficult to grasp large objects

Third surgery to deepen web space to allow grasping for large objects. The web space is skin grafted and the thumb is held maximally abducted with two Kirschner wires joining the thumb and index metacarpal.

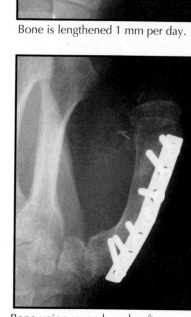

Bone is lengthened 1 mm per day.

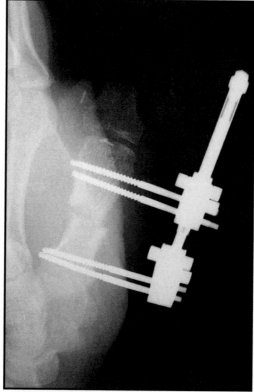

Osteotomy of thumb metacarpal with placement of lengthening external fixator (first surgery)

Bone union several weeks after second surgery to remove external fixator and placement of iliac crest bone autograft and plate/screw fixation

AMPUTATION IN THE HAND (Continued)

avulsed, it can be repaired with a grasping stitch in each slip and then sutured to the bone stump through a drill hole. If the sublimis cannot be repaired, there is little reason to preserve the middle phalanx, and disarticulation through the proximal interphalangeal joint should be considered. The nerves are carefully transected under tension and allowed to retract into the soft tissues. Bony spikes are removed, and the bone ends are smoothed to maximize function of the amputation stump. At this level, circulation to the residual skin flaps is usually quite good, and if there is any chance of preserving some function of the proximal interphalangeal joint, irregularly shaped flaps may be used to cover the stump to preserve length.

AMPUTATION OF FINGER AND RAY

Occasionally, an entire finger must be amputated because of severe injury, aggressive infection, or malignant tumor. Generally, the distal half of the respective metacarpal is resected as well—a procedure called a ray amputation. When the finger is amputated at the metacarpophalangeal level, leaving the metacarpal intact, a prominent stump persists in the palm. When the patient makes a fist, a hole is created through which objects can fall. The residual metacarpal is a significant problem after injuries of the index finger. If the index metacarpal is left in place, opposition of the thumb to the remaining long finger is difficult. Removal of most of the index metacarpal allows the thumb to lie closer to the middle finger, improving grip and overall function of the hand. Thus, when amputation is necessary at the metacarpophalangeal level, ray resection is often the treatment of choice. Central (long, ring) ray resection is accompanied by reconstruction of the intermetacarpal ligaments and bringing together the adjacent metacarpal heads to close the gap between the remaining fingers.

DEEPENING OF THENAR WEB CLEFT

The most important digit of the hand is the thumb, and all efforts should be made to preserve it and as much of its length as possible. Sometimes, it is even preferable to leave an insensate, motionless stump if the only alternative is complete amputation of the thumb. When all of the fingers have been amputated, gross gripping and prehension can be restored to some degree by deepening the thenar web space.

Deepening of the web space between the thumb and index metacarpals is accomplished by resecting a portion of the adductor pollicis muscle and the thenar half of the first dorsal interosseous muscle. A Z-plasty technique is used, and the skin is incised to provide access to the muscles for resection. Then, closure of the Z-plasty flaps creates a cleft in the web space. The residual adductor muscle is used to power the thumb metacarpal for gross prehension.

Plate 4.60

Hand and Finger

MICROSURGICAL INSTRUMENTATION FOR REPLANTATION

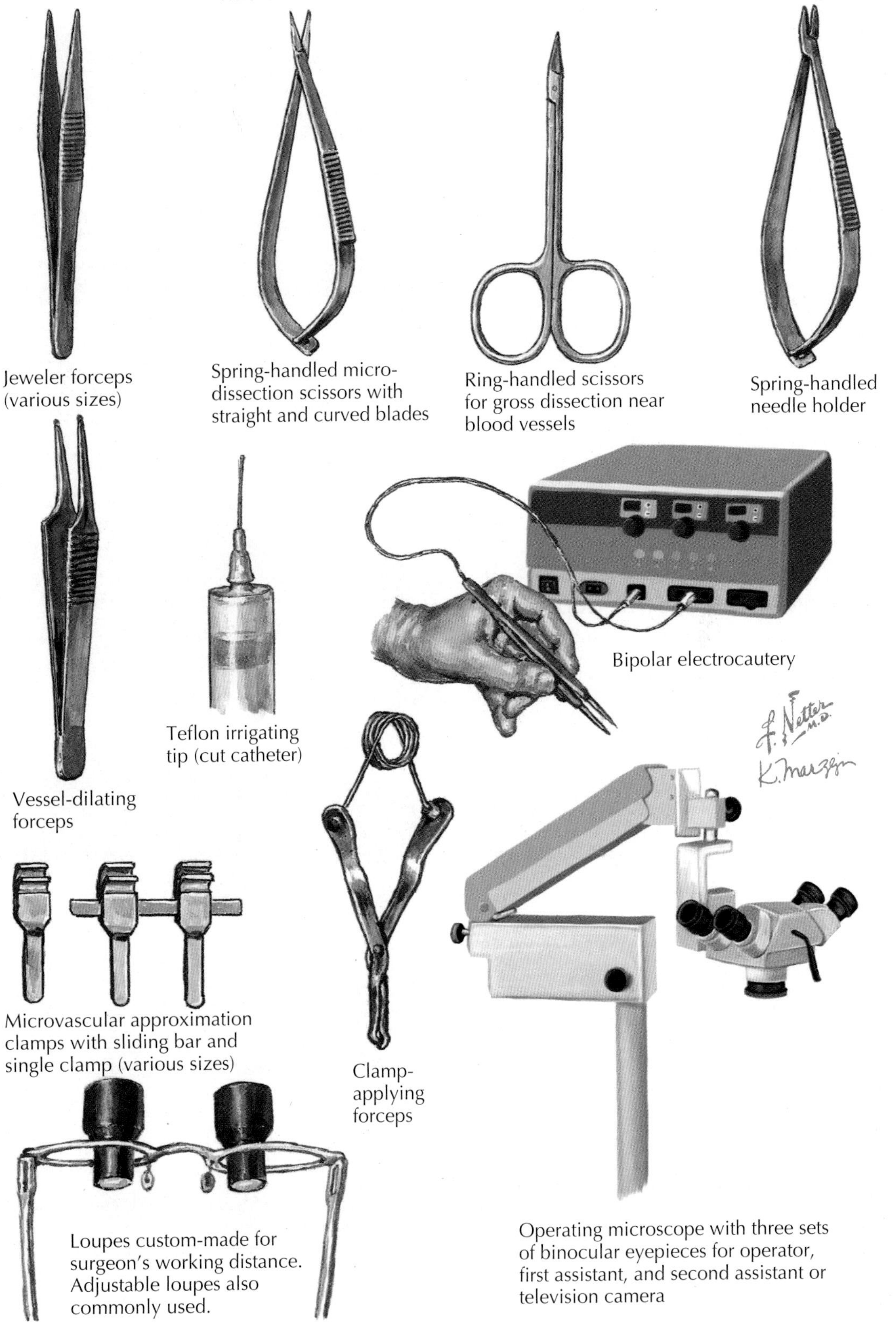

Jeweler forceps (various sizes)

Spring-handled micro-dissection scissors with straight and curved blades

Ring-handled scissors for gross dissection near blood vessels

Spring-handled needle holder

Vessel-dilating forceps

Teflon irrigating tip (cut catheter)

Bipolar electrocautery

Microvascular approximation clamps with sliding bar and single clamp (various sizes)

Clamp-applying forceps

Loupes custom-made for surgeon's working distance. Adjustable loupes also commonly used.

Operating microscope with three sets of binocular eyepieces for operator, first assistant, and second assistant or television camera

REPLANTATION

Replantation is defined as the reattachment of a completely severed part. The first successful replantation of an above-elbow amputation was reported in 1962 by Malt and McLehman. In 1965 Komatsu and Tamai reported the successful replantation of a thumb. The development of this type of microsurgery has been greatly aided by advances in optical instrumentation and especially in the manufacture of needles and sutures fine enough to repair vessels 1 mm in diameter or less.

Replantation is not suitable or possible for all patients with amputations. Great care must be given to the assessment of patients and their requirements. The surgical technique is exacting and the postoperative care prolonged and difficult. However, with an experienced team and a well-informed and motivated patient, the procedure can produce good functional and cosmetic results.

Amputations and replantations are categorized as major or minor. A major amputation involves muscle and is treated differently from a minor amputation, which involves tendons but no muscle. Because both types of amputation require great expertise and special surgical techniques, patients with amputations should be referred to centers where such resources are available.

INDICATIONS

The decision to undertake replantation of a severed part is influenced by many factors, especially the level and mechanism of the amputation and, equally important, the needs and desires of the patient. There are no hard-and-fast rules to help in this decision. The patient and the family must be fully informed about the possible outcomes and consequences of replantation in terms of hospitalization, postoperative care, and hand therapy.

In a child, replantation of any amputation should probably be attempted. In adults, replantation is indicated for amputation of the thumb, multiple digits, hand, distal forearm, or single digit distal to the insertion of the flexor digitorum superficialis tendon. Replantation should be considered whenever the amputated part is

crucial to hand function or when good functional restoration of the part can be expected.

CONTRAINDICATIONS

The only absolute contraindication to replantation is a health condition, either a preexisting illness or associated injuries that precludes a prolonged surgical procedure. Treatment of other severe injuries,

which often accompany a major amputation, obviously takes priority over the replantation effort. Relative contraindications are numerous and can be either patient related or injury related.

Systemic Illness

Diabetes, renal failure in a patient treated with dialysis, generalized vascular disorders of the upper limb, and advanced connective tissue disease all reduce the likelihood

Plate 4.61

Upper Limb: PART I

DEBRIDEMENT, INCISIONS, AND REPAIR OF BONE IN REPLANTATION OF DIGIT

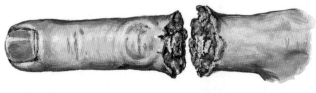

Digit traumatically amputated through proximal phalanx (before debridement)

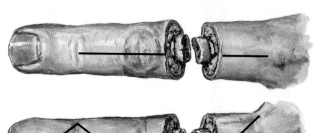

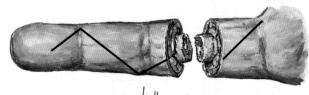

Debridement
Proximal and distal ends of amputation site cleaned and debrided, removing all nonviable tissue. Bone ends not yet shortened. Incisions: longitudinal on dorsal surface, zigzag on volar surface.

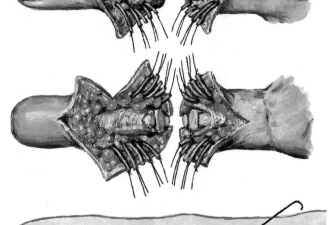

Trimming of bone
Bone ends shortened, flaps reflected, and structures to be joined identified and marked with sutures (one for veins and nerves, two for arteries)

REPLANTATION (Continued)

of a successful outcome because of associated microvascular damage and possible vessel thrombosis.

Multiple Level Injuries

Replantation is rarely successful when there is widespread vascular damage due to multiple level injuries. If the injury is both above and below the elbow, however, every attempt should be made to save the elbow because the presence of the joint improves the function of a prosthesis.

Extreme Contamination

Replantation is contraindicated when both the stump and the amputated part have been inoculated with soil bacteria (particularly with *Clostridium* species). This degree of contamination is common in some farm injuries and in war injuries.

Age

The patient's age alone is not a contraindication to replantation, but it must be considered. Although the tiny size of infants' vessels reduces the chance that the replanted part will survive, the function gained by a successful replantation is often quite good. In elderly persons, useful or functional recovery is not a realistic expectation. Even in patients with mild degenerative joint disease, postoperative edema and the required postoperative splinting lead to stiffness in the whole hand. Therefore replantation in an elderly patient must be carefully considered.

Amputation of Single Digit

Replantation of a finger amputated proximal to the insertion of the flexor digitorum superficialis tendon on the middle phalanx may be contraindicated because motion is limited by the severe scarring and tendon adhesions that develop after replantation. The index finger is not an essential finger; if the return of function or sensation after replantation is poor, the patient may prefer to use the normal adjacent middle finger for tasks usually accomplished with the index finger. A stiff

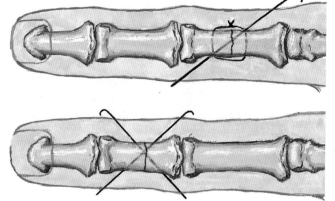

Repair of bone
Bone fixed with Kirschner wire inserted diagonally plus interosseous wire to prevent rotational displacement. Sometimes, 90-90 interosseous wires without Kirschner wires or two cross Kirschner wires are preferred. Unstable fractures may require plate/screw fixation.

little finger does not flex well in power grip, often catching in clothing. The benefits of replantation of either of these digits must therefore be carefully assessed.

Avulsion

The likelihood of successful replantation of digits or limbs torn from the body is poor because of the extent of injury and the amount of dissection needed to escape the zone of injury. A red line on the skin overlying the neurovascular bundle of a digit suggests an extensive avulsion of these structures and a poor chance of recovery. Ring avulsions are the most difficult avulsion injuries to replant. Even major vessel repair may not revascularize the devascularized flexor tendons and proximal

Plate 4.62

Hand and Finger

REPAIR OF BLOOD VESSELS AND NERVES

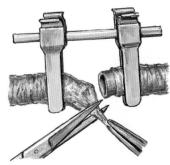

Vessel ends positioned in approximation clamps. Adventitia removed by pulling it down over vessel end, cutting it, and letting it retract.

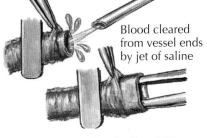

Blood cleared from vessel ends by jet of saline

Vessel ends dilated 1½ times normal diameter

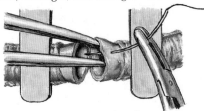

First stay suture applied with tip of forceps in lumen to protect back wall from needle and to provide counterpressure.

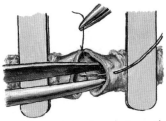

Second stay suture placed at one-third of vessel circumference away from first suture. This allows back wall to drop away, which protects it and facilitates later suturing.

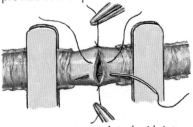

Gaps between stay sutures closed with interrupted sutures. Vessel turned over for suturing back wall. For large arteries, running suture may be used, carefully avoiding purse-stringing. In areas where clamp does not fit, back wall repaired first, with top of vessel and lumen in view at all times.

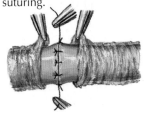

Veins anastomosed using similar technique; because they are very fragile, veins must be handled with great care. Clamps may be used but very cautiously.

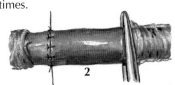

Test for patency and security of anastomosis. **1.** Nontoothed jeweler forceps applied just downstream of suture line. Second forceps applied just distal to first and slid farther downstream to milk blood from intervening segment. **2.** First forceps removed to allow flow of blood into empty segment; leaks noted.

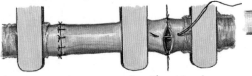

If vessel defect too long to permit anastomosis without tension, vein graft may be interposed. Graft harvested from dorsum of finger or volar aspect of wrist; for vein replantations in lower limb of structures larger than digit, graft obtained from saphenous vein.

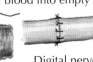

Digital nerves contain only sensory fibers and are repaired with simple sutures through epineurium only.

REPLANTATION (Continued)

interphalangeal joint; and although the finger may be successfully replanted, it often becomes stiff and atrophic. A revision amputation may be a better treatment choice, especially in the older patient.

Prolonged Ischemia

Either warm (32°C) or cold (5 to 10°C) ischemia seriously reduces the likelihood of a successful replantation. Unfortunately, studies have not yet shown what duration of warm or cold ischemia is critical. Most amputated parts sustain some warm ischemia until medical help arrives. Once the replantation procedure begins, the part goes through a second period of warm ischemia until vascular continuity is restored. Cooling (cold ischemia) to about 10°C clearly helps to preserve the amputated part. Given adequate cooling, major replantations have been successfully performed 8 to 16 hours after amputation, and minor replantations have been successful even after 18 to 30 hours.

PREOPERATIVE MANAGEMENT

Treatment at the scene of the accident and at first medical contact strongly affects the outcome of later replantation. Improper handling of the amputated part or stump can seriously compromise the final result. The initial assessment of the patient's status must exclude any life-threatening injuries, particularly if a major amputation is involved. The patient must be hemodynamically stable before either transportation or replantation is attempted.

Once the patient's safety is ensured, the stump is cleaned of gross contamination and protected with a sterile compression bandage. Bleeding after amputation is rarely a problem because fully transected vessels usually contract. If bleeding persists, however, it should never be stopped with the blind application of a hemostat, because this may further damage the neurovascular structures. Elevation of the stump usually stops the bleeding. A tourniquet should not be used because unregulated pressure increases the risk of ischemia and vascular damage.

The severed part is cleaned of any gross contamination and foreign material and cooled to reduce its metabolic rate. A severed digit should be wrapped in moist gauze and placed in a watertight plastic bag, which is then immersed in ice water. The amputated part must not be allowed to come into direct contact with any ice, and dry ice should never be used. Properly

cooled, a digit can be successfully replanted within 30 hours of amputation.

With a major amputation, preparation of the severed part is even more important. The amputated part is cleaned of all gross contamination, wrapped in a moist towel, and placed in a plastic bag. The part should be rapidly cooled to 10°C by immersing the plastic bag in ice

Plate 4.63

Upper Limb: PART I

POSTOPERATIVE DRESSING AND MONITORING OF BLOOD FLOW

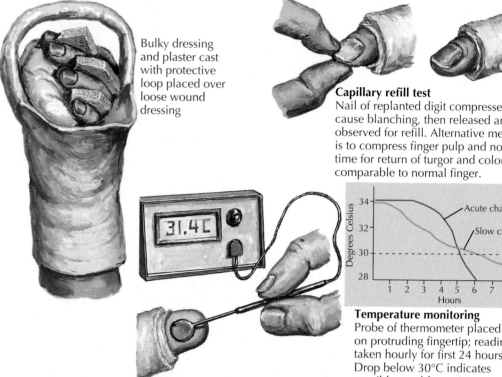

Bulky dressing and plaster cast with protective loop placed over loose wound dressing

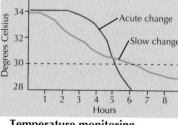

Capillary refill test
Nail of replanted digit compressed to cause blanching, then released and observed for refill. Alternative method is to compress finger pulp and note time for return of turgor and color comparable to normal finger.

Temperature monitoring
Probe of thermometer placed on protruding fingertip; readings taken hourly for first 24 hours. Drop below 30°C indicates possible need for revision surgery.

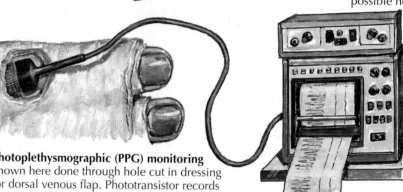

Photoplethysmographic (PPG) monitoring
Shown here done through hole cut in dressing for dorsal venous flap. Phototransistor records changes in blood volume near skin surface.

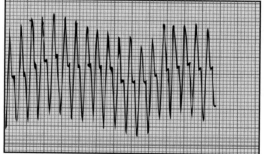

Normal PPG tracing

Tracing shows occluded blood supply

Pulse oxygen monitor

REPLANTATION (Continued)

water for 20 to 60 minutes. The part is then placed in an insulated container (but not in contact with the ice) and maintained at 10°C. Thus prepared, the amputated part is clearly labeled and rapidly transported to the replantation center.

Cold ischemia can preserve muscle up to 8 to 12 hours, after which irreversible changes may occur. Warm ischemia, which results from improper cooling, can lead to irreversible changes in as little as 4 to 6 hours, thus preventing successful replantation. Several attempts have been made to reduce ischemia time by perfusing the amputated limb with various substances such as oxygenated fluorocarbon solutions. At present, the most reliable fluid appears to be autologous arterial blood mixed with heparin. Perfusion plus cooling may make major replantations possible as much as 12 to 16 hours after injury.

In the emergency department, tetanus prophylaxis and a broad-spectrum antibiotic are administered as soon as possible. A complete history is obtained and a physical examination performed. Treatment options are thoroughly discussed with the patient and family. The decision to replant or to revise the amputation is based on the patient's wishes, age, health, and occupation; the type and level of the amputation; ischemia time; associated injuries; and the surgeon's experience.

TECHNIQUE FOR MINOR REPLANTATION

Repair of Bone and Tendon

Ideally, every replantation center should have two surgical teams available at all times. Once the decision to undertake replantation is made, the severed part is taken to the operating room. While one team prepares the patient for surgery, the other team thoroughly debrides the amputated part, viewing it under magnification. All devitalized and heavily contaminated tissue is excised, including frayed tendon ends, comminuted bone fragments, but only a small margin of skin, because coverage is important and skin is more resilient than deeper tissues. Frayed tendon ends are excised

because the damage to the exposed tendon surfaces greatly increases the risk that adhesions will subsequently form and restrict motion.

Bone is trimmed to (1) remove avascular bone that could initiate the development of osteomyelitis; (2) provide flat, congruent surfaces for stable bone fixation; and (3) provide the necessary skeletal shortening to

facilitate tension-free vessel anastomoses and nerve coaptations after debridement. At the digital or metacarpal level, the bone may be shortened about 1 cm. In the arm or forearm, the amount of bone shortening may be as much as 2 to 4 cm.

A severed part can be handled more easily while it is detached from the body. An interosseous wire or a

Plate 4.64

Hand and Finger

Replantation of avulsed thumb

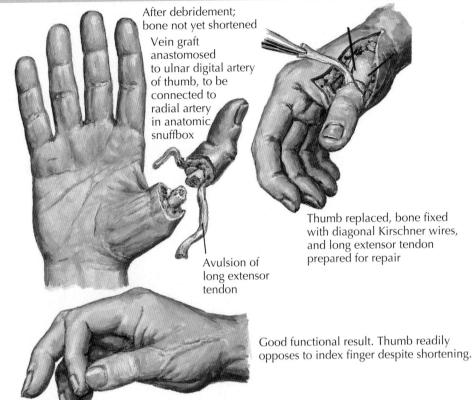

After debridement; bone not yet shortened

Vein graft anastomosed to ulnar digital artery of thumb, to be connected to radial artery in anatomic snuffbox

Avulsion of long extensor tendon

Thumb replaced, bone fixed with diagonal Kirschner wires, and long extensor tendon prepared for repair

Good functional result. Thumb readily opposes to index finger despite shortening.

REPLANTATION (Continued)

Kirschner wire can be placed in the bone of the amputated part to facilitate later fixation. A tendon suture of the Kirchmayr type (modified Kessler) can also be inserted at this time. The distal arteries, veins, and nerves are identified and tagged with fine sutures. Skin incisions are usually needed to expose these structures. The volar aspect of the finger is usually opened with a Brunner zigzag incision. A straight midline incision is made on the dorsal aspect. Only full-thickness skin flaps are reflected; the subcutaneous tissue and veins are left intact for later dissection under microscopic visualization.

While the amputated part is being prepared, the patient is transferred to the operating room and regional anesthesia is administered (preferably an axillary block). Regional anesthesia provides some sympathetic blockade and vasodilation as well as pain relief. The arm is cleaned with antiseptics, draped, and exsanguinated. The surgeon thoroughly debrides the stump, shortening the bone and tendon to permit easier anastomosis of vessels and coaptation of nerves. Use of a tourniquet facilitates the debridement. Once corresponding structures in the stump and the amputated part have been identified, replantation is begun. Because stability is essential for the vascular reconstruction, bone fixation is carried out first.

The technique of bone fixation should be appropriate for the type and level of amputation and provide stable fixation for early mobilization. Fixation devices include interosseous wires, Kirschner wires, and compression plates and should minimize further soft tissue disruption.

Replantation at the phalangeal level can be secured with interosseous wires with or without the added stability of a Kirschner wire; some surgeons prefer to use crossed Kirschner wires. Replantations at the joint level require a removable fixation device if the joint is to be preserved; otherwise, any standard technique for arthrodesis of small joints is suitable. At the metacarpal or more proximal level, a compression plate is preferred. If contamination is significant, however, an external fixator should be used to reduce the risk of infection. If possible, the periosteum is repaired to help bone healing and minimize adhesions to the flexor and extensor tendons. Kirchmayr (Kessler) sutures are used to repair flexor tendons, and interrupted figure-of-eight sutures are used for extensor tendons.

Replantation of midpalm

Amputation through metacarpals with thumb, index, and middle fingers on severed part, and ring finger longitudinally amputated. Debridement complete but bones not yet shortened.

Severed palmar metacarpal arteries from deep palmar arch to common digital arteries ligated to avoid hematoma.

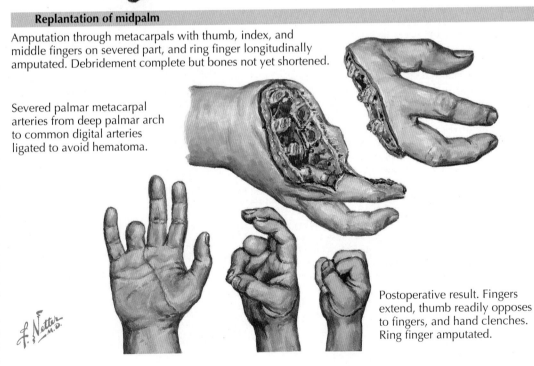

Postoperative result. Fingers extend, thumb readily opposes to fingers, and hand clenches. Ring finger amputated.

Repair of Blood Vessels and Nerves

After repair of bone and tendon, microvascular clamps are applied to the prepared arteries and veins, the tourniquet is released, and the blood flow is noted. This is the only way to assess arterial inflow. If arterial bleeding from the stump is not pulsatile after the arterial clamp is released, further resection of the artery is required to

Plate 4.65

Upper Limb: PART I

LATERAL ARM FLAP FOR DEFECT OF THUMB WEB

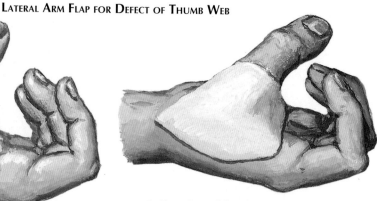

1. Defect after thumb replantation. Recipient vessels carefully dissected to receive flap vessels.

2. Template of flat, thin rubber (Esmarch) fashioned to conform to defect

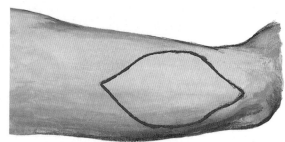

3. Template used to mark shape of skin flap on arm

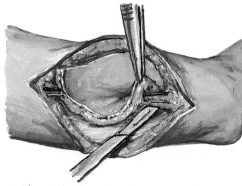

4. Flap with adequate subcutaneous tissue dissected free with vascular pedicle entering at one end and leaving at other

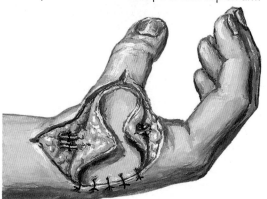

5. Flow-through flap placed in defect; pedicle anastomosed proximally and distally to revascularize thumb

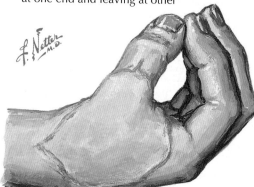

After healing, good cosmetic and functional results

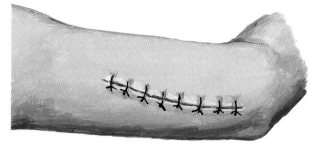

6. Donor site repaired with direct suturing

REPLANTATION (Continued)

bypass the zone of injury. The distal artery and vein must be resected to remove all damaged tissue. Vein grafts are inserted to bridge the gap produced by the resection if the vessels cannot be anastomosed without tension. When used for repairing arteries, vein grafts are reversed so that valves do not impede the flow of blood. Repairing rather than resecting injured and compromised vessels to avoid use of vein grafts almost always ends in failure because thrombosis occurs almost immediately in these injured vessels.

The surgeon's preference dictates whether repair of the arterial or the venous system is performed first. Generally, the arteries are repaired first to reduce ischemia time and to allow the surgeon to assess the adequacy of the venous debridement and determine which veins are best suited for repair. Ideally, both arteries and at least three veins are repaired in each digit.

Once the finger is revascularized, the nerves are repaired in standard fashion. Tendons are then repaired by tying the two core stitches in each end, adding a second core stitch and then an epitendinous repair. Then the skin is loosely approximated to avoid constriction of the vasculature when postoperative edema develops. Skin grafts or flap coverage should be used if primary closure is not possible and typically done secondarily within the initial hospital stay. For example, the lateral forearm rotation flap or free flow-through flap can be used to cover skin defects to the thumb after replantation. Use of normal skin and subcutaneous tissues from an uninjured zone brings excellent vascularity to the compromised digit.

Replantation of multiple digits is carried out in a similar sequence. One finger is completed at a time, while the other fingers are kept cold. However, nerve and tendon repair is often delayed until all digits are replanted and successfully perfused. If all the fingers are replanted together (i.e., bone fixation completed, then all tendons sutured, then blood vessels and nerves repaired), the prolonged duration of warm ischemia under the microscope lights may compromise the final result.

Postoperative Dressing

After replantation of fingers, a bulky dressing is applied to splint and protect the finger and hand in a position that enhances mobility, taking into account the delicate nature of the surgical repairs. The elbow should be flexed and the fingers pointing to the ceiling for edema control. The ideal position for postoperative immobilization is with the metacarpophalangeal joints in 70 degrees of flexion, with interphalangeal joints in neutral position, and with the thumb in maximal volar abduction. If this position is not possible, the alternative position used should come as close as possible to the ideal yet not stress or compress the vascular repairs. The dressing should be applied to allow easy visual inspection and temperature

Plate 4.66

Hand and Finger

TRANSFER OF GREAT TOE TO THUMB SITE

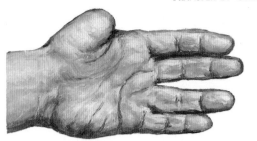

1. Hand with stump of previously amputated thumb

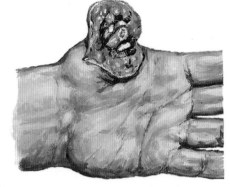

2. Incision, reflection of skin, and identification of structures

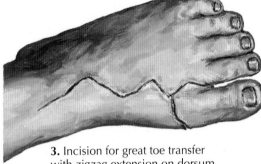

3. Incision for great toe transfer with zigzag extension on dorsum of foot for access to tendons

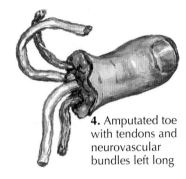

4. Amputated toe with tendons and neurovascular bundles left long

REPLANTATION (Continued)

monitoring of the finger yet guard against excessive manipulation of the finger itself.

SECONDARY RECONSTRUCTION

One-stage reconstruction (primary repair or grafting of all divided structures) is the preferred treatment because it avoids scarring from additional surgical procedures and because the patient can concentrate on rehabilitation after surgery. However, some procedures cannot be effectively completed at the time of replantation. Rarely, a replanted part is stiff, painful, useless, and ugly, and the patient may benefit from reamputation. Secondary reconstruction is much more common after major replantations than after minor replantations. The most common secondary procedures are bone grafting to treat a nonunion, soft tissue surgery to correct scar deformity at the amputation site, tenolysis to restore motion, and nerve grafting to improve sensation. Most often, however, patients require muscle and tendon transfers to restore function after poor recovery after nerve repair.

A toe-to-hand transfer is recommended when an additional digit would significantly improve hand function. Because the transplanted toe never functions as well as the original finger, patients must first appreciate the deficit created by the missing finger before they can accept the reconstructed digit.

RESULTS

Results of replantation must be interpreted with great care and compared not with normal function but with function with the best prostheses. Replantations often survive, but the more important outcome—subsequent hand and limb function—is not well reported. For example, the person who cannot return to work because a replanted finger is stiff and painful has a much greater disability than someone who has a well-performed revision amputation and can return to work 4 weeks after surgery.

5. Great toe transplanted. Bone, tendons, vessels, and nerves united, and skin loosely closed. Skin graft not needed in this patient.

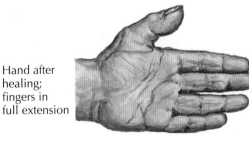

Healed foot after removal of great toe. Plantar skin turned up over end of amputation stump.

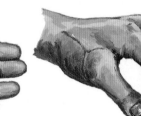

Hand after healing; fingers in full extension

"Thumb" (transplanted great toe) opposes index finger

Generally, functional recovery is determined by nerve regeneration, which tends to be better in patients younger than 35 years with more distal amputation sites. However, good recovery is often seen in young patients with more proximal amputations. Regarding nerve regeneration, different parts of the hand have different functional requirements. For example, the thumb and index finger require good sensation and stability, whereas the three ulnar digits require motion for power grip and are less involved in sensation. A comparison of functional assessments of replantations is difficult because patients' needs with respect to mobility and stability vary. However, most patients are satisfied with the replanted part and report that they would choose the procedure again.

Section 1 Shoulder

Banerjee R, Waterman B, Padelecki J, Robertson W. Management of distal clavicle fractures. J Am Acad Orthop Surg 2011;19:392–401.

Chen AL, Joseph TN, Zuckerman JD. Rheumatoid arthritis of the shoulder. J Am Acad Orthop Surg 2003;11:12–24.

Ecklund KJ, Lee TQ, Tibone J, Gupta R. Rotator cuff tear arthropathy. J Am Acad Orthop Surg 2007;15:340–349.

Elhassan B, Wagner E, Kany J. Latissimus dorsi transfer for irreparable subscapularis tear. J Shoulder Elbow Surg 2020;29:2128–2134.

Gerber C, Pennington SD, Nyffeler R. Reverse total shoulder arthroplasty. J Am Acad Orthop Surg 2009;17:284–295.

Green A. Chronic massive rotator cuff tears: evaluation and management. J Am Acad Orthop Surg 2003;11:321–331.

Iannotti JP. Full-thickness rotator cuff tears: factors affecting surgical outcome. J Am Acad Orthop Surg 1994;2:87–95.

Kucirek NK, Hung NJ, Wong SE. Treatment options for massive irreparable rotator cuff tears. Curr Rev Musculoskelet Med 2011;14:204–315.

McConville OR, Iannotti JP. Partial-thickness tears of the rotator cuff: evaluation and management. J Am Acad Orthop Surg 1999;7:32–43.

Millett PJ, Clavert P, Hatch GFR III, Warner JJP. Recurrent posterior shoulder instability. J Am Acad Orthop Surg 2006;14:464–476.

Nuber GW, Bowen MK. Acromioclavicular joint injuries and distal clavicle fractures. J Am Acad Orthop Surg 1997;5:11–18.

Pearl ML. Shoulder problems in children with brachial plexus birth palsy: evaluation and management. J Am Acad Orthop Surg 2009;17:242–254.

Piasecki DP, Verma NN, Romeo AA, Levine WN, Bach BR Jr, Provencher MT. Glenoid bone deficiency in recurrent anterior shoulder instability: diagnosis and management. J Am Acad Orthop Surg 2009;17:482–493.

Schenk TJ, Brems JJ. Multidirectional instability of the shoulder: pathophysiology, diagnosis, and management. J Am Acad Orthop Surg 1998;6:65–72.

Schlegel TF, Hawkins RJ. Displaced proximal humeral fractures: evaluation and treatment. J Am Acad Orthop Surg 1994;2:54–66.

Turkmen I, Koraman E, Poyanh O. Latissimus dorsi tendon transfers: a historical journey. SICOT-J 2021;7:9.

Wagner E., Elhassan B. Tendon transfers for rotator cuff pathologies. Curr Orthop Pract 2019;30:192–199.

Warner JJ. Frozen shoulder: diagnosis and management. J Am Acad Orthop Surg 1997;5:130–140.

Wiater JM, Fabin MH. Shoulder arthroplasty: prosthetic options and indications. J Am Acad Orthop Surg 2009;17:415–425.

Wolff AB, Sethi P, Sutton KM, Covey AS, Magit DP, Medvecky M. Partial-thickness rotator cuff tears. J Am Acad Orthop Surg 2006;14:715–725.

Section 2 Upper Arm and Elbow

Abboud JA, Ricchetti ET, Tjoumakaris F, Ramsey ML. Elbow arthroscopy: basic setup and portal placement. J Am Acad Orthop Surg 2006;15:312–318.

Beatty JH, Kasser JR, editors. Rockwood and Green's Fractures in Children. 6th ed. Lippincott Williams & Wilkins; 2006.

Bucholz RW, Heckman JD, Court-Brown CM, editors. Rockwood and Green's Fractures in Adults. 6th ed. Lippincott Williams & Wilkins; 2006.

Cheung EV, Adams R, Morrey BF. Primary osteoarthritis of the elbow: current treatment options. J Am Acad Orthop Surg 2008;16:77–87.

Cheung EV, Steinmann SP. Surgical approaches to the elbow. J Am Acad Orthop Surg 2009;17:325–333.

Flynn JM, Sarwark JF, Waters PM, Bae DS, Lemke LP. The surgical management of pediatric fractures of the upper extremity. Instr Course Lect 2003;52:635–645.

Hoppenfeld S, deBoer P, Buckley R, editors. Surgical Exposures in Orthopaedics: The Anatomic Approach. 4th ed. Lippincott Williams & Wilkins; 2009.

McKee MD, Veillette CJ, Hall JA, Schemitsch EH, Wild LM, McCormack R, et al. A multicenter, prospective, randomized, controlled trial of open reduction–internal fixation versus total elbow arthroplasty for displaced intra-articular distal humeral fractures in elderly patients. J Shoulder Elbow Surg 2009;18:3–12.

Morrey BF, Askew LJ, Chao EY. A biomechanical study of normal functional elbow motion. J Bone Joint Surg Am 1981;63:872–877.

Morrey BF, Sanchez-Sotelo J, editors. The Elbow and Its Disorders. 4th ed. Saunders; 2009.

Nesterenko S, Domire ZJ, Morrey BF, Sanchez-Sotelo J. Elbow strength and endurance in patients with a ruptured distal biceps tendon. J Shoulder Elbow Surg 2010;19:184–189.

O'Driscoll SW, Bell DF, Morrey BF. Posterolateral rotatory instability of the elbow. J Bone Joint Surg Am 1991;73:440–446.

O'Driscoll SW, Morrey BF, Korinek S, An KN. Elbow subluxation and dislocation: a spectrum of instability. Clin Orthop Relat Res 1992;280:186–197.

Pugh DM, Wild LM, Schemitsch EH, King GJ, McKee MD. Standard surgical protocol to treat elbow dislocations with radial head and coronoid fractures. J Bone Joint Surg Am 2004;86:1122–1130.

Sanchez-Sotelo J, Morrey BF. Total elbow arthroplasty. J Am Acad Orthop Surg 2011;19:121–125.

Sanchez-Sotelo J, Torchia ME, O'Driscoll SW. Complex distal humeral fractures: internal fixation with a principle-based parallel-plate technique. J Bone Joint Surg Am 2007;89:961–969.

Sarmiento A, Latta LL. Functional fracture bracing. J Am Acad Orthop Surg 1999;7:66–75.

Section 3 Forearm and Wrist

Beredjiklian PK. Kienböck's disease. J Hand Surg Am 2009;34:167–175.

Diao E, Andrews A, Beall M. Proximal row carpectomy. Hand Clin 2005;21:553–559.

Giannoulis FS, Sotereanos DG. Galeazzi fractures and dislocations. Hand Clin 2007;23:153–163.

Henry MH. Management of acute triangular fibrocartilage complex injury in the wrist. J Am Acad Orthop Surg 2008;16:320–329.

Herzberg G. Perilunate and axial carpal dislocations and fracture dislocations. J Hand Surg Am 2008;33:1659–1667.

Kawamura K, Chung KC. Treatment of scaphoid fractures and nonunions. J Hand Surg Am 2008;33:988–997.

Moss JP, Bynum DK. Diaphyseal fractures of the radius and ulna in adults. Hand Clin 2007;23:143–151.

Peterson B, Szabo RM. Carpal osteoarthritis. Hand Clin 2006;22:517–522.

Plancher KD, Piza PA, Bravo CJ. Treatment of hook of the hamate fractures in golfers. Atlas Hand Clin 2006;11:67–78.

Slutsky DJ, Nagle DJ. Wrist arthroscopy: current concepts. J Hand Surg Am 2008;33:1228–1244.

Williams DP, Lubahn JD. Reconstruction of extensor tendons. Atlas Hand Clin 2005;10:209–222.

Wulf CA, Ackerman DB, Rizzo M. Contemporary evaluation and treatment of distal radius fractures. Hand Clin 2007;23:209–226.

Section 4 Hand and Finger

Chesney A, Chauhan A, Kattan A, Farrokhyar F, Thoma A. Systematic review of flexor tendon rehabilitation protocols in zone II of the hand. Plast Reconstr Surg 2011;127:1583–1592.

Dorf E, Blue C, Smith BP, Koman LA. Therapy after injury to the hand. J Am Acad Orthop Surg 2010;18:464–473.

Henry MH. Fractures of the proximal phalanx and metacarpals in the hand: preferred methods of stabilization. J Am Acad Orthop Surg 2008;16:586–595.

Jalil A, Barlaan PI, Fung BK, Ip JW. Hand infection in diabetic patients. Hand Surg 2011;16:307–312.

Jupiter JB, Hastings 2nd H, Capo JT. The treatment of complex fractures and fracture-dislocations of the hand. Instr Course Lect 2010;59:333–341.

Kozlow JH, Chung KC. Current concepts in the surgical management of rheumatoid and osteoarthritic hands and wrists. Hand Clin 2011;27:31–41.

Patterson RW, Li Z, Smith BP, Smith TL, Koman LA. Complex regional pain syndrome of the upper extremity. J Hand Surg Am 2011;36:1553–1562.

Pike JM, Gelberman RH. Zone II combined flexor digitorum superficialis and flexor digitorum profundus repair distal to the A2 pulley. J Hand Surg Am 2010;35:1523–1527.

Rivlin M, Sheikh E, Isaac R, Beredjiklian PK. The role of nerve allografts and conduits for nerve injuries. Hand Clin 2010;26:435–446.

Scheker LR, Becker GW. Distal finger replantation. J Hand Surg Am 2011;36:521–528.

Sebastin SJ, Chung KC. A systematic review of the outcomes of replantation of distal digital amputation. Plast Reconstr Surg 2011;128:723–737.

Tang P. Collateral ligament injuries of the thumb metacarpophalangeal joint. J Am Acad Orthop Surg 2011;19(5):287–296.

Vermeulen GM, Slijper H, Feitz R, Hovius SE, Moojen TM, Selles RW. Surgical management of primary thumb carpometacarpal osteoarthritis: a systematic review. J Hand Surg Am 2011;36:157–169.

A

A1 pulley fibers, 198f
Abdominal compression test, 49f
Abductor digiti minimi, 130f
Abductor digiti minimi muscle, 132f, 156f, 157f, 163, 163f, 167f
Abductor pollicis brevis muscle, 129f, 132f, 163f, 166f, 168f
Abductor pollicis longus muscle, 124f, 125f, 127, 127f, 157f, 163
Abductor pollicis longus tendon, 123f, 124f, 125f, 126f, 162f, 169f, 178f
Above-elbow amputation, 61, 61f
Accessory cephalic vein, 79f, 83, 131f, 172
Accessory collateral ligament, 158f
Achilles tendon graft, 48f
Acromial anastomosis, 18f
Acromial angle, 2f, 69f
Acromial end, 4f
Acromial facet, 4f
Acromial plexus, 18f
Acromioclavicular dislocation, 33
Acromioclavicular injection, 62f
Acromioclavicular joint, 8f, 12f
    arthritis, 41, 41f
    capsule, 5f
    injury to, 33f
Acromioclavicular ligament, 9f, 13f
Acromion, 2f, 3f, 5f, 8f, 9f, 10f, 11f, 12f, 13f, 14f, 16f, 18f, 35f, 36f, 58f, 62f, 66f, 69f, 75f, 76f
    normal, 41f
    prominent, 28f
Acute tendonitis, needle rupture of deposit in, 36f
Acute traumatic full-thickness subscapularis tears, 49
Adducted retroposed thumb, 178
Adductor pollicis muscle, 132f, 156f, 163, 163f, 164, 164f, 165f, 167f, 206f
    fascia of, 164f, 165f
    oblique head, 156f
Anatomic neck, 22f, 69f
    of humerus, 3f
    of scapula, 2f
Anatomic snuffbox, 116f, 157f
Anatomic total shoulder arthroplasty, 54f
Anconeus muscle, 74f, 76f, 78, 78f, 82f, 124f, 125f, 145f
Animal bites, infection in, 195
Annular ligament, of radius, 72f, 73, 73f, 145f
Ansa pectoralis, 14f
Antebrachial cutaneous nerve
    lateral, 123f, 125f, 128f, 131f
    medial, 125f, 128f, 129f
    posterior, 131f
Antebrachial fascia, 125f
Anterior axillary fold, 8f
Anterior circumflex humeral artery, 11f, 14f, 16f, 17f, 18f, 66f, 75f, 83f, 84f
Anterior closed space, 173
Anterior dislocation of glenohumeral joint, 28–30
    pathologic lesions, 29–30
Anterior fat pad, 87f
Anterior inferior capsule, 29f
Anterior inferior portal, 66f
Anterior interosseous artery, 84f, 124f
Anterior interosseous nerve, 103f, 129f
Anterior joint
    capsule, 66f
    tenderness, 51f
Anterior scalene muscle, 14f, 18f
Anterior sternoclavicular dislocation, 33
Anterior sternoclavicular ligament, 5f
Anterior superior portal, 66f
Anterior ulnar recurrent artery, 84f, 123f
Anterosuperior labrum, 13f
Aponeurosis, 206f
Arcade of Frohse, 103f
Arcade of Struthers, 103f

Arcuate ligament, 103f
Arm, median nerve in, 129
Artery of Liang, 17f
Arthritis
    of elbow, 100–102, 100f, 101f, 102f
    of hand, 175–177
    of wrist, 150, 150f
Arthrodesis, 180f, 181
Arthroplasty
    of flexible implant resection, 183f
    modular *versus* implant resection, 184f, 188f
Arthroscopy, portals in, 114f
Articular capsule, 72
Articular cartilage, 13f, 72f, 173f, 198f
Articular cavity, 173f
Articular surfaces, 69, 72
Ascending cervical artery, 18f
Axilla, 8f, 16
    dissection, 14f
    posterior wall and cord, 15f
Axillary artery, 9f, 13f, 14f, 16f, 17f, 61f, 83f, 84f
Axillary fascia, 16f
Axillary fold, adhesions obliterating, 37f
Axillary lymph nodes, 16f, 171–172, 172f, 196f
    apical group of, 172
    central group of, 171
    lateral group of, 171
    pectoral group of, 171
    subscapular group of, 171
Axillary nerve, 11f, 14f, 15f, 16f, 19f, 21f, 48f, 59f, 76f, 80f, 81f, 82f, 129f
    anterior branch, 15f
    branches, 15f
    posterior branch, 15f
Axillary vein, 9f, 13f, 16f, 61f, 83

B

Balanitis, 177f
Balloon arthroplasty, 47, 47f
Bankart lesion, 29f
Basal joints, surgery for, 179–180
Basic shoulder-strengthening exercises, 64–65, 64f, 65f
Basilic vein, 14f, 68f, 77f, 79f, 83, 116f, 131f, 171, 171f, 172, 172f
Bennett fracture, 202, 202f
Biceps brachii muscle, 3f, 8f, 13f, 14f, 15f, 16f, 68f, 74f, 75–76, 77f, 81f, 83f, 104f, 123f, 127f, 128f
    long head of, 15f, 16f, 62f, 66f, 74f, 75, 75f, 77f, 83f
        tendon, 15f, 29f, 39f
    short head of, 9f, 11f, 13f, 15f, 16f, 62f, 66f, 74f, 75, 75f, 77f, 83f
        tendon, 15f
Biceps brachii tendon, 16f, 46f, 72f, 73f, 75f, 83f, 84, 122f, 123f
Biceps groove, 37f
Biceps labral complex, 9f
Biceps tendon, 66f, 78f
    long head, 6f, 7f, 9f, 13f, 23f, 26f, 45f, 46f, 49f, 60f
    rupture of, 106, 106f
    tears, 39–40, 39f, 40f
Bicipital aponeurosis, 75f, 76, 78f, 83f, 84, 122f, 128f, 131f
Bicipitoradial bursa, 75–76
Bier block anesthesia, 197–198, 197f
Bipolar electrocautery, 215f
Blauth classified thumb hypoplasia, 152, 153, 153f
Bone
    avulsion of, 206f
    of elbow, 68–69, 70f
    of forearm, 116–119, 116f, 117f
    resorption, 109f
    suture anchor in, 46f
    tamp, 25f
Boutonnière deformity, 178, 178f, 185
    reconstructive surgery for, 186f

Brachial artery, 14f, 17f, 18f, 75f, 77f, 78f, 83, 84f, 122f, 123f, 128f
    ascending (deltoid) branch, 84, 84f
    muscular branch of, 83f
    in situ, 83f
Brachial fascia, 74, 77f
Brachial plexus, 14f, 19, 61f
    cords of, 81f, 129f
    lateral cord of, 16f, 81f, 83f
    medial cord of, 16f, 81f, 83f
    posterior cord of, 15f, 16f, 81f, 82
Brachial trunks, 15f
Brachial veins, 14f, 77f
Brachialis muscle, 2f, 14f, 74f, 75f, 76, 77f, 78f, 81f, 82f, 83f, 104f, 122f, 123f, 127f, 128f
    insertion of, 72f
Brachialis tendon, 78f
Brachioradialis muscle, 68f, 74f, 75f, 76f, 78f, 82f, 83f, 116f, 122, 122f, 123f, 124f, 125, 125f, 127f, 128f
Brachioradialis tendon, 123f, 125f
Bursitis, 36f

C

C2 nerve, 20f
C3 nerve, 20f
C4 nerve, 20f
C5 nerve, 20f
C6 nerve, 20f
C7 nerve, 20f
C7 vertebra, spinous process of, 10f
C8 nerve, 20f
Calcific deposit, 36f
Calcific tendonitis, 36
Camper chiasm, 160f, 161f, 200f
Capillary refill test, 218f
Capitate, 118f, 119, 126f, 132f, 156f, 157f
    head of, 150f
Capitohamate ligament, 120f
Capitulum, 69, 69f, 70f, 71f, 78f
    fractures of, 90, 90f
Capsular lesion, 29f
Capsular ligament, 5f, 12f
Capsule, 36f
Capsulodesis, 179
Carbuncle, 191f
Carpal articular surface, 116, 117f
Carpal bones, 117–119, 118f, 156f, 157f
Carpal instability, 142
Carpal tunnel syndrome, 132, 132f, 133, 133f
Carpometacarpal (CMC) joint, 158, 159f
    1st, 175f
    arthritis, ligament replacement and tendon interposition arthroplasty for, 180f
    dislocation of, 206–207, 206f
    hyperextension of, 178f
    injuries, 206–207
    radial styloid, 161f
Cellulitis, 191, 191f
Central compartment, of palm, 170
Central tendon, 173f, 181f, 187f
Cephalic vein, 8f, 13f, 14f, 16f, 66f, 68f, 77f, 78f, 79f, 83, 116f, 131f, 171, 171f, 172f
Charcot arthropathy, 59, 60f
Chronic tendonitis, 36f
Circumflex scapular artery, 14f, 16f, 17f, 18f, 75f, 84f
Clamp-applying forceps, 215f
Clavicle, 3f, 4, 5f, 8f, 12f, 14f, 15f, 16f, 18f, 41f, 62f
    end of, 41f
    fractures of, 34–35, 35f
    right, 4f
    shaft, 4f, 27f
        anterior, 4f
        posterior, 4f
    sternal end of, 4f
    trapezoid line of, 4f

Clavicular head, 8f
Cleland ligament, 190f
Closed reduction, of fingers, 204f
Closed-chain active-assisted strengthening, 65f
Club stump, 213f
Colinear intact Maloney line, 57f
Collar button abscess, 195, 195f
Collateral ligaments, 72, 158f, 159, 160f, 187f, 198f
Colles fractures, 135, 136f
Common extensor tendon, 74f, 78f, 124f, 127f
Common flexor sheath, 132f, 164f, 165f, 166f, 193f
Common flexor tendon, 74f, 78f
Common interosseous artery, 84f
Common palmar digital arteries, 163, 164f, 165f, 166f, 198f
Common palmar digital nerves, 130f, 164f, 166f, 167f, 168f
Common palmar digital vein, 198f
Condylar fractures, 205, 205f
Congenital dislocation, of radial head, 110, 110f
Congenital radioulnar synostosis, 111, 111f
Conjoined tendon, 75f
Conjunctivitis, 177f
Conoid ligament, 4f, 5f, 12f
Conoid tubercle, of clavicle, 4f
Conservative humeral head surface replacement, 55f
Coracoacromial ligament, 5f, 6, 12f, 16f, 62f, 75f
Coracobrachialis muscle, 3f, 9f, 11f, 13f, 14f, 15f, 16f, 61f, 62f, 74f, 75, 75f, 77f, 81f, 83f, 128f
Coracobrachialis tendon, 15f
Coracoclavicular ligament, 4f, 5f, 6, 12f
Coracohumeral ligament, 5–6, 5f, 62f
Coracoid process, 2f, 5f, 12f, 13f, 14f, 15f, 16f, 18f, 35f, 49f, 53f, 62f, 69f, 75f, 83f
Coracoid transfer, 30f
Coronoid fossa, 69, 69f, 70f
Coronoid process, 70f, 71, 71f
Costal cartilage, 5f
    6th, 8f
Costoclavicular ligament, 4f, 5f
Costocoracoid ligament, 16f
Costocoracoid membrane, 16f
Cubital fossa, 68, 68f, 84
Cubital lymph nodes, 171, 172f
Cubital tunnel release, 133f
Cubital tunnel syndrome, 103–104, 103f, 104f
Cutaneous nerves, of elbow, 79–80, 79f, 80f, 131, 131f
Cysts, 55f

D

de Quervain disease, 137, 148, 148f
Deep artery of arm, 17f
Deep back muscles, 61f
Deep brachial artery, 83
Deep compartments, infection of, 194–195, 195f
Deep dorsal dissection, 162f
Deep fascia, 169f, 170
Deep lymphatics, 172
Deep palmar arch
    arterial, 163
    severed palmar metacarpal arteries from, 219f
Deep transverse metacarpal ligaments, 158, 158f, 163, 163f
Deformities
    of interphalangeal joint, 185–188
    of metacarpophalangeal joints, 181–184
    of thumb joints, 178–180
Deltoid muscle, 2f, 3f, 4f, 8, 8f, 9f, 10f, 11f, 12f, 13f, 14f, 15f, 16f, 36f, 48f, 58f, 61f, 66f, 68f, 74f, 75f, 76f, 77f, 82f, 83f, 128f
Deltoid tuberosity, 2f, 3f, 68, 69f
Deltopectoral groove, 68f
Deltopectoral node, 172f
Deltopectoral triangle, 8f, 9
Diabetes, 38f
Digital artery, 166f, 190f
Digital block, 198, 198f
Digital fibrous sheaths, 158f
Digital movement, muscle actions in, 161
Digital nerve, 166f, 174, 189f, 190f

Digits, 173–174
    anterior closed space, 173
    nails, 173
    small arteries of, 173–174
DIP joint see Distal interphalangeal (DIP) joint
Dislocation, of carpus, 142–143, 142f, 143f
Distal anterior closed space, 173f
Distal biceps tear, 106f
Distal digital crease, 156f
Distal forearm, 161f
Distal humerus, fractures of, 88–90, 88f
    complex intraarticular, 88–89, 88f
    total elbow arthroplasty for, 89, 89f
Distal interphalangeal (DIP) joint, 158f, 159f, 161f, 175f, 176f, 177f
    deformities of, 186
    radiograph of, 175f
    site of, 157f
Distal lumbrical tendons, 161f
Distal palmar crease, 156f, 159f
Distal phalanges, 156f, 157f, 167f, 173f, 174f
    amputation in, 212f, 213
    base, 156f, 157f
    branches of, 166f
    dorsal branches to dorsum of, 168f
    dorsum of middle, 166f
    fracture of, 210
    head, 156f, 157f
    shafts, 156f, 157f
    tuberosity, 156f, 157f
Distal pole, 138f
Distal radius, 150f
    fracture of, 134–137, 134f, 135f
        of articular margin, 134–135
        closed reduction and pin fixation of, 136
        closed reduction and plaster cast immobilization of, 135–136, 136f
        complications of, 137
        extension/compression of, 134, 134f
        external fixation, 136
        open reduction and internal fixation, 136–137, 137f
        of styloid process, 135
Distal triceps tear, 106f
Dorsal carpal (arterial) arch, 162f
Dorsal digital artery, 162f, 173f
Dorsal digital nerves, 130, 131f, 171, 171f, 173f
Dorsal digital veins, 131f, 171, 171f
Dorsal dislocation, 208–209, 208f
Dorsal fascia, of hand, 164f
Dorsal hood
    line of incision through, 181f
    sagittal fibers of, 182f
Dorsal interosseous fascia, 164f
Dorsal interosseous muscle, 130f, 157f, 162, 163f, 164f, 167f
    1st, 163f, 165f, 169f, 174f
Dorsal metacarpal arteries, 162f, 166
Dorsal metacarpal veins, 83, 131f, 171, 171f
Dorsal ramus, 19f
Dorsal retinaculum, 161f
Dorsal scapular artery, 14f, 18f
Dorsal scapular nerve, 14f, 16f, 19f, 82f
Dorsal subaponeurotic space, 164f
    probe in, 171
Dorsal subcutaneous space, 164f
Dorsal surface, 158f
Dorsal (Lister) tubercle, 117f
Dorsal veins, 83
Dorsal venous arch, 83
Dorsal venous network, 125f
Double pneumatic tourniquet, 197f
Dupuytren contracture, 189–190, 189f
Durkan test, 132

E

Elastic bandage, 197f
Elbow, 67–114
    anastomoses around, 84f
    aspirations at, 112f
    basic rehabilitation for, 112
    blood supply to, 84

Elbow (Continued)
    bones of, 70f
    cross-sectional anatomy of, 78f
    cutaneous nerves of, 79f, 80
    dislocation of, in children, 98
    injections at, 112, 112f
    injury to, 87, 87f
        in children, 96–98
    ligaments of, 72–73
    muscles of, 74–78, 74f, 75f
    nerve supply to, 82
    neurovascular injury to, 99
    physical examination of, 85, 85f
    radiographs of, 71f
    superficial veins of, 79f
    surgical approaches to, 113–114, 113f, 114f
    tendon and ligament disorders at, 105–107
    topographic anatomy of, 68f
Elbow flexion test, 104f
Elbow joint, 70–71
    dislocation of, 94–95, 94f, 95f
    lateral (Kocher) approach to, 113f
    posterior approach to, 114f
    posterior dislocation of, 97f
Epicondylitis, 105, 105f
Epidermal abscess, 191
Epiphyseal fracture, 202, 202f
Epiphysis, 173f
Epitrochlear lymph nodes, 196f
Eponychium, 173f, 191f
Esmarch bandage, 197f
Essex-Lopresti fracture, 92
Extension (dorsiflexion), 159f
Extension block splint, 209f
Extensor carpi radialis brevis muscle, 68f, 76f, 78f, 82f, 116f, 124f, 125f, 126, 127f, 157f
Extensor carpi radialis brevis tendon, 124f, 125f, 162f, 169f
Extensor carpi radialis longus muscle, 124f, 125–126, 125f, 127f
Extensor carpi radialis longus muscles, 68f, 74f, 76f, 78f, 82f
Extensor carpi radialis longus tendon, 124f, 125f, 157f, 162f, 169f
Extensor carpi ulnaris muscle, 76f, 82f, 116f, 125f, 126, 127f, 145f
Extensor carpi ulnaris tendon, 124f, 125f, 157f, 162f
Extensor digiti minimi muscle, 124f, 125f, 126, 162f
Extensor digiti minimi tendon, 124f, 125f
Extensor digitorum communis, 157f
Extensor digitorum muscle, 76f, 78f, 82f, 124f, 125f, 126, 161, 162f
Extensor digitorum tendon, 116f, 124f, 157f, 174f, 198f
Extensor expansion, 160f, 174f, 198f
    tendinous slips to, 163f
Extensor indicis muscle, 124f, 127
Extensor indicis tendon, 116f, 124f, 157f, 162f, 174f
Extensor mechanism, 173f
Extensor muscle, 125–127, 125f
    deep layer, 126–127
    superficial layer, 125–126
Extensor pollicis brevis muscle, 124f, 126f, 127, 127f, 157f
Extensor pollicis brevis tendon, 123f, 124f, 125f, 162f, 169f, 174f, 178f
Extensor pollicis longus muscle, 124f, 127, 127f, 157f
Extensor pollicis longus tendon, 116f, 124f, 125f, 157f, 162f, 164f, 169f, 174f, 178f
Extensor pollicis longus tendons, 178f
Extensor retinaculum, 124f, 125f, 162f, 169f
    superficial branch of, 171f
Extensor tendon, 160f, 164f
External oblique muscle, 8f, 15f
External occipital protuberance, 10f
External rotation, range-of-motion exercises and, 64f
External rotator muscles, 22f
Extraarticular transverse fracture, 202f

F

Fascial closure, 61f
Fascial space, infection of, 192f, 193–194, 193f

Fat pads, 72f
  lesion of, 87f
Felon, 191f, 192
Fibrous arcade, 133f
Fibrous sheath, 164f, 165f, 173f
Fight bite, 201f
Finger flexion, 159f, 160f
Fingers, 155–221
  5th, 165f, 182f
  amputation in, 214
  dorsum of, 172f
  extensor mechanism of, 161
  flexor and extensor tendons in, 160f
  infected wounds of, 194f
  injury to, 203–205
    rehabilitation after, 211, 211f
  joints, deformities of, 182
  midlateral approach to, 190f
  surgical approach to, 190f
  vascular supply of, 166
  volar approach to, 190f
Fingertip
  amputation in, 212–213, 212f
  injuries to, 210, 210f
Flexible implant resection arthroplasty, 181
Flexion, 159f
Flexion contracture, of small fingers, 189f
Flexor carpi radialis muscle, 75f, 78f, 83f, 122f, 123, 123f, 125f, 127f, 128f, 129f
Flexor carpi radialis tendon, 116f, 123f, 125f, 126f, 128f, 132f, 156f, 164f, 165f
Flexor carpi ulnaris muscle, 76f, 78f, 104f, 116f, 122f, 123f, 124, 124f, 125f, 127f, 128f, 130f, 133f
Flexor carpi ulnaris tendon, 116f, 123f, 126f, 132f, 156f, 163, 165f
Flexor digiti minimi brevis muscle, 130f, 132f, 156f, 163, 167f
Flexor digiti minimi tendon, 182f
Flexor digitorum profundus muscle, 123f, 124, 125f, 126f, 127f, 128f, 129f, 130f
Flexor digitorum profundus tendon, 126f, 132f, 156f, 158f, 160f, 161f, 164f, 173f, 174f, 190f, 198f, 200f, 212f
  avulsion of, 199f
  insertion of, 165f
Flexor digitorum superficialis muscle, 78f, 103f, 122f, 123, 123f, 124, 125f, 126f, 127f, 129f, 156f, 161, 161f, 190f
Flexor digitorum superficialis tendon, 116f, 122f, 126f, 128f, 132f, 156f, 158f, 160f, 161f, 164f, 173f, 174f, 198f, 200f
  insertion of, 165f
Flexor muscles, 123–125
  deep layer, 124–125, 124f
  superficial layer, 123–124, 123f
Flexor pollicis brevis muscle, 132f, 156f, 163, 163f, 166f, 167f
  deep palmar branch of, 166f
  superficial head of, 168f
Flexor pollicis longus muscle, 123f, 125, 125f, 127f, 128f, 129f, 163
  tendinous sheath of, 164f, 165f, 193f
Flexor pollicis longus tendon, 123f, 126f, 132f, 174f, 178f
  in tendon sheath (radial bursa), 164f
Flexor retinaculum, 123f, 128f, 132f, 165f
  transverse carpal ligament, 163f, 164f, 166f
Flexor tendon sheaths, 165f, 190f, 198f
Flexor tendons, 182f, 190f, 207f
  to 5th digit, 164f
  accessories and, 160–161
  repair, 199–200
Flexor-pronator muscle mass, 104f
Flow-through flap, 220f
Fluid contrast, material, 45f
Forearm, 115–153
  blood supply of, 128
  fracture of both, 144, 144f
  median nerve in, 129
  muscles of, 122–127, 122f, 123f, 124f, 125f, 126f
    origins and insertions of, 127f
  radial longitudinal deficiency in, 152, 152f, 153, 153f
  ulnar nerve in, 130
Forequarter amputation, 61, 61f
Forward elevation, range-of-motion exercises and, 64f

Fracture
  complications of, 99
  of distal radius, 134–137, 134f, 135f
    of articular margin, 134–135
    closed reduction and pin fixation of, 136
    closed reduction and plaster cast immobilization of, 135–136, 136f
    complications of, 137
    extension/compression of, 134, 134f
    external fixation, 136
    open reduction and internal fixation, 136–137, 137f
    of styloid process, 135
  of hamulus of hamate, 141, 141f
  management of, 203
  of scaphoid, 138–140, 138f, 139f, 140f
    acute displaced fractures, 140
    acute nondisplaced fractures, 139–140
    nonunion, 140
Fracture line, 53f
Frozen shoulder, 37–38, 38f

G
Galeazzi fracture, 146, 146f
Ganglion cyst, 59f, 147, 147f
Gatching type of strengthening, 65f
Glenohumeral arthroscopic anatomy, 6f
Glenohumeral joint, 5f, 7
  capsule of, 76f
  contrast, 45f
  normal, 31f
  osteoarthritis of, 51–52, 52f
  posterior dislocation of, 31–32, 31f, 32f
  rheumatoid arthritis of, 54–55, 54f, 55f
  section through normal, 29f
Glenoid, 3f, 9f, 11f, 13f, 29f, 31f, 53f, 54f, 66f
  center of, 51f
Glenoid cavity, 29f, 31f, 35f
  of scapula, 12f, 69f
Glenoid cyst, 54f, 58f
Glenoid labrum, 12f
Glenoid rim, anterior inferior capsule, 29f
Glenosphere, 27f
Golfer's elbow, 105, 105f
Gout, 177
Gouty arthritis, 177, 177f
Grayson ligament, 190f
Great toe transfer
  incision for, 221f
  thumb site, 221f
Great vessels, ligation of, 61f
Greater tubercle, 2f, 69f, 75f
  crest of, 3f, 69f
  of humerus, 3f, 5f, 16f
Greater tuberosity, 22f, 26f, 27f, 29f, 31f, 46f
  displaced fracture of, 22f
  tendon, 45f

H
Halves of central tendon, 187f
Hamate, 118f, 119, 132f, 157f
Hamulus of hamate, 138f
  fracture of, 141, 141f
Hand, 155–221
  after healing, 221f
  amputation in, 212–214, 212f
  arthritis in, 175–177
  bones of, 156–157, 156f, 157f
  dorsal venous network of, 171
  fascia of, 170–172
  flexor and extensor tendons of, 160–161
  infections of, 191–196, 194f
  injury, rehabilitation after, 211, 211f
  innervation of, 167–169
  joints of, 158–159, 175f
  motion, definitions of, 159f
  movement of, 159
  muscles of, 162–165
  skin and subcutaneous fascia of, 170f
  spaces, bursae, and tendon sheaths of, 164–165, 164f
  surgery, anesthesia for, 197–198

Hand (Continued)
  tendon disorders in, 199–200
  topographic anatomy, bones, and origins and insertions of, 156f, 157f
  vascular supply of, 166
Hawkins impingement sign, 42f
Heberden nodes, 175f
Hemostasis, 194f
Herpes simplex cellulitis, 191f, 193
Hill-Sachs lesion, 29f, 30f
Hook of hamate, 118f, 123f, 126f, 156f, 158f, 166f
Horseshoe abscess, 192f
Human bite, infection in, 195
Humeral circumflex artery, ascending branch of, 18f
Humeral head, 2f, 3f, 7f, 11f, 13f, 26f, 29f, 31f, 54f, 74f, 103f, 128f
  articular surface of, 6f, 7f, 66f
  avascular necrosis of, 53
  bare area of, 7f
  center of, 51f
  coracoacromial arch, 57f
  cuff tear arthropathy with, 56
  fracture
    complex, in articular head, 26f
    percutaneous method of reduction of, 25f
  posterosuperior portion of, 7f
  prominent, 28f
  prosthesis, 57f
  rounding off of, 57f
  severe posterior subluxation of, 51f
  split, 26, 26f
  superior migration of, 58f
Humeral shaft, 11f, 13f, 26f
  fractures of, 86, 86f
Humeral stem, in medullary canal, 53f
Humeroulnar head, of flexor digitorum superficialis muscle, 74f
Humerus, 3, 46f, 61f, 68, 70f, 71f, 72f, 73f, 77f, 83f, 87f
  anterior and posterior views of, 69f
  anterolateral approach to, 113f
  head of, 69f
  supracondylar fractures, in children, 96–97, 96f
Hypothenar eminence, 156f
Hypothenar fascia, 170
Hypothenar muscles, 130f, 164f, 165f, 166f, 167f, 170f

I
Impingement syndrome, 42–43, 42f, 43f
Implant, distal stem of, 182f
Inconstant contribution, 16f
Inferior angle
  of humerus, 3f
  of scapula, 2f
Inferior capsule, diminished volume of, 37f
Inferior glenohumeral ligament, 5
Inferior glenoid labrum, 7f, 58f
Inferior lateral brachial cutaneous nerve, 21f, 76f, 79, 79f, 80f, 82f
Inferior thyroid artery, 18f
Inferior ulnar collateral artery, 83f, 84, 84f
Infraglenoid tubercle, 69f
Infraspinatus fascia, 10f
Infraspinatus muscle, 2f, 10f, 11f, 12–13, 12f, 13f, 16f, 18f, 29f, 31f, 45f, 46f, 59f, 61f, 74f, 76f, 82f
Infraspinatus rotator cuff tears, 48f
  imaging of, 45, 45f
  irreparable, surgical management of, 47–48, 47f, 48f
  physical examination, 44
  surgical management of, 46, 46f
Infraspinatus tendon, 7f, 12f
Infraspinous fossa, 2f, 69f
Intercapitular veins, 131f, 171, 171f
Intercostobrachial nerve, 14f, 21f, 79f, 80, 80f, 128f
Intermediate bursa, 193f
Intermediate supraclavicular nerves, 79f
Intermetacarpal joints, 158
Intermuscular septa, 74
Internal fixation, 25f
Internal rotation, range-of-motion exercises and, 64f
Internal rotation lag sign, 49f

Internal thoracic artery, 18f
Interosseous artery, 128
     recurrent, 84f, 124f
Interosseous border, 117f
Interosseous cubital bursa, 75–76
Interosseous membrane, 117f, 125f
Interosseous muscle wasting, 104f
Interosseous muscles, 126f, 160f, 164
Interosseous tendon slip, 160f
Interphalangeal joints, 159
     deformities, 185–188
     surgery for, 188
Interphalangeal ligaments, 158f
Intertendinous connections (juncturae tendinum), 160
Intertubercular sulcus, 3f, 69f
Intertubercular tendon sheath, 5f, 16f, 75f
Intraarticular fracture, 205f
Intrinsic muscles, 162–164
Irreparable supraspinatus tear, surgical management of, 47–48, 47f, 48f

J
Jersey finger, 199f
Jeweler forceps, 215f
Joint capsule, 9f, 11f, 13f, 66f, 72f, 73f, 78f, 126f, 158f, 174f
Joint fluid, 9f, 54f, 78f
Joint injection, 198
Joint ligaments, 190f
Joint space, loss of, 57f
Joint stiffness, 99, 99f
Joints
     of forearm, 116
     hand, 158–159, 175f

K
Kanavel's four cardinal points, 192f
Kienböck disease, 151, 151f
Kineplasty, 61f
Kirschner wire, 219

L
Labrum, 11f
Lacertus fibrosus, 78f, 103f
Lag sign, 44f
Lateral antebrachial cutaneous nerve, 75f, 77f, 79f, 80, 80f, 81, 81f, 84, 123f, 125f, 128f, 131f, 167f
Lateral bands, 160f, 173f
Lateral border, of scapula, 2f, 3f
Lateral condyle, 69f, 70f
     fractures of, 88f, 89–90
     in children, 97, 97f
Lateral cutaneous nerve of forearm, 122f
Lateral epicondyle, of humerus, 69f, 70f, 71f, 72f, 75f, 76f, 123f, 124f
Lateral epicondylitis, 105, 105f
Lateral intermuscular septum, 74, 75f, 76f, 77f, 82f, 123f, 124f
Lateral pectoral nerve, 14f, 16f
Lateral portal, 66f
Lateral supraclavicular nerves, 79f
Lateral supracondylar ridge, 69f, 70f
Lateral tendon, 181f
Lateral thoracic artery, 14f, 17f, 18f, 84f
Latissimus dorsi muscle, 2f, 3f, 8f, 9f, 10f, 11, 11f, 14f, 15f, 16f, 48f, 74f, 75f, 83f
Latissimus dorsi tendon, 77f, 83f
     transfer, 48, 48f, 50, 50f
Lesser tubercle, 69f, 75f
     crest of, 3f, 69f
     of humerus, 3f, 5f, 16f
Lesser tuberosity, 22f, 26f, 27f, 29f, 31f
Levator scapulae muscle, 2f, 10f, 11, 16f, 18f, 60f, 82f
Lichtman classification, 151
Ligament of Struthers, 103f
Ligaments
     of elbow, 72–73
     of shoulder, 5–7
     of wrist, 120, 120f
Lister's tubercle, 116f
Local anesthesia, 198

Long extensor tendon, 160f, 181f
     avulsion of, 219f
     slips of, 160f
Long radiolunate ligament, 120f
Long thoracic nerve, 14f, 21f, 60f
Loupes custom-made, 215f
Lower subscapular nerve, 14f, 15f, 16f, 19f, 82f
Lower trapezius tendon (LTT), 48f
Lumbrical fascial sheath, 1st, probe in, 165f
Lumbrical muscle, 132f, 160f, 161f, 163f, 164, 167f, 193f, 195f
     1st, 129f, 166f, 168f, 174f
     2nd, 129f, 165f, 166f, 174f, 198f
     3rd, 130f, 165f
     4th, 165f
     in fascial sheaths, 164f
Lunate, 118, 118f, 120f, 126f, 138f, 156f, 157f
Lunate fossa, 121f
Lunotriquetral ligament, 120f, 126f
Lunule, 173f
Lymphangitis, 196, 196f
Lymphatic drainage, 171, 172f

M
Mallet finger, 210, 210f
Maloney line, 53f
     loss of, 58f
Malunion, 205, 205f
Manubriosternal synchondrosis, 5f
Manubrium, 5f
MCP joint *see* Metacarpophalangeal (MCP) joint
Medial antebrachial cutaneous nerve, 14f, 19f, 77f, 79f, 80, 80f, 81f, 83f, 84, 125f, 128f, 129f, 162f, 167f
Medial border, of scapula, 2f, 3f
Medial brachial cutaneous nerve, 14f, 19f, 77f, 79f, 80, 81f, 83f, 128f, 129f
Medial condyle, 69f, 70f
Medial cubital vein, 79f, 83, 84
Medial cutaneous nerve, of arm, 21f
Medial elbow instability, 107, 107f
Medial epicondyle, 69f, 70f, 71f, 72f, 75f, 76f, 78f, 82f, 83f, 103f, 104f, 122f, 123f, 124f, 130f
     avulsion of, 97f
     fractures of, 90
     in children, 97–98
Medial epicondylitis, 105, 105f
Medial intermuscular septum, 74, 75f, 76f, 77f, 83f, 103f, 104f, 123f, 124f
Medial pectoral nerve, 14f, 16f, 19f
Medial supraclavicular nerves, 79f
Medial supracondylar ridge, 69f, 70f
Medial suture row, 46f
Median antebrachial vein, 79f, 83, 131f, 172
Median basilic vein, 83, 131f
Median cephalic vein, 78f, 83, 84, 131f
Median cubital vein, 68f, 116f, 172f
Median nerve, 14f, 19f, 75f, 77f, 78f, 81f, 83f, 122f, 123f, 125f, 128f, 129, 129f, 132f, 163, 165f, 166f, 168–169
     articular branch of, 129f, 130f
     branch of, 166f
     common palmar digital branches of, 165f
     communicating branch of, 166f
     cutaneous branch, 166f
     digital branches of, 168
     dorsal branches of, 162f
     palmar branch of, 80f, 122f, 125f, 129f, 168
     palmar cutaneous branch of, 168f, 170f
     palmar digital branches, 80f, 168f
     palmar digital nerves from, 166f
     proper palmar digital branches of, 80f
Meleney ulcer *see* Necrotizing fasciitis
Meniscus allograft, 55f
Meniscus homologue, 120f, 126f
Meso os acromiale, 43f
Metacarpal bone, 118f, 156–157, 156f, 157f, 158f, 160f, 161f, 174f, 181f, 195f
     1st, 123f, 124f, 126f, 132f, 156, 169f, 198f
     2nd, 124f, 156
          base, 126f
     3rd, 156, 198f

Metacarpal bone (Continued)
     4th, 156
     5th, 123f, 124f, 157
     amputation through, 219f
     base, 156f, 157f
     fracture of, 201–202, 201f
          reduction of, 203f
     head, 156f, 157f
     ossification of, 157
     shaft, 156f, 157f
Metacarpal head, 173f
Metacarpal neck, fracture of, 201
Metacarpal shaft, fracture of, 201, 201f
Metacarpophalangeal (MCP) joint, 158–159, 158f, 159f, 161f, 184f
     arthritis of, 181
     arthrodesis of, 183f
     arthroplasties, 184f
     dislocation of, 207
     implant resection arthroplasty for, 181f, 182f
     injuries, 206–207, 207f
     site of, 156f, 157f
     surgery for, 179, 184
Metacarpophalangeal ligaments, 158f
Microvascular approximation clamps, 215f
Mid forearm, 161f
Middle collateral artery, 17f, 76f, 77f, 84, 84f
Middle digital crease, 156f
Middle glenohumeral ligament (MGL), 5, 13f
Middle phalanges, 156f, 157f, 161f, 167f, 173f, 181f, 187f
     amputation in, 212f, 213–214
     base, 156f, 157f
     depressed, arthritic volar half, 209f
     dorsal branches to dorsum of, 168f
     fracture of, 203
          base, 203f
          management of, 204f
          neck, 203f
          special problems in, 205f
     fracture-dislocation of, 208f
     head, 156f, 157f
     insertion of extensor tendon, 160f
     shafts, 156f, 157f
Midpalmar space, 164f, 165f, 193f, 195f
     infection of, 194–195, 195f
     probe in, 165f
     replantation of, 219f
     septum separating thenar from, 165f
Minute arteries, 173f
Minute fasciculi attach palmar aponeurosis, 170f
Modular PIP joint arthroplasty, 188f
Monteggia fracture, 145, 145f
Motor weakness, 104f
Multiple metacarpal fractures, plate fixation of, 201f
Muscle wasting, 104f
Muscles
     of elbow, 74–78, 74f, 75f
     of forearm, 122–127, 122f, 123f, 124f, 125f, 126f
     of hand, 162–165
     of shoulder, 8–13
Musculocutaneous nerve, 14f, 19f, 75f, 77f, 81, 81f, 83f, 123f, 128f, 129f, 167f
     anterior branch of, 81, 81f
     articular branch of, 81f
     cutaneous innervation of, 81f
     lateral antebrachial cutaneous nerve, 162f, 168f
     posterior branch of, 81, 81f

N
Nail bed, 173f
Nail matrix, 173f, 212f
Nail pits, 176f
Nail plate, 173, 173f
Nail root, 173f
Nails, 174
Neck, 35f
     of humerus, 3f
     of radius, 117f
     of scapula, 2f

Necrotizing fasciitis, 196, 196f
Neer impingement sign, 42f
Neurovascular compartment, 77f
Neurovascular injury, 99, 99f
Neurovascular relationships, of shoulder, 14–16
Neviaser portal, 66f
Nonunion, 140
    treatment of, 205
Nonviable tissue, 194f
Nursemaid elbow, 98
Nutrient humeral artery, 84

O
Oblique cord, 117f
Oblique fractures
    of fingers, 204, 204f
    treatment of, 205
Olecranon, of ulna, 68f, 70f, 71, 71f, 76f, 82f, 104f, 116f, 117f, 124f, 133f
    fractures of, 93, 93f
Olecranon bursa, aspiration at, 112f
Olecranon bursitis, 105, 105f
Olecranon fossa, 69, 69f, 70f, 71f
Olecranon osteotomy, posterior approach with, 114f
Omohyoid muscle, 3f, 8f, 14f, 16f, 18f
Onycholysis, 176f, 177f
Open reduction and internal fixation (ORIF), 136, 137f
Operating microscope, 215f
Opponens digiti minimi muscle, 130f, 132f, 156f, 163, 167f
Opponens pollicis muscle, 129f, 132f, 163, 163f, 166f, 168f
Os acromiale lesions, 43f
Ossification
    of radius, 116, 119
    of ulna, 71
Osteoarthritis, 175, 179f
    advanced hand involvement, 176
    of glenohumeral joint, 51–52, 52f
    hand involvement in, 175f
Osteochondritis dissecans, of elbow, 108, 108f
Osteochondrosis, of elbow, 109
Osteophyte, 51f, 55f
Osteotomy, of thumb metacarpal, 214f

P
Palmar aponeurosis, 122f, 124, 126f, 131f, 164f, 165f, 170, 170f, 195f
    septa from, 165f
Palmar carpal arterial arch, 163
Palmar carpal ligament, 122f, 123f, 130f, 131f, 132f, 167f, 170f
Palmar carpometacarpal ligaments, 158f
Palmar digital artery, 165f, 166f, 170f
    dorsal branches of, 173f
    to neighboring digit, 173f
Palmar digital nerves, 129, 130, 165f, 166f, 167f, 170f
    to 5th finger and medial half of 4th finger, 165f
    branches of, 166
    dorsal branches of, 171, 171f
    from superficial branch of ulnar nerve, 170f
    of thumb, 165f
Palmar digital veins, 83
Palmar dislocation, 208f
Palmar infections, 195f
Palmar interosseous fascia, 164f
Palmar interosseous muscles, 130f, 162, 163f, 164f, 167f
    1st, 174f
    2nd dorsal, 174f
Palmar ligaments, 158f, 159, 160f, 200f
    plates, 160f, 161f, 173f
    volar plate, 158f
Palmar metacarpal arteries, 163, 166f
Palmar metacarpal ligaments, 158f
Palmar plate, 198f
Palmar radiolunate ligament, 120f
Palmar surface, 158f
Palmaris brevis muscle, 130f, 133f, 167f, 170f
Palmaris longus muscle, 78f, 122f, 123, 125f, 127f, 129f
Palmaris longus tendon, 116f, 122f, 125f, 132f, 156f, 165f
Panner disease, 109

Paresthesias, 104f
Paronychia, 191f, 192
Partial fasciectomy, 190
Passive external rotation, 38f
Passive forward flexion, 38f
Pectoralis major fascia, 16f
Pectoralis major muscle, 3f, 4f, 8f, 13f, 14f, 15f, 16f, 48f, 61f, 66f, 68f, 74f, 75f, 77f, 83f
    abdominal part, 8f
    clavicular head, 8f
    sternal head of, 60f
    sternocostal head, 8f
Pectoralis major tendon, 77f, 83f
Pectoralis minor fascia, 16f
Pectoralis minor muscle, 3f, 13f, 14f, 15f, 16f, 61f, 62f, 83f
Pectoralis minor tendon, 14f, 16f, 75f
Pectoralis muscle, 8–9
Pectoralis transfer, 50, 50f
Perforating veins, 79f, 131f
Periosteum, 212f
Peripheral capsule, adhesions of, 37f
Peripheral nerves, 20–21, 81
Phalanges, 129f, 157
    amputation in, 212f
    fractures of
        reduction of, 203f
        special problems in, 205
    ossification of, 157
Phalen test, 132
Photoplethysmographic (PPG) monitoring, for replantation, 218f
Phrenic nerve, 14f, 19f
PIP joint see Proximal interphalangeal (PIP) joint
Pisiform, 118, 118f, 122f, 123, 123f, 132f, 133f, 156f, 158f, 163, 165f, 166f, 170f
"Popeye" deformity, 39, 39f
Port of Wilmington, 66f
Positive lift-off rest, 49f
Posterior antebrachial cutaneous nerve, 76f, 77f, 79f, 80, 80f, 82f, 131f, 162f, 171
Posterior antebrachial fascia, of extensor retinaculum, 171
Posterior axillary fold (pectoralis major), 8f
Posterior brachial cutaneous nerve, 76f, 79–80, 80f, 82, 82f
Posterior circumflex humeral artery, 9f, 11f, 14f, 16f, 17f, 18f, 76f, 83f, 84f
Posterior circumflex humeral nerve, 9f
Posterior circumflex humeral vein, 11f
    superficial branches of, 79f
Posterior (subacromial) dislocation, 31f
Posterior dislocation of glenohumeral joint, 31–32, 31f, 32f
Posterior fat pad, 87f
Posterior glenoid bone, 32f
Posterior glenoid rim fracture, 32f
Posterior glenoid wear, 51
Posterior interosseous artery, 84f, 124f
Posterior interosseous nerve, 103f, 124f
Posterior labrum, 13f
Posterior portal, 66f
Posterior ulnar recurrent artery, 78f, 84f, 123f, 124f
Posterolateral rotatory elbow instability, 107, 107f
Posterolateral soft spot, 68
Postural deformities, 178–179
Prestyloid recess, 120f, 126f
Princeps pollicis artery, 166f
Profunda brachii artery, 14f, 76f, 77f, 83f, 84f
Profundus flexor tendons
    to 3rd digit, 164f
    common flexor sheath (ulnar bursa) containing, 165f
Pronator quadratus muscle, 123f, 125, 126f, 127f, 129f, 163f, 164f
Pronator teres muscle, 75f, 78f, 83f, 122f, 123, 123f, 124f, 125f, 127f, 128f, 129f
Proper dorsal digital arteries, 166
Proper palmar digital nerves, 168f
Prosthesis, function of, 61f
Proximal biceps tendon tear, 39f
Proximal digital crease, 156f
Proximal extensor forearm musculature, 68
Proximal flexor pronator musculature, 68
Proximal forearm, 161f

Proximal humeral fractures
    humeral head split with a classic four-part fracture-dislocation, 26
    Neer classification, 22, 22f
    reverse total shoulder replacement, 27
    two-part greater tuberosity fracture, 23, 24, 24f
    valgus-impacted four-part fracture, 25
Proximal interphalangeal (PIP) joint, 158f, 159f, 161f, 175f, 177f
    dislocation of, 208–209, 208f
    dorsal dislocation of, 208f
    site of, 157f
    surgery for, 186–188
Proximal palmar crease, 156f
Proximal palmar plate, 174f
Proximal phalanges, 156f, 157f, 161f, 174f, 181f
    base, 156f, 157f
    fracture of, 203
        management of, 204f
        special problems in, 205f
    head of, 156f, 157f, 187f
    shafts, 156f, 157f
    thumb, 174f, 187f
Proximal pole, 138f
Proximal radioulnar articulation, 73
Pseudoparalysis, in shoulder, 44, 57
Psoriatic arthritis, 176–177, 176f
Pull elevation, loss of, 55f
Pulse oxygen monitor, for replantation, 218f
Purulent drainage, 191f
Pus, in web space, 195f
Pyoderma, 191f, 192–193
Pyrolytic carbon-coated implant arthroplasty, 184f

Q
Quadrangular space, 16f
Quadrate ligament, 72f, 73

R
Radial artery, 83f, 84f, 122f, 125f, 126f, 128, 132f, 163f, 165f, 166f
    in anatomic snuffbox, 162f, 169f
    branch, 163f
    to deep arch, 169f
    dorsal carpal branch of, 169f
    palmar carpal branches of, 166f
    superficial palmar branch of, 163f, 166f
Radial collateral artery, 17f, 76f, 77f, 84, 84f
Radial collateral ligament, 72f, 73, 73f, 78f, 174f, 182f
Radial deviation, 159f
Radial dysplasia, 152
Radial fossa, 69, 69f, 70f
Radial groove, 2f
Radial head, 116f
Radial longitudinal crease, 156f
Radial longitudinal deficiency, 152–153, 152f, 153f
Radial nerve, 14f, 15f, 16f, 19f, 21f, 69f, 76f, 77f, 78f, 80f, 81f, 82, 82f, 84, 103f, 123f, 128f, 129f, 169
    communicating branches of, 171, 171f
    dorsal digital branches of, 80f, 168f, 169f
    lateral branch, 169f
    medial branch, 169f
    palsy, 99
    posterior antebrachial cutaneous nerve, 168f
    superficial branch of, 80f, 124f, 131f, 162f, 167f, 168f, 169f, 171, 171f
Radial notch, of ulna, 70f, 71, 117f
Radial recurrent artery, 83f, 84f, 123f
Radial splint, of fingers, 204f
Radial styloid process, 118f
Radial tuberosity, 70f, 71f, 75f, 78f
Radialis indicis artery, 166f
Radiate sternocostal ligament, 5f
Radiocarpal destruction, 150
Radiolunate ligament, 120f
Radioscaphocapitate ligament, 120f, 150f
Radius, 70f, 71f, 72f, 73f, 117f, 118f, 125f, 127f, 145f, 163f
    dislocation of, 98f
    distal parts of, 116–117
    fracture of shaft of, 146, 146f

Radius (Continued)
    head of, 70f, 71f, 75f, 117f
        fractures of, 91–92, 91f, 92f, 98
        subluxation of, 98, 98f
    neck of, 70f, 71f
        fractures of, 91–92, 91f, 98
Range-of-motion exercises, active-assisted, 63–64, 63f, 64f
Ray, amputation in, 214
Recurrent radial artery, 103f
Regional anesthesia, for hand, 197
Reiter syndrome, 177, 177f
Replantation, 215–221
    of avulsed thumb, 219f
    contraindications of, 215–217
        age, 216
        amputation of single digit, 216
        avulsion, 216–217
        extreme contamination, 216
        multiple level injuries, 216
        prolonged ischemia, 217
        systemic illness, 215–216
    debridement, 216f
    indications of, 215
    microsurgical instrumentation for, 215f
    minor, technique for, 218–221
    postoperative dressing, 220–221
    preoperative management of, 217–218
    repair of
        blood vessels and nerves, 217f, 219–220
        bone and tendon, 216f, 218–219
    results, 221
    secondary reconstruction, 221
    trimming of bone, 216f
Resection interposition arthroplasty, 181
Resting hand splint, 211f
Resurfacing joint replacement, 181
"Reverse" Hill-Sachs lesion, 31f
Reverse total shoulder replacement, 27, 57–58, 57f, 58f
Rheumatic disease, 175
Rheumatoid arthritis
    of glenohumeral joint, 54–55, 54f, 55f
    of hand, 175–176, 176f
    of wrist, 149, 149f
Rhomboid major muscle, 2f, 10f, 16f, 60f, 82f
Rhomboid minor muscle, 2f, 10f, 16f, 60f, 82f
Rhomboideus muscle, 11
Rib, 61f
    1st, 5f, 14f, 19f
        synchondrosis of, 5f
    2nd, 5f
Ring fingers, flexion contracture of, 189f
Ring-handled scissors, 215f
Rolando fracture, 202, 202f
Rotational dislocation, treatment of, 208–209
Rotator cuff, 12–13, 42–43, 42f, 46f
    muscle of, 13f
    posteriormost insertion of, 7f
    radiologic and arthroscopic imaging, 43f
Rotator cuff tears
    arthropathy, 56f
    arthroscopic surgery for, 46f
    open surgery for, 46f
    surgical management of, 45–48, 45f, 46f
Rotator cuff tendons, 45f, 46f
Rotator cuff–deficient arthritis (rotator cuff tear arthropathy),
    56–58, 56f, 57f, 58f
Rotator interval, 22f
Russe bone graft, for nonunion of scaphoid, 139f

S
Scaphocapitate ligament, 120f
Scaphoid, 117–118, 118f, 126f, 156f, 157f, 169f
    fracture of, 138–140, 138f, 139f, 140f
        acute displaced fractures, 140
        acute nondisplaced fractures, 139–140
        nonunion, 140
    tubercle of, 118f
Scapholunate interosseous ligament disruption
    (SLAC), 150

Scapholunate ligament, 126f
Scaphotrapeziotrapezoid ligament, 120f
Scapula, 2–3, 2f, 3f, 36f, 61f
    anastomoses around, 18f
    body of, 16f
    drooping of, 60f
    fractures of, 34–35, 35f
    inferior angle of, 10f
    medial border of, 10f
    spine of, 10f, 12f, 16f, 18f, 48f
    superior border of, 12f
    winging of, 60f
Septa forming canals, 164f
Serratus anterior muscle, 8f, 14f, 15f, 21f, 60f, 61f, 68f
Serratus muscle, 9
Sesamoid bones, 156f, 174f
Short radiolunate ligament, 120f
Shoulder, 1–66
    acromioclavicular and sternoclavicular dislocation, 33
    acromioclavicular joint arthritis, 41, 41f
    amputation of, 61
    anterior dislocation of glenohumeral joint, 28–30
    anterior muscles of, 8f, 9f
    avascular necrosis of the humeral head, 53
    biceps tendon tears and SLAP lesions, 39–40, 39f
    brachial plexus, 19
    calcific tendonitis, 36
    clavicle, 4
    common surgical approaches to, 66, 66f
    cutaneous nerves of, 79
    disarticulation of, 61f
    exercises for range of motion and strengthening,
        63–65, 63f
    fractures of the clavicle and scapula, 34–35
    frozen, 37–38
    humerus, 3
    impingement syndrome, 42–43, 42f
    injections, 62, 62f
    ligaments, 5–7
    muscles of, 8–13
    neurologic conditions of, 59–60
    neurovascular relationships, 14–16
    osteoarthritis of the glenohumeral joint, 51–52, 52f
    peripheral nerves, 20–21
    posterior muscles, 10, 11f
    proximal humeral fractures
        Neer classification, 22, 22f
        two-part greater tuberosity fracture, 23
        valgus-impacted four-part fracture, 25
    rheumatoid arthritis of glenohumeral joint, 54–55,
        54f, 55f
    rotator cuff tears, physical examination, 44
    rotator cuff–deficient arthritis (rotator cuff tear
        arthropathy), 56–58
    scapula, 2–3
    sensory distribution and neuropathy in, 21f
    supraspinatus and infraspinatus rotator cuff tears
        imaging of, 45, 45f, 46f
        irreparable, surgical management of, 47–48,
            47f, 48f
        surgical management of, 46, 46f
    upper arm, 12–13
    vascular anatomy of, 17–18
Shoulder joint, deltopectoral approach to, 66f
Shrug sign, 44f
Silastic arthroplasty, 183f, 188f
Skin closure, 61f
Skin graft, use of, 213f
SLAP lesions, 39–40, 39f, 40f
Snuffbox contents, 169f
Space of parona, infection in, 195
Spinal accessory nerve, 60f
    palsy, 60f
Spine, of scapula, 2f
Spinoglenoid notch, 2f
Sporotrichosis, 192f, 194
Spring-handled microdissection scissors, 215f
Spring-handled needle holder, 215f
Squeezing tennis ball, 211f

Stable intraarticular fractures, 205
Sternal head, 8f
Sternoclavicular dislocation, 33
Sternoclavicular joint, 5f, 6–7, 8f
    articular cavities of, 5f
    articular disc of, 5f
    posterior dislocation of, 33f
Sternoclavicular ligaments, 5f
Sternocleidomastoid muscle, 4f, 8f, 14f, 15f
Sternocostal (synovial) joint, 5f
Sternohyoid muscle, 4f
Sternum, 8f
Stimson maneuver, 28f
Student's elbow, 105f
Styloid process, of ulna, 117f, 157f
Subacromial balloon, 47f
Subacromial bursa, 62f, 75f
    subdeltoid bursa fused with, 12f
    technique for injection of, 62f
Subacromial contrast, 45f
Subacromial injection, 62f
Subacromial space
    loss of, 57f, 58f
    palpation of, 42f
Subchondral bone plate, irregularity of, 53f
Subchondral cyst, 58f
Subchondral fracture line, 53f
Subchondral sclerosis, 179f
Subclavian artery, 14f, 18f
Subclavian groove, 4f
Subclavian vein, 14f
Subclavicular dislocation, 28f
Subclavius fascia, 16f
Subclavius muscle, 4f, 5f, 10, 14f, 15f, 16f
Subcoracoid dislocation, 28f
Subcutaneous abscess, 191f, 192–193
Subcutaneous olecranon bursa, 73f
Subdeltoid bursa, 12f, 36f
Subglenoid dislocation, 28f
Sublabral foramen, 13f
Sublabral recess, 9f
Sublime tubercle, 70f
Subscapular artery, 14f, 16f, 17f, 18f, 84f
Subscapular fossa, 3f
Subscapularis muscle, 3f, 9f, 12f, 13, 13f, 15f, 16f, 22f, 29f, 31f,
    45f, 46f, 49f, 61f, 62f, 66f, 74f, 75f, 83f
Subscapularis tears, management of, 50
Subscapularis tendon, 5f, 12f, 13f, 16f, 23f, 31f, 66f
    upper border of, 6f
Subungual hematoma
    fracture of, 210
    from trauma, 210f
Subungual space, 173f, 191f
Superficial flexor muscles, 122f
Superficial head, of flexor pollicis, 129f
Superficial palmar arterial arches, 128f, 132f, 165f, 166f
    distal limit of, 166f
Superficial radial nerve, 103f
Superficial transverse metacarpal ligaments, 131f, 170f
Superficial veins, 172
    of elbow, 79f
    of upper arm, 79f, 83
Superficialis flexor tendons
    to 3rd digit, 164f
    common flexor sheath (ulnar bursa) containing, 165f
Superior angle, 2f, 3f
Superior border, 2f, 3f
Superior capsular reconstruction, 47, 47f
Superior glenohumeral ligaments, 5
    confluence of, 6f
    rotator interval, 6f
Superior glenoid bone loss, 58f
Superior labrum biceps tendon complex, 6f
Superior lateral brachial cutaneous nerve, 15f, 76f, 79, 79f,
    80f, 82f
Superior lateral cutaneous nerve, 16f, 21f
Superior thoracic artery, 14f, 17f, 18f, 84f
Superior transverse scapular ligament, 5f, 9f, 15f, 16f
Superior ulnar collateral artery, 77f, 83f, 84, 84f, 124f

Supinator muscle, 74f, 78f, 103f, 123f, 124f, 125f, 126, 127f, 128f, 145f
Supraclavicular nerves, 21f, 79, 80f, 82f
Supracondylar fractures, of humerus, 96–97, 96f
Supracondylar process, 103f
Supraglenoid tubercle, 69f
Suprascapular artery, 9f, 13f, 14f, 16f, 18f
  infraspinous branch of, 18f
Suprascapular foramen, 18f
Suprascapular nerve, 9f, 13f, 14f, 16f, 19f, 53f, 59f
Suprascapular notch, 2f, 3f, 5f, 9f, 53f, 59f
Suprascapular vein, 9f
Supraspinatus muscle, 2f, 3f, 9f, 10f, 12, 12f, 13f, 15f, 16f, 18f, 22f, 45f, 46f, 53f, 59f, 62f, 74f, 76f, 82f
Supraspinatus rotator cuff tears
  imaging of, 45, 45f
  surgical management of, 46, 46f
Supraspinatus tendon, 5f, 12f, 13f, 16f, 36f
  anterior edge of, 6f
Supraspinous fossa, 2f, 69f
Surgical neck, of humerus, 3f, 22f, 69f
Suspensory ligament, of axilla, 16f
Sutures, 46f
Swan neck deformity, 178, 185–186
  reconstructive surgery for, 186f
Synovial membrane, 12f, 72f, 73, 173f
Synovial tendon sheath, 161f, 164f, 173f, 193f
Synovitis, 37f, 54f

T
T1 nerve, 20f
T2 nerve, 20f
T12 vertebra, spinous process of, 10f
Teflon irrigating tip, 215f
Temperature monitoring, for replantation, 218f
Tendinosis, 105, 105f
Tendinous sheath of flexor pollicis longus
  (radial bursa), 165f
Tendon adhesions, treatment of, 205
Tendon deformities, 179
Tendon disorders
  in hand, 199–200
Tendon sheath, 132f
  injections, 198
Tendon tear type, defined, 45
Tendon transfer, path of, 60f
Tendons, 68f
  amputated toe with, 221f
  repair of, 200f
  suture line, 212f
Tennis elbow, 105, 105f
Tenosynovitis, 192f, 193–194, 193f
Teres major muscle, 2f, 3f, 10f, 14f, 15f, 16f, 17f, 18f, 74f, 75f, 76f, 77f, 82f, 83f, 84f
Teres major tendon, 76f
Teres minor muscle, 2f, 10f, 11f, 13, 13f, 15f, 16f, 18f, 45f, 74f, 76f, 82f
  branch to, 15f
  tear of, 48f
Teres minor tendons, 12f, 76f
Terrible triad injury, 92f
TFCC see Triangular fibrocartilage complex
Thenar eminence, 116f, 156f
Thenar mass, 174f
Thenar muscles, 126f, 129f, 165f, 168f
  branches of median nerve to, 163f
  recurrent (motor) branch of median nerve, 166f, 170f
Thenar space, 164f, 165f, 193f
  infection of, 195, 195f
Thenar web cleft, deepening of, 213f, 214
Therabands, 64f
Thoracoacromial artery, 14f, 16f, 17f, 18f, 84f
  acromial branch of, 13f, 14f, 17f, 18f
  clavicular branch, 14f, 17f, 18f, 84f
  deltoid branch of, 8f, 14f, 17f, 18f
  pectoral branch, 84f
  pectoral branch of, 14f, 17f, 18f
Thoracoacromial vein, acromial branches of, 79f, 84f

Thoracodorsal artery, 14f, 16f, 17f, 18f, 84f
Thoracodorsal nerve, 14f, 15f, 16f, 19f
Three-part O'Brien test, 39f
Thumb
  amputation in, 213f, 221f
  avulsed, replantation of, 219f
  carpometacarpal articulation of, 175f
  carpometacarpal injection, 198f
  carpometacarpal joint, 157f
  carpometacarpal osteoarthritis, 179f
  joints, deformities of, 178–180
  lengthening post amputation, 214f
  ligament injury and dislocation, 206f
  metacarpal of, fracture of base of, 202
  metacarpophalangeal deformities, 178f
  nerves of, 166f
  palmar digital nerves of, 165f
  radial longitudinal deficiency in, 152
  replantation, 220f
  transplanted great toe, 221f
Thumb metacarpal base, fracture of, 202f
Thumb opposition, range of, 159f
Thumb web, lateral arm flap for defect of, 220f
Thyrocervical trunk, 18f
Tinel sign, 104f
Tophaceous gout, chronic, 177
Total elbow arthroplasty
  for distal humerus fractures, 89, 89f
  imaging of, 102
  options of, 101
Transverse carpal ligament, 126f, 133f, 165f
Transverse cervical artery, 14f, 18f
Transverse fasciculi, 170f
Transverse head, 156f
Transverse humeral ligament, 5f
Transverse ridges, 176f
Transverse scapular ligament, 18f
Trapeziectomy, 180f
Trapeziocapitate ligament, 120f
Trapeziotrapezoid ligament, 120f
Trapezium muscle, 118, 118f, 126f, 132f, 156f, 157f, 158f, 169f, 174f, 198f
  tubercle of, 118f
Trapezius muscle, 3f, 4f, 8f, 9f, 10, 10f, 14f, 15f, 16f, 48f, 49f, 60f, 74f
Trapezius transfer, 48
Trapezoid, 118–119, 118f, 126f, 132f, 156f, 157f
Trapezoid ligament, 4f, 5f, 12f
Trauma, immobilization after surgery, 38f
Traumatic posterior dislocation, 32
Triangle of auscultation, 10f
Triangular aponeurosis, 160f
Triangular fibrocartilage complex (TFCC), 120, 121f, 126f
  tear, 121f
Triangular space, 16f
Triceps brachii muscle, 2f, 8f, 10f, 14f, 15f, 68f, 74f, 76–78, 77f, 104f, 124f, 127f
  lateral head of, 10f, 18f, 68f, 76–77, 76f, 77f, 82f
  long head of, 10f, 15f, 18f, 68f, 74f, 76–77, 76f, 77f, 82f, 83f
  medial head, 15f
  medial head of, 74f, 76–77, 76f, 77f, 82f, 83f, 103f
  tendon, 10f
Triceps brachii tendon, 73f, 76f, 77f, 82f, 124f, 127f
Triceps muscle, 78f
  lateral head, 13f
  long head, 11f
Triceps tendon, 78f
  rupture of, 106, 106f
Trigger finger, 199, 199f
Triquetrocapitate ligament, 120f
Triquetrohamate ligament, 120f
Triquetrum, 118, 118f, 121f, 126f, 138f, 156f, 157f
Trochlea, 69, 69f, 70f, 71f, 78f
Trochlear notch, 71, 71f, 117f
Tubercle, 138f
Two-part greater tuberosity fracture, 23
  and dislocation of the humeral head, 24, 24f

U
Ulna, 70f, 71f, 72f, 73f, 78f, 87f, 117f, 118f, 125f, 127f, 145f, 163f
  distal parts of, 116–117
  fracture of shaft of, 145, 145f
  tuberosity of, 75f
Ulnar artery, 78f, 83f, 84f, 122f, 123f, 126f, 128, 128f, 132f, 163, 165f, 166, 166f, 170f
  deep palmar branch of, 163, 165f, 166f, 170f
  dorsal carpal branch of, 162f
  palmar carpal branches of, 166f
Ulnar collateral ligament, 72, 72f, 73f, 78f, 126f, 174f
  injury to, 206
  posterior bundle of, 78f
  ruptured, 206f
  torn, 206f
Ulnar deviation, 159f
Ulnar digital nerve, 189f
Ulnar head, 74f, 103f, 126f, 128f
Ulnar intrinsic tendon divided, 181f
Ulnar nerve, 14f, 19f, 76f, 77f, 78f, 80f, 81f, 83f, 103f, 122f, 123f, 124f, 125f, 126f, 128f, 129f, 130, 130f, 132f, 133f, 163f, 165f, 166f, 167, 167f
  branches from deep branch of, 163f
  communicating branches of, 166f, 167f, 171, 171f
  deep branch of, 130f, 163, 166f, 167f, 170f
  deep palmar branch of, 165f, 166f
  deep terminal branch of, 167
  dorsal branch of, 80f, 124f, 128f, 130f, 131f, 162f, 167, 171, 171f
  dorsal digital branches of, 80f
  groove for, 69f, 70f
  palmar branch of, 130f, 131f, 167f, 168, 170f
  palmar carpal branch, 163, 163f
  palmar cutaneous branch, 166f
  palmar digital branches, 167f
  palmar digital nerves from, 166f
  proper palmar digital branches of, 80f, 128f
  submuscular transposition of, 104f
  superficial branch of, 123f, 128f, 130f, 165f, 166f, 167f, 170f
  superficial terminal branch, 167
  ulnar artery with venae comitantes, 165f
Ulnar notch, of radius, 116
Ulnar recurrent artery, 123f, 128
Ulnar splint, of fingers, 204f
Ulnar styloid process, 116f, 118f, 126f, 157f
Ulnar tuberosity, 117f
Ulnar tunnel, 133f
Ulnocapitate ligament, 120f
Ulnolunate ligament, 120f
Ulnotriquetral ligament, 120f
Unstable transverse fractures, of fingers, 204f
Upper arm, 67–114
  amputation of, 61
  blood supply of, 83–84
  cross-sectional anatomy of, 77f
  cutaneous nerves of, 79–80, 79f
  injury to, 86
  muscles of, 75f, 76f
    elbow, 74–78, 74f
    shoulder, 12–13
  physical examination of, 85
  superficial veins of, 79f, 83
  surgical approaches to, 113–114, 113f, 114f
  topographic anatomy of, 68f
Upper limb
  cutaneous innervation of, 80f
  dermatomes of, 20f
Upper subscapular nerve, 14f, 15f, 19f
Upper trapezius atrophy, 60f
Urethritis, 177f

V
Valgus-impacted open reduction, 25f
Vascular leash of Henry, 103f
Vein graft, anastomosed, 219f
Venae comitantes, 165f

Venous arches, 165f
Vertebral artery, 18f
Vertical shear, 138f
Vessel-dilating forceps, 215f
Vincula longa, 160f
Vincula tendinum spring, 160
Vinculum breve, 160f
Volar carpal ligament, 133f
Volar dislocations, treatment of, 209
Volar fragment, depressed, 209f

Volar interossei, 156f
Volar plate, 207f
   arthroplasty, 209f
   stretched, 180f

W
Wedge flaps, 213f
Winging of scapula, 21f
Wrist, 115–153, 176f
   anatomy of, 126f

Wrist (Continued)
   arthritis of, 150, 150f
   arthroscopy, 121, 121f
   arthroscopy of, 121, 121f
   bones of, 116–119, 116f, 117f
   ligaments of, 120, 120f
   radiograph of, 119, 119f

Z
Z-plasty, incision of, 213f